The MidLife Health Guide for Men

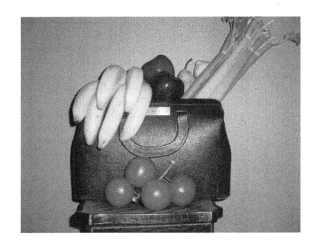

Works pending publishing:

Diet for Life

The Midlife Health Guide for Women

The Health Guide for Children

Renaissance (fiction)

The MidLife Health Guide for Men

Chris G. Rao, M.D,

board-certified Family Doctor and Fellow of the
American Academy of Family Physicians
Chief Medical Officer of Unison Pro-Youth Medical
Institute, Florida.

iUniverse, Inc.
New York   Lincoln   Shanghai

The MidLife Health Guide for Men

Copyright © 2007 by Christopher G Rao, MD

iUniverse books may be ordered through booksellers or by contacting:

iUniverse
2021 Pine Lake Road, Suite 100
Lincoln, NE 68512
www.iuniverse.com
1-800-Authors (1-800-288-4677)

Because of the dynamic nature of the Internet, any Web addresses or links contained in this book may have changed since publication and may no longer be valid.

The information, ideas, and suggestions in this book are not intended as a substitute for professional medical advice. Before following any suggestions contained in this book, you should consult your personal physician. Neither the author nor the publisher shall be liable or responsible for any loss or damage allegedly arising as a consequence of your use or application of any information or suggestions in this book.

Edited by Reiza S. Dejito
Reviewed by Elmer J. Mangubat

ISBN: 978-0-595-42176-3 (pbk)
ISBN: 978-0-595-86514-7 (ebk)

Printed in the United States of America

In memory of Dad

If you want to beat Mother Nature, you must learn to play her game.

—Chris G. Rao, MD

Contents

List of Illustrations

Preface

"Do you see anything wrong with the print on this newspaper?" I asked my wife. "Well, are you sure? It's all blurry!" After rushing off to an ophthalmologist friend, I learned the coldhearted truth I was denying all along. Having finished examining this forty-four-year-old, he casually said, "Chris, you're just simply getting old and need reading glasses." Wow, all in one day. Wham! Nowadays I have specs all around the house, yet I can never seem to find them. "I need my OPGs!" I often call out. (Around our house, that means old people's glasses.) I used to joke, "Maybe I lost my hair … but at least, I still have great vision." Well, there goes that quip. A few weeks before that, I was getting into some heavy yard work. (Yes, doctors do that occasionally.) Working at the breakneck pace I've kept since my youth, I found myself huffing and puffing like an old man. I had to then lie down to keep from almost passing out. When getting dressed to go out later that night, I had to shuffle through all my pants to find the few that still fit—size thirty-four. Slowly but surely, middle age was wrapping around me like a kudzu vine alongside an old blacktopped Mississippi highway.

Facing the truth of getting older was even scarier. This can't be happening to me. As a doctor, I'm constantly reminded of the ravages Father Time deals the elderly every day—pneumonia, osteoporosis, stroke, dementia, and so on. It's definitely better to be on the outside looking in as opposed to being on the inside looking out. All these thoughts and nuances had been working on me for a while. I've always tried to practice what I preach to my patients. I always ate right and got some exercise but had fell off the health wagon the past few years.

In medical school only ten years before, I had jogged my way to first place for my age group in a 5 km run. Achieving many awards in residency, I worked diligently to integrate many of the modern technologies into health-care delivery. I got invited to join the think tank in helping to design the Disney Institute and Celebration Health in Orlando, Florida. Though it may seem ironic to some, I've always stressed how the average person can stay healthy without having to visit doctors. Pills were never my first, or only, recommendation. My focus has always been on preventing them from getting sick in the first place. Later, as a clinical professor at Tulane and Louisiana State University medical centers, I enjoyed passing on this knowledge to many eager medical students and stressing the importance of being a healthy role model to their patients. Soon, this exposure, along with my entertainment background, got me regularly writing health-related editorials.

One night, I woke up with this vision of one place where people could go and get the best of both worlds—medical and complementary methods. Since patients would now be on one track to better health, I aptly named the facility Unison Pro-Youth Medical Institute. After all, I'm not really into *antiaging*. That would be like wanting people to die early, right? Instead, I want to help them be physiologically younger and healthier—thus the term *pro-youth*. Eventually, I landed my own radio show, *In the Know with Dr. Rao!* It was quite a success; however, the coverage was only about ten square miles. After much coaxing from others, I felt the desire to write about all I've learned and to spread this mantra to many more.

So why write a book about middle age? This period of a man's life presents what I see as a *window of opportunity*. It's unique in its changes and many challenges. It's a time when most men are at the top of their game, yet early disease may be progressing undetected. Some friends or siblings in their forties or fifties may have already suffered a bout with a severe illness. With a more proactive, preventative approach to health, this need not happen to you. Look at things this way. If you only had one car to drive your whole life, wouldn't you take extra special care of it? Similarly, midlife is a time when our original genetic warranty has expired. We need to protect what's left. As the famous comedian George Burns wisely commented when he was quite elderly, "If I knew I was going to live this long, I would've taken better care of myself!"

Granted, there's been a lot of focus in the past on all the other periods of one's life, i.e., pediatrics or geriatrics; however middle age has oddly been ignored. Yet it's our health in middle age that mostly determines how well we do in our golden years. Furthermore, we baby boomers desire more *quality* of life than just the *quantity* of life our parents wished. Despite modern medicine improving on the latter, there's, unfortunately, more morbidity and suffering at life's end.

Our generation wants to be more proactive and revolutionary in this regard too. We demand a more integrative and functional approach—one that focuses on prevention and more natural means. We refuse to suffer the ills of our parents or take eight to twelve medications. We don't want to become a mere victim of multiple surgical procedures and specialists. It's really what you and your doctor don't know that *can* hurt you!

Most physicians, including myself, spend the majority of our careers treating the very sick, nearly dead, or the aged with advanced multiple diseases. Having my choice of any specialty, I chose my original passion of becoming a true doctor, a family physician. Preventative, holistic medicine with established long-term patient relationships are what I enjoy most. Unfortunately, today's insurance environment doesn't correlate with that. Less than five cents of our national health-care dollar is spent on prevention. Now, patients often see a "health-care provider" in a six-minute time slot. Given all the confusion going on, I felt the need to provide middle-aged men with the resources and information to take the wheel and make their lifetime vehicle shine, go fast, and last a long time. Now is the time, guys.

Today, we have the ability to retain a healthy forty-year-old functioning level well into his eighties! Many baby boomers are expected to live until 120! As promising as this may seem for us proactive ones, I am very disheartened by the improper lifestyle and subsequent poor health of our children. One needs to only look at the young to see our future national health-care costs. The contemporary medical approach reacts with multiple drugs and surgical procedures that merely treat the *symptoms* of aging. This Band-Aid approach results in having just older, sicker people. Instead, there needs to be a better focus on disease *prevention*.

The *Midlife Health Guide for Men* starts off explaining why and how we age in the first place. This is followed by the current and future research being done to determine ways to slow down the heavy hands of time. Next, the basics are covered concerning diet and exercise, the proven ways to lower insulin and cortisol—the aging hormones. Helpful dietary tips and various fad diets are reviewed for their benefits and shortcomings. The ways to start a comprehensive, effective exercise program are also included. As a method to complement these, various supplements and important fluid intake are reviewed as well as recommendations on how to survive today's toxic environment.

There's a lot of controversy concerning testosterone and human growth hormone (HGH) replacement in men. Are these magical, youthful elixirs? When is their use appropriate and safe? Historical points, scientific literature, and practical guidelines are given concerning *all* these men's hormones including melatonin, thyroid, and cortisol. Additionally, insights into dealing with midlife stress and getting the proper rest are presented. Lastly, special concerns for the midlife male are covered, including prostate health, erectile dysfunction, hair loss, mood disorders, chronic pain, and more.

This book and its upcoming sister book, *The Midlife Health Guide for Women* explain this much-needed paradigm shift in health care. Introductions, explanations, and resources will be given for further reading on discussing these novel modalities. It is my hope this book will provide you with the tools necessary to be proactive and responsible for your own health. As I say, "The best health insurance is to be healthy in the first place!" You are the main player and should be the one most in charge of your own health. As your most important asset, you'll only get out of it what you put into it. This book will get you on the proper path to arrive at optimal health.

MAG

Let me introduce you to MAG, Middle-Aged Guy. As a teen, he lettered in football and track. He's the average midlifer I see in the office. Now forty-five, he's starting to feel the early symptoms of aging. MAG has gained that middle-age spread and lost some of the muscle strength and endurance he used to crow about. Being in sales, he feels stressed at work, often brings work home, and feels challenged by his younger coworkers. MAG has two young kids and a wife. He often feels guilty about the time he spends away from his children. As far as the marriage … well, let's say it's more of a convenience now. There's not much passion or lovemaking, a far cry from when they first began chirping as two lovebirds. He wouldn't be surprised one day if she said it was all over. At times, he finds it hard to control his emotions—sometimes crying and sometimes yelling and cussing. MAG sleeps poorly and drinks more than he feels he should. He's been to his family doctor and got some baseline lab work and a full exam. The nurse practitioner told him all his labs were great, except he may want to lose weight, as he did have mildly elevated cholesterol and sugar. MAG told her he didn't feel great, though. After getting a rectal, he was told he could be referred to a psychiatrist or started on some medications.

MAG wanted to try natural things first. He's heard some friends talking about herbs that may be safer. Some coworkers that hang out at the gym said he should get on some testosterone and supplements. MAG, having good sense, steered away from that and tried things the old-fashioned way; he got back to dieting and exercising. He's tried this for a few weeks and finds he does feel better but only lost a few pounds—nothing near where he needs to get. MAG feels like giving up. He heard of Dr. Rao and comes in for a consultation. At the end of each chapter, we'll give MAG the bottom-line advice he has to follow. Do you know anyone like MAG? These tips offer simple ways to stay healthier and avoid medications and operations later on in life.

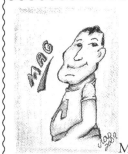

MAG will be given the bottom-line advice to avoid the ravages of aging.

Acknowledgments

I would like to thank all the Age-Management Medicine doctors I've had the pleasure of learning from throughout the years.

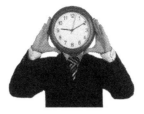

I.

An Introduction: Why and How Do We Age?

Aging is a tug of war that we can win!

—Michael Fossel, M.D.

While this may seem to some like a pipe dream or quackery, it's nonetheless a real possibility. This book will give insight into this changing view, or *paradigm shift*. Traditional thinking believes this is absurd or impossible. Yet, many scientists and research now say this can be a reality, although it demands a more proactive approach by both doctors and patients. If we truly desire to enjoy our golden years, we must better understand what causes aging in the first place.

What is age? Let's start by understanding the difference between *chronological age* and *physiological age*. Chronological age is simply your age in years since you were born. We cannot reverse the clock. For example, if you were born thirty-seven years ago, you're chronologically thirty-seven years old—nothing can change that. *Physiological age* is different though. All of us will age at an individual, physiological rate. This is simply a combination of your overall conditioning and functioning level. Think about this for a moment, because this perspective is quite new and a very important one to grasp. Like it or not, we have all been to family or high school reunions and had to face up to those that seem to somehow age better than others. Some old girlfriends may seem as if they were "rode hard and put up wet" a few times too many. You may also have an elderly aunt that looks better preserved than that '55 T-Bird at the big annual car show. She's quite an ageless classic. To some, life just seems unfair. To others, life is great! Personally and scientifically, we need to find out just why is this so that we can tilt things to our favor.

Of course, how we physiologically age is determined by many factors. We shall review the various theories of aging and then identify the proven ways we can manipulate to our favor. The latter will result in a younger physiological age. Rediscovering the Fountain of Youth that Ponce de Leon bragged about is doable, but it has to be a journey from the inside out! The Tool Guy wouldn't patch a moldy stain without fixing the leaky pipe inside the wall, right? Your woman wouldn't be totally happy to have a face like Kate Moss's, but a figure like Kate Smith's. (You may have to ask your parents who that was.) So it's true; youth starts from within. Let's take a wild trip through these theories.

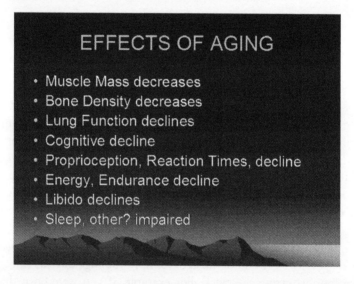

Figure 1.1. A few biomarkers, or measurable health parameters, which generally decline as we chronologically age and comprise our *physiological* age. Many are additive, which lead to more severe consequences. (C. Rao, 2006)

Chronological age—your age in years since your original birthday suit—"can't touch this" until we discover how to go back in time.

Physiological age—your overall level of functioning. You're as young as you feel!

A. The Genetic Theory. As famously elucidated by Watson and Crick in 1953,[1] the double helix configuration of deoxyribonucleic acid (DNA) contains the encrypted codes for our many genes. These genes, found on the twenty-three paired chromosomes found in a human cell's nucleus, determine our many inherited traits. In fact, the human genome, the entire genetic map, has now been qualified and quantified since the mid-1990s. There are about 3.5 billion DNA base pairs that determine the blueprints for who and what we are. Although we have identified about 35,000 different genes and have come a long way, genetic therapies are still far from being perfected. Let's not wait until then, though. We can actually do our *own* genetic manipulation cheaply and safely today. Yes, you *can* try this at home! Here are some background and techniques.

We all hope that if our parents lived a long and healthy life, we will too. Unfortunately, this is not always the case. Let me explain with a few examples. If fortunate enough to have healthy parents, we do have some selective advantage for a longer, healthier life. This does make common sense, and scientific evidence backs this up. However, let's take an example of somebody that may have had great genes from the start, yet abused his health. He smoked, drank too much alcohol, didn't exercise, and ate an unhealthy diet. He would probably start to suffer from many mild or frank diseases by middle age. As you will read later, these may include diabetes, hypertension, high cholesterol, obesity, emphysema, back pain, fatigue, sexual problems, and so forth. This will ultimately result in his premature disability and death. So having great genes is like a lottery check that gets cashed in by middle age if you don't invest wisely. Basically, your original factory warranty has run out, and now Mother Nature has to do her recycling thing. (Sorry, she doesn't offer extended warranties at this time.)

Another analogy may be the soapbox derby car you raced as a young Boy Scout. Remember how your dad and you invested the time to make sure it was all shiny and put together right? Sure, having it all aligned on that hill with your back to the wind was a great head start. That's really all he could do for you at that point. It was then up to you to steer the right course and win. If you didn't, you might have lost a wheel or crashed into a tree. Well, midlife is very similar, guys. At this important *fork in the road,* it's all up to you to steer the right course for a healthy finish!

Lastly, an alarming example is the onset of adult diabetes in our younger population. Here, the not-so-good genes are being expressed at a much earlier age. We're now in a

---

1   In 1962, Watson and Crick were awarded the Nobel Prize for their discovery. There were many other researchers that pioneered discoveries leading up to this final compilation. Visit http://www.geneticengineering.org for more background information.

pandemic of diabetes nationally, if not worldwide. There is an increasing number of preteens with what's been coined *early-onset* adult diabetes. As I like to succinctly put it, diabetes represents *premature aging of the body*. With diabetes, instead of getting the many age-related complications in the seventies, we experience them in our fifties. Unfortunately, today's diabetic teenagers are suffering the same fate as their diabetic grandparents, but at a much earlier age—many in their twenties! This is probably due to their lack of regular exercise, a simple starch-based diet, and more factors that will be discussed later. They never enjoyed the healthier childhood we had that would help them delay these deleterious metabolic changes. They got off on the wrong path from the get-go. Their beneficial, protective genes are, in effect, being repressed. I cannot stress how important it is for us to set the example of proper diet and exercise for our children. In the end, our genes, and jeans, will fit much better!

All we middle-aged men should undergo a full assessment of our health and behavior to make sure we are on our healthiest track. This, of course, will help prevent early-disease risks from worsening. An example is the increase of visceral fat, or the middle-age spread, we guys get. Insulin and cortisol are increasing, therefore increasing risks for hypertension, diabetes, inflammation, and decreased immune function. Cholesterol streaks may be silently progressing to inflamed plaques in the coronary and peripheral arteries. These subacute, hidden changes are quite subtle. Yet, these set the course for us to acquire more severe diseases later, such as dementia, osteoporosis, frailty syndrome, rheumatological diseases, and more that we will present later. Let's prevent these problems before they happen. Let's not wait for a mad scientist to get in our genes and do it for us. At the very least, we will have better genes later on when genetic manipulation may be perfected.

> No matter what genetic predisposition you may have, you can *express* the beneficial genes and *repress* the not-so-good ones by being proactive with a healthier lifestyle. So far, scientific genetic manipulation has had not much success. But as the above suggests, you can do your own genetic manipulation cheaply, safely, and effectively with healthier behavior. Avoid smoking, boozing, and just hangin' out. Get moving! Having great genes is a good head start, but you still must be proactive to help ensure a healthy middle and older age. Much research has proven this. The time to act is now. Get moving on the right path!

B. The Wear 'n' Tear Theory.
This basically became popular in the early 1960s. This is based on a lot of the work on free radical theory done by Denam Harman in the late 1950s. He basically hypothesized that one's life span is determined by the amount

of cumulative mitochondrial damage that takes place. (The mitochondria are much like the batteries within the cell.) According to his theory, aging is mostly considered a process of repeated, additive damage to the many cellular molecular structures and the resulting dysfunction. In other words, we age when this damage gradually outpaces the repairs we can make. More damage and fewer repairs equal advanced aging. This damage results from the production of *free radicals*.

> Accordingly, aging occurs when the rate of damage exceeds the rate of repair.

Free radicals are also called reactive oxygen species (ROS). As a background, chemical compounds can be either stable or unstable. Unstable molecules are more *reactive*. This stability is determined by the amount of paired electrons or *shared* electrons in an element or compound respectively. Basically, nature prefers compounds to have a completed outer shell of electrons in order to be balanced. If a compound has an unpaired electron in the outer shell, it will then try to *scavenge* an electron from a nearby compound. When this electron is then stolen, the donating compound becomes damaged. It then, in turn, becomes an ROS, trying to complete its outer shell and causing a chain reaction of damage. Please see diagram below:

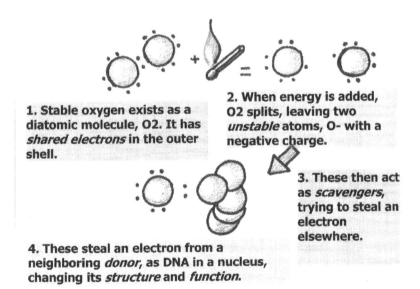

1. Stable oxygen exists as a diatomic molecule, O2. It has *shared electrons* in the outer shell.

2. When energy is added, O2 splits, leaving two *unstable* atoms, O- with a negative charge.

3. These then act as *scavengers*, trying to steal an electron elsewhere.

4. These steal an electron from a neighboring *donor*, as DNA in a nucleus, changing its *structure* and *function*.

Fig 1.2. Free radicals and reactive oxygen species (ROS) can cause damage like fire. Antioxidants help put the fire out. (C. Rao, 2007)

Most of us are familiar with oxygen. The elemental gas O2 exists as paired oxygen molecules, which has a complete outer shell of electrons. Normally, oxygen is quite stable when possessing paired electrons as in water, H2O. But when the oxygen molecule is split, it becomes an ROS and then tries to scavenge electrons from surrounding structures. Now, these structures may be the cellular membrane, nucleus, mitochondria, or other important cellular components. This damage is microscopic, but it's real and snowballs into the observable, degenerative changes we commonly observe with aging. Indeed, rapid oxidation causes fire. If we look at how these damages occur on a *biochemical* or *cellular* level, we can understand what happens at the next higher *tissue* level. This in turn gives us a clue into what's going on at the larger *organ* or *system* level. Ultimately, this should give insight into what happens to the organism as a whole. As exclaimed by a pioneer in this field Dr. Michael Fossel back in 1999, "Aging is a tug of war that we can win!" I opine that we can slow down or postpone many aspects of aging. It's seems much easier to extinguish a small fire before we become engulfed in the insidious inferno of illness and incompetence.

For example, if we could find out what abnormally happens biochemically inside an aging neuron, we could then start to understand what is going on in the aging brain with mild cognitive impairment or dementia. Armed with this knowledge, we can hopefully find newer ways to slow down or, better yet, prevent this degeneration. Likewise, when we find ways to improve the longevity of the individual heart muscle *cell*, then we can help prevent myocardial infarction and congestive heart failure of the heart *organ*. These benefits then spread to an overall healthier circulatory *system*, both cardiac and peripherally. Because of the mind-body connection, this approach ultimately and synergistically leads to a better-functioning, happier individual as a whole.

This damage is very important to understand from a structural and functional standpoint. If you recall from high school biology, the cell's *membrane* basically determines what comes *into* and what goes *out* of the cell. Additionally, there are many receptors *on* the membrane that determines the many metabolic consequences occurring *in* the cell. There are receptors that can stimulate the cell to grow and produce various hormones, products, or messengers, either beneficial or harmful. It can also trigger apoptosis (its own cellular death) and trigger reactions in the mitochondria and nucleus. ROS cause damage to the mitochondria, causing an impairment of cellular energy production and mitochondrial DNA. In the nucleus, ROS cause damage to the most important DNA or RNA, the blueprints for the cell. It must be appreciated that damage to any of the cellular components predisposes the cell to early degeneration, death, or even cancer. We certainly don't desire any of these outcomes, but they variably occur with increasing frequency as we age. If one abuses their body by overwhelming it with smoking, alcohol, and other unhealthy acts, then this degeneration is further accelerated. Frequently living life in the fast lane with fast food will only get you there sooner.

So what do we do about this? It is known that *antioxidants* act as scavengers of the ROS. These effectively act as buffers and donate their electrons so that the needed normal-functioning cellular constituents don't have to become damaged. Out of such necessity, the body makes a lot of these naturally. Glutathione, peroxidases, and many others naturally flourish in our younger body. As we age, besides the increasing damage to deal with, we naturally produce less of these scavengers. Therefore, taking supplements may be an added benefit in helping to limit the degeneration as we age.

We will discuss supplements later, but I will give a brief introduction. I believe, and most others do too, that there is no one magic supplement that prevents the ravages of age. Rather, a nice consortium of these probably benefits us more than taking megadoses of only a few. For example, it is probably better to take a daily low-dose multivitamin than it is to take only megadoses of vitamin C or E. Some recent research as the HOPE-TOO trial reinforces this view. Additionally, it is more important to have the proper diet and exercise than to merely rely on a few magic potions to compensate for our misbehavior. At any rate, the *convergence of evidence* I reviewed suggests that taking a multivitamin may help prevent some of the degeneration and conditions we acquire as we gracefully mature. Supposedly, 70 percent of Americans are deficient in at least one vitamin.

> The wear 'n' tear theory suggests most age-related inflammation and degeneration result from the damage caused by free radicals at the cellular level. This can then spread like fire throughout the body. Antioxidants may offer some benefit, but they are no replacement for a proper lifestyle.

C. The Neurohormonal Theory of Aging.

This was promoted by Dr. Daniel Rudman's groundbreaking research in 1990 that concluded, "The overall deterioration of the body that comes with growing old is not inevitable … we now realize that some aspects of it can be prevented or reversed." It's just a sad fact of life that as we age, the hormones we wish would go up, *go down*. And the ones we would like to go down, *go up!* Tony Soprano might say that this is how *normal* aging tries to whack us out! Think of the hormones as the musicians in an orchestra that must all play in harmony to keep us humming throughout life. Nature uses these chemical messengers to regulate the millions of duties the body performs. They must play the right song, key, tempo, and be in a dynamic balance. They're also like the legs on the chair you're sitting on; they should be optimally balanced and upright as when new. If not, you may one day scream, "I've fallen and I can't get up!"

As we age, insulin and cortisol go up; and thus the risk for hypertension, diabetes, obesity, osteoporosis, arthritis, and more follow. The hormones that diminish usually include dehydroepiandrosterone (DHEA), pregnenolone, melatonin, testosterone, thyroid, and human growth hormone. (Of course, menopause causes a marked decrease in estrogen and progesterone for women—the aptly named change of life.) These changes cause risks for many other conditions such as the frailty syndrome, hypercholesterolemia, fatigue, depression, insomnia, and many others. It would then make sense that restoring these hormones to optimal levels would help ward off these complications. As we will review later, most of the scientific literature reflects the fact that hormonal replacements do have such dramatic health benefits in the middle-aged, healthy individual. This is ideally when prevention should take place.

I fully believe if you want to beat Mother Nature at her game, then you must learn to play *her* game in order to win. The only true ways to slow down aging would be to undo her modus operandi. The hormones, being the chemical messengers in the body, dictate whether we are anabolic (building up and repairing ourselves) or catabolic (breaking down, a.k.a. aging). Today, there are lots of professionals and industries touting natural remedies when, in fact, they're not when you really think about it. Antiaging is big business with big profits. We must remember that any herb or supplement is still in pill form, made somewhere in some factory, and therefore not truly *natural*. When was the last time you saw pills growing as a leaf or a root on a tree? As that old Parkay Margarine commercial boasted, "It's not nice to fool Mother Nature!" So you must first have a greater appreciation of the scientific facts of aging and its causes to then recognize the many proven, safe methods of achieving optimal health. Right on, brother!

As we age, insulin and cortisol levels tend to increase; and thus the risks for hypertension, diabetes, obesity, osteoporosis, inflammation, and infection. The hormones that variably diminish include DHEA, pregnenolone, melatonin, testosterone, thyroid, and human growth hormone. These changes cause risks for the above and many other conditions such as the frailty syndrome, hypercholesterolemia, fatigue, depression, and insomnia, It then makes sense that restoring these hormones would help ward off these complications.

D. Let's Expand on the Age-Management Medicine Paradigm.

To some, slowing down or reversing aging may still seem like quackery. Novel thinking and modalities are commonly met with such skepticism and mockery; so don't feel bad if you're still a little leery. For example, until the late 1970s, the only successful treatment for gastric ulcers was surgery. Many well meaning surgeons believed that if it's bad or defective, simply cut it out and it's cured." There was little appreciation for why divineness may have put that organ there in the first place. Thousands, as my darling uncle Steve, received the typical vagotomy and antrectomy procedure for treating duodenal ulcers.[2] Their ulcer was now gone, but they suffered some lifelong consequences, as well. The antral portion of the stomach is responsible for the absorption of B_{12}, folate, and iron. Many who received these operations suffered from vitamin deficiencies and the so-called dumping syndrome. The latter caused them to have diarrhea soon after eating. In the end, many lifestyles were often more interrupted from the cure than from the actual disease itself. Then, one of the first *miracle drugs*, Tagamet, came into the scene. This was a novel medical treatment that basically replaced the surgery. It effectively reduces the acidity of the stomach and was first greeted with skepticism and reluctance, but eventually gained popularity. Nowadays, it's considered quite safe and is now available over the counter (OTC)—no prescription needed; and you can add your own knife to enjoy.

When we look at gastric ulcer research in the 1990s, we again encounter reluctance with the idea ulcers can be caused by a bacterial infection. Initially, the contemporary medical establishment laughed at this because of the long-held belief that bacteria simply cannot survive in the stomach's acidic environment. It was ridiculous to consider an infection causes an ulcer and even increases risk for stomach cancers. Yet, now, after years and much further research, it's now accepted that

---

2   The vagus nerve is cut for less excitation to the stomach to produce acid; and the antral portion of the stomach is removed resulting in fewer glands to make acid and risk for an ulcer.

Helicobacter pylori causes the majority of ulcers in people who do not partake of alcohol or aspirin-like products. Patients with ulcer symptoms typically receive endoscopy with gastric biopsies and cultures to rule out this infection, as many can now be cured permanently with proper antibiotic treatment. For many today, there's no longer a need for lifelong Tagamet therapy.

Historically, many doctors that presented novel diagnostic and treatment options were initially ridiculed. Dr. K. McCully first suggested homocysteine was a modifiable risk factor for coronary disease. He subsequently suffered enormous harassment from his colleagues and even lost his tenure and position. (You'll read more on this topic in the supplement chapter.) There's also the noted obstetrician-gynecologist that help introduced laparoscopy as a less-invasive surgical procedure. Initially scoffed by his contemporaries that used open-type surgeries, he endured challenges from his peers as well. Yet, laparoscopy has now evolved into the preferred method for most surgeries. Anything else would be like operating in the Stone Age at Megasaurus Memorial in Fred Flintstone's town of Bedrock. So you can see it's quite common for novel thinking to be initially ridiculed, even rejected. There may also be some confusion and abuse by inexperienced doctors that initially go along with novel techniques until the proper niche is found. Much is the current state of affairs with using hormonal replacements. Although mostly scientifically proven to help prevent and treat many conditions of aging, there's still much confusion, abuse, and needed debate.

As with all medical doctors, I was trained on the hospital floors and had to work my way up to the top. In medical school, all students learned first about normal physiology followed by the pathophysiology of diseases—like if the Fox Network did a "When Good Organs Go Bad" special. We spend six of our eight years of training studying *sickness* and *disease*. Patients we see are typically in their last six months, or even six days, of life's journey. Therefore, the main exposure is treating the very sick or very elderly. It's then no wonder that these processes are considered a normal part of life. There's relatively little time spent on *prevention* or how to *optimize* a patient's health. As a family physician, I did select a specialty where prevention does play a larger role. Treating the person as a whole, I also enjoy the long-term rewarding relationships. That's not to denigrate the breadth and depth of training that a modern medical school and residency provides an MD. I believe there is no better replacement; however, there needs to be more taught on nutrition, exercise, and disease prevention. My passion, since such formal education, has been on learning more about the nonmedical means to achieve healthier aging.

Most medical training has taken place in large university settings that have long been overwhelmed with treating the very sick and disabled. In order to survive, they have promoted a Band-Aid, pass-the-buck mentality that now permeates all levels of health care. Reinforced by drug firms that sponsor most academic research, this reactive view has been cross-pollinated by our political leaders and corporate profits. It's been an expensive, bitter pill to swallow with many side effects. Overall, America's health today is unacceptable. It's time for a change, although this new paradigm of curing yourself will be met with resistance on many fronts.

The big paradigm shift I'm talking about requires that we look at aging as a *syndrome* itself. As opposed to treating the many complications of aging, let's treat the root cause! Let me explain with a few analogies. Most people are now familiar with AIDS.[3] As a brief review, this disease is a viral infection that compromises the immune system and is usually transmitted via blood or other body fluids. It's progressive, and there's currently no real cure. Many lives have been claimed by HIV since its appearance in the early 1980s; it's now a global epidemic. Yet, when a person gets HIV, he doesn't actually die from the virus itself. Rather, he dies from the *complications* brought on by HIV. This is a very important point to grasp. The viral infection eventually progresses to become AIDS. Now, the immune system is nil, and he suffers from the frailty syndrome[4] and probably dementia, too. There are many other abnormalities such as the wasting syndrome, *Pneumocystis pneumoniae* infection, lymphoma, or other cancers. He may survive one bout of pneumonia today but may encounter a severe case of diarrhea or other malady weeks later.[5] As you can deduce, treating merely the complications doesn't really *effect* a cure. Rather in many instances, this only prolongs the sickness and the inevitable. Of course, the best *cure* for HIV would be to *prevent* the viral infection in the first place by a vaccine or other primary prevention method. But once the

---

3   A medical resident in 1994, I was chosen to help revamp the Florida Medical Association's CME course on HIV/AIDS. That same year, my uncle Steve eventually succumbed to the ravages of AIDS.

4   The frailty syndrome closely resembles advanced age or the neglect of a healthy lifestyle. More will be covered in the hormonal chapters. In actuality, human growth hormone replacement has been used to fight the frailty syndrome of AIDS.

5   HIV (human immunodeficiency virus); AIDS (acquired immunodeficiency syndrome). There are many complications of AIDS. This disease is briefly presented as an analogy to the aging syndrome.

person is infected with HIV, the only cure would be to eliminate the virus or its replication—the root cause of the disease.

Another case for this paradigm shift can be made with the disease progeria. In this poorly understood, rare disease, children age at a much faster rate. While only in their teens, they begin to suffer arthritis, heart disease, dementia, and all the other maladies we normal people get much later in life. Given what was presented above, how would we then devise the best cure for progeria? Would we want to treat the many *outcomes* of such premature aging? Or would we try to identify and treat the *true underlying cause* in the first place, say a gene mutation? Of course, the latter makes more sense.

With those examples as a preface, let's delve into what this paradigm shift means to the middle-aged man trying to fight off old age. In today's world, doctors treat you for the *many outcomes* of aging. As you mature, cholesterol generally goes up, so you are prescribed a cholesterol pill. Along with the weight and fat gain, maybe hypertension and diabetes result in three more pills—right into the breadbasket. You then may need inhalers because your lungs got the wind knocked out of them. Maybe depression and back pain has now got you bent over, so that adds a few more pills. Because of their side effects, you may be prescribed more pills. You then get sucker punched by artery disease that demands a bypass, angioplasty, or other quick fix. You may even rebound after a few bouts with pneumonia. Then, you'd stagger to get up from arthritis. As frailty increases, you are forced to chug down an osteoporosis pill. You've not tossed in the towel yet. Then there are the final rounds with dementia, Parkinson's disease, urosepsis,[6] hip fracture, and so on—all the experienced fighters are now ganging up on you.

Despite being punch-drunk, you keep getting tossed back in the ring by your many doctors. You begin to see the spotlights, only they're the ones in the OR. You feel the heat. It's really a fever. The crowd is screaming, but you realize that it's the Code Team working on the patient next to you. The stench of the arena intoxicates you … well, that's really *your* stench, and you're actually overmedi-cated. Don't you wish you had a coach like Rocky Balboa had in *Rocky II* about now? Becoming too weak to hold your guard up, you may prefer to get TKO'd than to risk getting paralyzed and winding up in a retirement home.

---

6   Urosepsis is a urinary tract infection that spreads to the blood (sepsis) and is probably the second-biggest infection cause of death in the elderly after pneumonia.

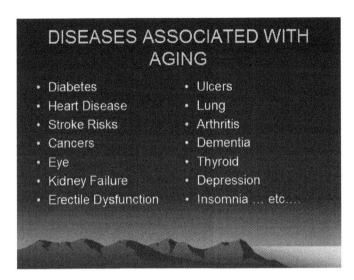

Figure 1.3. Listed above are diseases occurring with increased frequency as we age. In most instances, one disease causes many other conditions to appear and, thus, has a snowballing effect. For example, diabetes causes at least four times risk of heart and peripheral vessel disease, cancers, dementia, and kidney failure. (C. Rao, 2007)

In summary, our current healthcare model of individually treating all these outcomes of *normal* aging is not the best. We now have the research and know-how to promote a new paradigm, but such change on a large scale is inherently slow. We have identified a lot of what occurs as we age: the changes in genetic expression, the degeneration, the decrease in immune function, the increase in inflammation, the increase in frailty, and so on. The frailty and metabolic disorders result from the decrease in bone and muscle mass and the increase in fat mass. The increase in inflammation causes arthritis, dementia, heart disease and peripheral vascular disease, and more. All these conditions are then worsened by what's currently accepted as normal age-related neurohormonal changes. Yet, what can we do to fight back and regain the power to control our destiny? By reading this book, you can grasp your health by the wheel and steer clear of many of life's missiles, much as you did as a kid playing the video game Space Invaders!

It's far better in the long run to treat the true underlying abnormalities than merely trying to alleviate the many increasing symptoms of what prematurely ages us. Since most all pills merely treat the symptoms of chronic diseases, prevention is key.

As introduced in the preface, I feel midlife is a very important yet grossly under-appreciated stage of a man's life. Personally, we all may want to deny it to some degree, maybe even spend a lot of money and time trying to hide from it. Yet, we should embrace it as the window of opportunity it really represents. Yeah, yeah, yeah, we have all heard about pediatrics, adolescent medicine, geriatrics, and gynecology, but no medical specialty has focused on middle-age health as a priority. There's even less focus on men's health and the importance of fatherhood. I would also venture to state that middle age now represents the longest stage in modern men's lives. (This makes sense, especially given the fact that we generally don't live as long as women.) I think a tremendous opportunity to get things healthier is currently being ignored. Midlife is a time when most of us guys are at the top of our game at the workplace. Yet, the warranty that we were given when we were young and disease-free is about to wear out. We may have even lost some friends in their forties or fifties, who died from an unexpected, sudden disease. This can be quite alarming and eye-opening. Ironically, we still may trudge along doing the same daily grind. We put on the blinders and earplugs ourselves in a way, just working for the weekend. Meanwhile, we may be ignoring the many early warning signs of disease. What you don't know *can* hurt you!

Mostly undetectable from the outside, there may be many signs of progressive disease festering inside. This is the opportune moment to effect a lifestyle change that will help you later in life. I do believe that how proactive you are about your optimal health in midlife determines how well you do in the latter half of life. It *can* be the golden years! But you *have* to be proactive about it now. In my practice, I see some men, forty-five years old, that possess the *physiological* age of someone in their early thirties. Yet, I also see some of the same chronological age that, because of having many of the mostly preventable problems mentioned above, their physiological age is over sixty! Ultimately, it's up to *you* to have great health because the other players involved in this decision making are either upside-down or have other agendas.

> In most midlifers, there are often signs of subtle, early disease. These are usually ignored by the person or undetected by doctors until they progress to frank, overt disease later on. Then, it may be too late.

The current health care system we have also contributes to this reactive, fix it only when it's broken mentality. Most people have health insurance during their employable years, which works similar to the following scenario: You must have a complaint, thus a *diagnosis code*, for insurance to pay for your doctor's visit. So actually, you *do* have to first be *sick* to be seen by a doctor. If you visit the doctor too much, you will then get a lot of diagnosis codes listed on your record, and you subsequently may be dropped for being high risk. This works as any other insurance, be it car or home. Or your business or job may change, and then your new policy states all these *prior conditions* aren't covered. You may now find you're in quite a bind. As an example, one time I saw a middle-aged dentist who wanted to know if he had arthritis. I warned him that if we ordered a sedimentation rate, a lab test for inflammation, I would have to put down "joint pain" as a diagnosis code for the insurance to pay for it. As it turned out, the test was negative—luckily, rheumatoid arthritis was effectively ruled out. However, a few months later, he called up, complaining that his disability insurance had dropped him because he now had a history of arthritis!

The current state of the health-care system is indeed distorted at many levels. If a guy is truly concerned about his health and desires some lab work and a few doctor visits, he then gets a lot of diagnoses written down in his health record. This is actually seen as *negative* behavior, and he is usually penalized in some way by the insurance company because they had to lay out more money for such proactivity. On my side of things, with the decreasing reimbursements for decades by insurance companies, doctors' offices now have to see more patients per day to meet the bottom line. The staff's time is very limited and the patients are put on a strict time schedule—even overbooked, much like in the airline industry. These restraints cause less time for a lengthier evaluation and when combined with the current malpractice insurance crisis, may often result in the overordering of tests to cover the doctor's butt or the likelihood of unnecessary procedures in order to cost shift. This adds to more referrals to specialists and often leads to more frustration and expense. Yet, insurance firms are exempt from antitrust laws and can simply raise their premiums to reflect their increased operating costs. The doctor usually can't, despite office costs skyrocketing over the past ten years. Most of the doctors' fees are decreasing and are unrealistically set by Medicare, with insurances then unfairly paying only a fraction of that. All this sets the stage for spiraling costs with little hope for preserving a good doctor-patient relationship. Some would call that the *perfect storm*.

Included in all this is the possibility of increased medication errors because of the limited time available for the counseling of *nonmedical* ways to treat or prevent disease. According to the October 18, 2006, *JAMA* (*Journal of the American Medical*

Association), an estimated seventy thousand Americans are seen annually in the ER because of adverse reactions from prescribed medications. Patients are now being seen more often by lesser-trained so-called health-care professionals. It's all about *volume*, not *service* anymore. It's a shame less than 5 percent of the health-care dollars spent in this country is for prevention. I believe the only way to truly *contain* health-care costs in this country is to have a *healthier* nation as a whole, including the very young and old. That should be a no-brainer, right? Lastly, I find it very frustrating to regularly see many diseased individuals that could be enormously helped by even minimally improving their lifestyle habits. They too may be looking for the one magic pill or an operation as an easier way out. There must be better ways; and there are—the more proactive, safer, and integrative approaches methods expressed in this book. "The *best* health insurance is to healthier in the first place!" I always say.

> Being proactive about your health now will result in less insurance premiums as you age and lower the risks of taking multiple medications. It's a win-win!

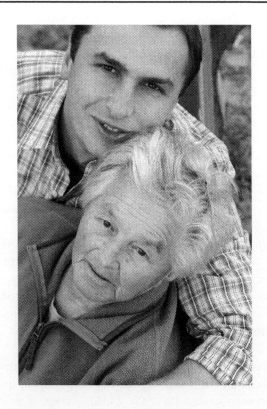

Now for some tongue-in-cheek good news; no one has died from "old age" since 1951. Wouldn't it be great if we did, in fact, find a cure for old age back then! Unfortunately, this is not the case. Rather at that time, federal and state law dictated that a physician can no longer put the immediate cause of death on the death certificate as "old age." Now most of the time the elderly patient has multiple comorbidities, namely, COPD (emphysema), hypertension, coronary and peripheral vascular disease, risk for blood clots, immune compromise, and many others. This makes it virtually impossible for a physician to know what the elderly patient at home exactly died from. So we basically *guesstimate* what did him in. Research and autopsies have shown at least half of the time what the physician lists on the death certificate doesn't match what the patient actually died from. Not so surprising, heart attack and stroke appears to be the first and third biggest killer overall. Cancer, all ages combined, happens to be the second biggest killer. However, it's important to note that for people under the age of eighty-five, cancer is the biggest killer. We will find in later chapters that the age-related increase in inflammation which causes a decrease in immune function, as well us living in a more toxic environment contribute to these statistics.

> The paradigm shift in age-management medicine is that aging is a syndrome, a collection of related conditions, which varies by severity and onset for each individual. By identifying the root causes of why and how we age, we can find out better ways to help prevent or delay many of its complications.

Let's explore the important concepts of *health span* and *life span*. *Life span* is basically the same as physiological age; it's solely about how long you live. Take for example our grandparents' generation that was born in the early 1900s; they had a life expectancy of only about forty-seven years. Yet, the ones alive today have survived more than double this estimate. Some researchers now suggest that increasing numbers from our generation may live between 110 to 120 years! I don't know about you, but if I live to 120, I don't want to live, act, or feel it. As The Who sang, "Hope I die before I get old!"

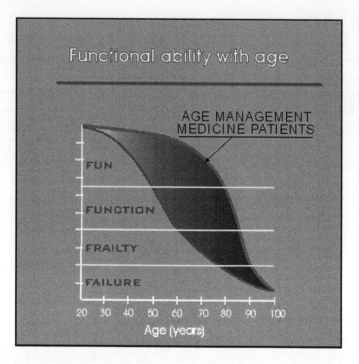

Figure 1.4. Health span curves. How well you take care of yourself determines which of the above curves you will follow as you age. Which curve do you want to ride? (Adapted from Cenegenics©)

Health span is basically how *well* you live. It's not mere quantity, but more important, it's the *quality of life*. From talking with many elderly patients, I'm amazed to find most have generally accepted their eventual demise without fear. What's scary to them is *how* they spend their later years. All of us want to live a long time but realize it's more important to live healthier. If you look back a few generations, you'll see most of our forefathers did enjoy a healthy life. This is due in part to their lifestyle. They probably had less stress or learned better ways of dealing with it. Indeed, Gramps had more manually laborious activities combined with a healthier diet. There was less pollution too. For example, my grandfather lived a healthy life up until he was sixty-two. At such time, he probably suffered a stroke or heart attack and suddenly died. Yet, he lived happily at home and was healthy his entire life. He *lived* until the day he died. Not on any pills or suffering from any known medical conditions, he never had any operations. His health span would be represented by curve A in figure 1.5.

This is exactly what Mother Nature selected for him and, for that matter, all of us men. We're basically selected and evolved to live to reproduction age and pass on our genes—to ensure life continues on. Maybe, she'll add a few more years to help raise our young, so they can survive better. At this point, we're done as far as Mother Nature is concerned. We've done all our duties by middle age; now it's best for us to be well … recycled. Why have bunches of old men just hanging around, doing nothing, and using up valuable resources? While this may be good for the survival of the species as a whole, we baby boomers probably aren't ready to be all that altruistic.

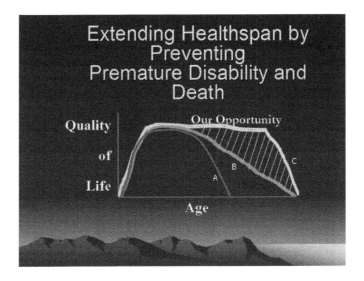

Figure 1.5. Extending health span. Where are you now? Where do you want to go from here?

Now, we come to our parents' health span, curve B. Here, quantity beats quality, man! With all the medical innovations in the past few decades, people are, indeed, living a *longer* time. But are they necessarily enjoying an entirely *better* life? Some do, but many don't. Although we now have effectively increased *life span*, I believe we haven't improved the *health span* as much as we could. I'll tell you what I mean. Granted, a lot of older people have received antibiotics or an operation, which allowed them to live a somewhat longer time. Included in this has been an increased morbidity, or sickness, in their later years. People are living a longer life-time but a longer *sick-time* as well. Today, most nursing homes and assisted-living facilities are full to capacity. We often read how the health-care system is becoming more strained. Additionally, no one really wants to become dependent on others or be a burden to family. Giving up one's home and spending one's last few years on Earth debilitated among strangers in a nursing home is quite a depressing ending to life, but it's becoming a common reality. This would be represented by the last part of curve B above. Although a number of years were added, they're more sickly years of declining function and more dependence.

Curve C is really where we should be headed. It represents what I promote—increasing health span as well as life span. Here, we keep the optimal health and functioning of a forty-year-old while in our seventies! In this scenario, the sickly portion of the curve is limited to the very end. This paradigm combines the best parts of the previous two curves and limits the bad. This approach is very aptly called *morbidity compression*. It's all about *living* until the day you die. I think most would rather follow curve C. Believe it or not, this thinking is quite new. The health-care delivery system and the insurance industry don't appreciate it or are willing to support it. Instead of crooning Tim McGraw's catchy tune, "Live Like You Were Dying," I'd rather sing, "Die like you were really living!"

Reinforcing this paradigm were recent findings from the renowned Framingham Heart Study.[7] Basically, men and women who reached fifty with the fewest risk factors for disease had a better chance of a healthier, longer life. Researchers found dramatic increases in cardiovascular disease risk and length of life between participants who reached age fifty with two or more risk factors. Those with two risk factors lived a decade less. "Reducing risk factors to one or none is very achievable," encouraged the author. He added that exercising, maintaining a healthy weight and proper diet, and not smoking may make a difference in life span, risk for disease, and long-term quality-of-life measures. I can find volumes of research that parallel these conclusions. It makes common sense that midlifers enjoying a healthier diet and staying more active would end up keeping their muscle and bone mass up and fat mass down. This also limits inflammation and boosts their immune system. They'll ultimately fare much better than their less-proactive cohorts.

Staying Alive! Elizabeth "Lizzie" Bolden, the world's oldest person according to the Gerontology Research Group, recently died in a nursing home in Memphis on December 12, 2006.[8] There supposedly existed a woman in Chechnya whom many believed reached 124! Before Lizzie, the longest living American was Maude Farris-Luse who reached 115. What was her secret to having such a long life? "Not moping around!" Supposedly, the world's oldest *man* died at 114 in Japan in

---

7   D. Lloyd-Jones, "Reach fifty with as few risk factors," *Circulation* (2006): 113.

8   Before that, a Japanese woman, believed to be the world's oldest person according to the *Guinness Book of World Records* also reached 116.

2003. He was a teetotaler who drank a glass of milk per day. His predecessor was an Italian that swore his secret to longevity was a daily glass of red wine. Family members stated both men led a very stress-free life.[9] Well, that sounds like good advice from those, besides maybe Star Trek Captain Kirk, that have gone where no man has before. Keep your life stress-free, yet stay busy. Some tea and wine may help out too.

Additionally, the health ministry of Japan announced in 2003 they had well over twenty thousand centenarians. As expected, the vast majority, 84 percent, were women. Japan also holds the record for the world's longest life expectancy—almost eighty-five years for women and seventy-eight for men. However, this accolade is causing the country some problems. It's estimated that one person will be over sixty-five for every two working by 2025, a situation that is bound to place a strain on the economy.[10] I have to add that the Japanese and Okinawans have some of the healthiest lifestyles, including a less inflammatory diet consisting of more omega-3 fats. (You'll read more about that, later.)

The World Health Organization (WHO) recently reported life expectancy in the United States has reached another all-time high, 77.6 years. The average life span was 74.8 years for men and 80.1 years for women, and has been rising steadily since 1900. This increase is mostly due to the advances made in sanitation, antibiotics, and childbirth. The WHO added that deaths from heart disease, cancer, and stroke continue to drop, albeit with some precautions. Apparently, half of the older baby boomers aged fifty-five to sixty-four have high blood pressure; and two out of five are obese. Basically, we are in worse shape than those born a decade earlier. Dr. Julie Gerberding, director for the Centers for Disease Control in Atlanta, reminds us it's never too late to adopt a healthier lifestyle and enjoy a longer, healthier life; yet middle age is a crucial time to focus on disease prevention. This same group is expected to rise from twenty-nine million in 2004 to forty trillion by 2014. Interestingly, the number of those with hypertension and obesity are higher; but because of the many anticholesterol drugs we now have available, the rate of hypercholesterolemia has supposedly dropped.[11] Meanwhile, expenditures on health care rose 7.7 percent to 1.6 trillion dollars in 2002—well over

9   http://www.guardian.co.uk, accessed July 30 and September 30, 2003.
10 http://www.reutershealth.com, accessed September 9, 2003.
11 From U.S. Centers for Disease Control, WHO, as reported in *Associated Press* (2006).

$5,000 per person![12] That's almost 50 percent more than the next biggest spender, Switzerland. Prescription drugs were the fastest-growing expenditure, rising 11 percent in 2003. Most data indicate baby boomers can expect to live a longer time due to medical innovation, but not necessarily a healthier time in their later years. Smoking, alcoholism, drug use, violence, AIDS, and the fact that our children are becoming more obese with chronic complications as diabetes, will continue to bring on greater personal and societal burdens unless needed changes are made.

This gets down to what I'm talking about. Thanks to many medical innovations, we can now prolong life span. However, because of worsening social, personal, and environmental factors, health span hasn't followed. This is particularly true during the later years of life. In a way, we've exchanged quality for more quantity of life. Nowadays, we have to be concerned about many age-related complications our parents never heard of—dementia, osteoporosis, frailty syndrome, erectile dysfunction, and so on. This adds up to an enormous expense, both socially and personally. By the 1990s, buying the average sixty-five-year-old an extra year of life costs society $145,000.[13] Most of this is largely for futile end-of-life care. Unless we identify and treat what causes the syndrome of aging in the first place, we're left with merely treating its many complications. This only delays and worsens the inevitable, at best. Additionally, the personal choices we make for a sedentary lifestyle and improper diet result in an earlier onset and increased severity of these complications. As a reflection of the above, death rates from falls in older men have increased almost 50 percent in the past ten years.[14] We guys need to bone up on prevention and personal responsibility if we are to have an optimal quality of life in our later years.

We can extrapolate this even further. As mentioned, scientists today predict middle-aged persons may live to be 120! It's not too far of a stretch to expect these outcomes when genetic engineering, stem cell therapies, and even replacing worn-out body parts with longer-lasting prosthesis become a reality. Personally, I am planning to harvest my bone marrow sometime this year in anticipation. Some predict that with these advancements, people may be able to live even hundreds of years old! Naturally, I have some healthy skepticism about that; yet I keep an open mind. If I live to be that old *chronologically*, I certainly don't want to feel that ancient!

---

12 Health Affairs Report by Center for Medicare and Medicaid Services, January 8, 2004.
13 D. Cutler, *NEJM* (October 2006).
14 Stevens J. *CDC Morbidity and Mortality Report*, November 16, 2006.

When it comes down to it, there is no *one* theory that fully explains how we age; it is a combination of all of them. Accordingly, I offer an encompassing view, a better *paradigm*, for looking at our number one asset, our health. However, this new paradigm *must* be accompanied by a change in behavior in order to affect any real good—especially in middle age. One's health *can* truly be an asset, if optimized, or a *liability*, on the other hand. It takes a commitment on your part as *you* are ultimately the one most responsible for how well you age. Look around you next time you're at the drugstore that's having an adult diaper two-for-one sale. Do you want to age normally, or *optimally*?

Everything old may be new again, after all. A lot of what I present in this book will have its roots in many old-time sayings. I will then proceed to reinforce this by recent medical literature. It's comforting to know these two reflect what I will continually refer to as the *convergence of evidence*: "If you don't use it, you lose it" and "An ounce of prevention is worth a pound of cure." Ironically enough, the lack of healthy behavior is causing many problems with the current state of health affairs, both individually and socially. It's an *energy crisis* all right—only it's being caused by the lack thereof! Take action and be an example. As one of the '60s anthems goes, "You're either part of the solution or part of the problem." Who knows exactly what the future will hold? Yet we *do* know having a healthier midlife will only improve your chances in later life. As I see it, this *window of opportunity* is the best time. At times, I joke that if you do all the things I say in this book, you'll still eventually die, but you'll feel and look a heck of a lot better! Live your life to its fullest.

Chapter 1. MAG feels enlightened and hopeful this book will steer him in the right direction. He definitely wants to avoid getting diabetes and hypertension. MAG wants to become a role model for his kids and wife. Health span and avoiding multiple drugs is what he's all about.

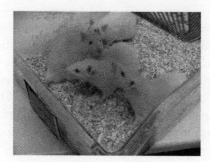

II.

Current Research and the Future ... of Mice and Men

There's tons of information on these topics, so only a few interesting ones will be mentioned. I've also included tips on how to interpret scientific research and news.

As explained, I believe if we're going to live a longer time, we need to focus on ways to optimize our *health span*. After all, it's not *how* long you live; it's how *well* you live, right? Most research involves trying to express the good genes or repress the bad ones. Investigators are trying to discover new disease markers that may allow us to uncover abnormalities and offer earlier, better-tolerated treatments. Currently, many antioxidants are being scientifically investigated for their safety and disease-fighting effects. For the time being, genetic manipulation and stem cell research has come up short. Despite this, I believe this modality will become a reality within the next twenty-five years. So for now, you'd better take good care of your genes; that washed-out look won't work here. Lastly, the *miniaturization* of mechanics and solid-state components will allow us to replace many worn-out parts. Remember the Six Million Dollar Man? What would he cost today? Back then, a new Cadillac would set you back just five grand. Dr. Langer of MIT stated in the *New York Times* in 2004, "Someday, every human part will be replaceable, even if that day is centuries away." Just where will all these discoveries eventually lead us? Read on, my friend.

The antioxidant Resveratrol, commonly found in wine, grapes, and nuts, may prove to be an elixir for health and longevity, after all. According to *Nature* (November 2006), Harvard researchers studied "middle-aged" mice and found palatable amounts of the compound reduced many of the aging effects of a high-calorie, high-fat diet. There was also a 31 percent death reduction in older mice; and they had preserved motor skills and metabolic parameters and had exhibited less fatty liver disease. One author is already taking this supplement. Though most prior studies were on nonmammals, the surprised researchers cautioned about the extrapolation to humans. How similar are all men to rats, anyway? Regardless, we do know the French are a healthy bunch, by and large, and do seem to get away with consuming wine and fatty foods.

Many current drugs that were originally designed to treat one disease may help cure another one. This may be especially true for those that lower the age-related increase in inflammation. An example is research on a drug class called the glitazones, such as Avandia. While limiting the effects of insulin and diabetes, this drug may also inhibit tumor growth. This was presented by Richard Pestell, director of Lombardy Comprehensive Cancer Center. Back in 2003, they found the glitazones inhibited tumor growth by possibly turning *off* cancer-causing genes and turning *on* some of the cancer-protective genes.

There are other examples of drugs that may prevent conditions that they were not originally designed to cure. There are also drugs that can have ill effects on other conditions that were not fully appreciated when originally marketed, i.e., Vioxx. I'll present some of the former. Let's look at some drugs that may prevent dementia, as that's understandably a big concern as we age. This makes sense if we're planning to live a longer time as almost half of people above eighty-five get dementia. What now can one do to help prevent dementia? Of course, the obvious thing your parents said, "If you don't use it, you lose it." As medications or supplements are concerned, possibly low-dose Advil, moderate doses of vitamin E, and fish oil may help.[15]

There is also some evidence that Zocor, a statin drug by Merck, may also help prevent the onset of dementia. This was suggested by a research by Nymox Pharmaceuticals and published in the January 8, 2004, issue of *Neurons*. This review stated that there may be up to a 70 percent lower prevalence in incidence of Alzheimer's disease in subjects taking statin drugs. Although such evidence may be considered by some to be weak, as to date, there is no cure for dementia—a progressive, debilitating and humiliating disease for the patient, family, and society.

---

15   D. Press and M. Alexander, "Prevention of dementia," *Up To Date in Family Practice* (October 2003).

An equally debilitating disease, osteoporosis, is usually helped by the bisphos-phonates, i.e., Fosamax. Originating from the soap scum inhibitors used to clean pipes, these drugs chelate the calcium back into brittle bones. Some current research suggests the drug may also chelate out the calcifications seen in diseased coronary and peripheral vessels. However, the jury is still out on this one.

A favorite topic of mine that's politically hot is *stem cell research*. There's a lot of news sensationalism that clouds the real issues here, as well. There's a lot of valid, remarkable research that's still in the infantile stages. I don't know any current, valid clinical human studies that have had beneficial results without some del-eterious ones. Reinforcing this was Professor Lindvall who, in a meeting of more than five hundred stem cell experts in London in September 2003, stated, "I'm convinced that stem cell technology can become, in the future, a cure for condi-tions leading to brain injury; but I think we have a long way to go." Stem cell research seems promising in the future for treatment of Parkinson's disease; this professor's research studied how rats' brain cells migrated to the area of a stroke in order to affect repair. This could open up the possibility of developing drugs that encourage the brain to repair itself when damaged by stroke, trauma, or disease. There are also promises of even fat cells, called *stromal* cells, being used to help collateral heart vessels grow. They may offer stem cell—like abilities too. At the very least, it would be easier getting fat cells from people than bone marrow cells.

There are many *cancer genes* getting discovered. One of the most studied is the mutation of the BRCA1 tumor suppressor gene, involved with an estimated fifty percent of inherited breast cancers. Interestingly enough, we must first under-stand how the regulating mechanisms of a cell cycle actually work—what signals the growth phase, resting phase, and replicating phase. Basically, a cancer can be caused by the unregulated growth of any type of cell. Without the proper rate of growth, or death (*apoptosis*), the cell continues to divide, causing the resulting tumor to grow and spread, resulting in the overconsumption of nutrients and many other complications. Getting back to the breast cancer genes mentioned above, in actuality only a very small percentage of breast cancers are genetically based. Most of are de novo from mutations of breast tissue. Inflammation, xeno-hormones, pesticides, smoking, diabetes, and other factors play more important roles. (There's more on simpler, proven ways to prevent breast and prostate cancer later.)

The National Cancer Institute and the National Human Genome Research Institute in October 2006 began sequencing the genes to three cancers—lung, brain, and ovarian. The three-year project will use large-scale genomic analysis technologies to hopefully develop better ways to prevent, diagnose, and treat these. There's also considerably a lot of research on the p53 gene, one of the first genes found to be implicated with cancer regulation. Basically though, any acquired or inherited mutated gene can cause a cancer, although it may take a few hits. If that gene happens to be one that codes for a cancer-causing or cancer-protective gene, then problems occur. In addition, any acquired mutations to the genes that code for immune function, membrane, nuclear or mitochondrial DNA can induce cancer.

In a hope to invent a health pill for dummies, British scientists in 2003 invented what they called the poly pill. This combination pill combined six medications. It contained aspirin, a statin drug, folic acid, an ACE inhibitor drug, a beta blocker, and a diuretic. They claimed this pill could prevent more than 80 percent of heart attacks and strokes for heart patients, diabetics, and everyone over fifty-five. Talk about your one-size-fits-all approach! Most professional organizations, including the American Heart Association, issued caution and expressed doubt of its effectiveness and safety. More promising and practical is the shift in focus to HDL cholesterol lipoprotein in lipid management. Most know LDL is the bad cholesterol lipoprotein. However, HDL (high-density lipoprotein) actually scavenges away LDL (low-density lipoprotein), thereby reducing risks for plaques and vascular disease.

In the past, doctors' main focus has only been on lowering LDL. Granted, the statin drugs' effect has been quite impressive. I believe this one-prong approach was partly due to the big push and sponsored research made by the major drug firms that held patents to these expensive pills. There's really no trade name drug that raises HDL appreciably. Exercise, niacin, and fish oil would be the most effective modalities. These don't require a prescription, are quite cheap, and without serious side effects. Amazingly, only a 6 percent increase in HDL has been shown to lower risk for coronary disease by up to 35 percent! Gemfibrosil, a generic drug, and Omacor, a new prescription form of fish oil, also help. Several drug firms are investigating drugs that raise HDL, although Pfizer just halted research of its drug Torcetrapib. There may also be various vaccines and even gene therapies in the pipeline. The latter came from a finding that relatives in a northern Italian village discovered in the 1980s had virtually no coronary disease yet had low HDL. The presumably responsible gene called Apo A-I Milano may code for a *supercharged* HDL.

A high *myeloperoxidase* level may help identify patients in the ER with an increased risk of heart problems, needed cardiac intervention procedures, and even death within six months. According to a study in the October 2003 issue of the *New England Journal of Medicine*, this enzyme's production is increased when arteries are exhibiting fatty deposits, which are likely to rupture and cause either thrombus or embolus. Additionally, a gene called MEF2A plays a role in protecting artery walls against building up plaque that leads to a heart attack. Dr. Eric Topol of the Cleveland Clinic states that people having a mutation in this gene are destined to have heart disease. Interesting enough, this finding was isolated from an extended Iowa family that had been plagued for generations with severe coronary artery disease.

However, based on all the research I've read, this has to be taken in the proper context. Family history, personal risk factors, CRP-hs, and other clotting factors may also help us decide with whom to be more aggressive when it comes to prevention and treatment options. Additionally, I believe other inflammatory factors, or lipoprotein subfractions, *H. pylori*, and *Cytomegalovirus* titers may help identify those at increased risk. These are discussed in the men's special topics chapter. Decode Genetics and Roche Diagnostics recently announced a landmark discovery that may help develop DNA-based diagnostic tests for common diseases like atherosclerosis. Both companies seem committed to futuristic discoveries. Given the genetic diversity worldwide, there are probably many other genes that promote heart disease.

I must digress some to talk about the nuances of research so that you can discern the news from the noise for yourself. I will use some examples to illustrate my points. What's especially important in middle age is the *prevention* of diseases. In the case of coronary vessel disease, it's far better to *prevent* forming enlarged, inflamed plaques than having your chest cracked open for a bypass. For cancer, it's better to prevent *carcinogenesis* in the first place, than to get numerous bouts of near-lethal, toxic injections. "An ounce of prevention is worth a pound of cure." When President Nixon declared a war on cancer back in the 1970s, a lot of research and money was spent on ways to *treat* cancer. Too bad, more of it wasn't spent finding ways to *prevent* carcinogenesis in the first place.

I must also add that one must understand the difference between the modalities that are used for *prevention* and the ones for the *treatment* of a particular disease. Let's say for the sake of argument, I had a patient complaining of angina come into my office. (Angina is chest pain that's due to an acute coronary vessel blockage.) If I then told this patient to immediately start exercising, quit smoking, and consume a better diet, he may suffer an acute heart attack, possibly even die. Is that to say that if the patient had practiced a healthier lifestyle before, he probably wouldn't have heart disease today? Probably, he wouldn't. However, recommending something that's safe and proven to prevent heart disease would actually put this patient at increased risk of death once the disease progressed to this very severe, unstable state. So something that's proven safe and effective to *prevent* a disease could cause unintentional harm to this person with *unstable*, severe disease. It's the right treatment, but at the wrong time.

Let's take this point one step further. Would it be correct to say that starting a good exercise and diet program wouldn't help this patient avoid acute coronary events in the future *once* the established disease is stabilized? Of course, it would. As a matter of fact, cardiac rehabilitation is a very important step in helping someone with coronary disease and congestive heart failure. This latter example illustrates how some safe and proven modalities that could make *established* disease worsen are, in fact, beneficial once the disease is adequately controlled. In other words, we must look at all distinct stages of a disease and then tailor its unique treatments. What's proven to prevent a disease? Then, what should we do, or don't do, once that disease is present? Lastly, what could we do to prevent the return of that particular disease? As explained, it's not necessarily the same recommendations in all three scenarios.

That's precisely what was covered when I went to a daylong seminar this past year in Miami sponsored by the H. Lee Moffet Cancer Center and the American Institute for Cancer Research. It covered the latest advice concerning diet and supplements for cancer survivors, who made up the majority of the audience. Even most of the speakers were nurses that personally battled breast cancer. The crowd mostly wanted to know what *they* can do themselves to better their odds of a recurrence. They are very confused by the many contradictory reports given in the media. What seems good for you one month is bad the next! As a point of interest, there are about ten million cancer survivors in America, and most of these had breast cancer. Unfortunate and eluded above, most research has focused only on the treatment of disease, far less on prevention, and even less so on what to do once a cancer is in remission. Just what is best to prevent a recurrence? You would think that since so much effort has gone into curing cancer somebody would've looked at what happens next. Anyway, there were a lot of great questions, but not many scientifically proven answers.

I will develop this further in the introductory chapter and have more examples. But next, let me explain what I mean by the *convergence of evidence.* This is very important to understand. Imagine, if there were one hundred different experiments that tested the effectiveness of a new medical treatment, you would expect 90 percent to reach the same conclusions, right? The remaining 10 percent, when analyzed more closely, should show why they didn't. In other words, the vast majority of research that questions a particular topic or treatment should agree; the *evidence* should *converge* or point toward one logical, practical conclusion. Now, to fully explain this would take up too much space in this book, but you need to understand many other factors when evaluating research. How was it designed? What was the population studied? Did the conclusion match the original design and hypothesis? Who sponsored the research? Were the researchers free of financial incentives? Was it a crossover, double-blind prospective study? How long was the study? What were the P and Q values? This way, we can tell if the conclusions are valid or perchance. You can see that scientific research is often hard to design, and it may take time to intelligently interpret the results for practical use.

Even the adding to this complication is what I call *science by press.* This occurs when the media sensationalizes the premature results of a trial. Usually, there's no scientific basis or completeness, but the story has to be entertaining and gotten out sooner than the other networks. It has to have some sound bites too. "This is the fast, easy way to cure … (just add a ridiculous symptom, like ball ache!). The new, easy thing we promoted last month happens to be the worst thing you could ever do!" No wonder the general public is confused about virtually everything. A quick, easy example is the recent *science by press* release about how low-fat diets may not be healthy, after all. This was according to data pulled from the Women's Health Initiative (WHI) trial. (Yes, the same one that stated hormonal replacement therapy in menopausal women is taboo.) You should always ask yourself in these instances if the news story actually makes any common sense. Does it agree with what's been proven for decades? Does it disagree with common practices or health beliefs that have been passed down for generations? Another complication from such *science by press* is that it promotes malpractice lawsuits. Because of such, doctors are often scared into not practicing in a way totally in line with their better judgment or training. Examples may be silicone breast implants or hormonal therapies.

Even medical journals aren't exempted from such misinformation. In the April 15, 2006, issue of the *Family Practice News* is an article entitled "Homocysteine's Role in CVD Risk Appears Dead." There's a bold box in the middle of the article that gives a summary for those docs not wanting to read the full article: "Supplements with Folic Acid and B Vitamins Do Not Reduce Cardiovascular Events in High-risk Populations with Established Vascular Disease."[16] Using the very simplified definitions I presented above, let's see if all these statements agree. By just looking at the population studied, we can see if this is in line with the article's conclusion. The author, Mitchel Zoler, uses two trials to arrive at this. One is the Heart Outcomes Prevention and Evaluation-The Ongoing Outcomes (HOPE-TOO, or HOPE-2) which used patients fifty-five or older *with* vascular disease and diabetes or multiple other complicating diseases. The second, the Norwegian Vitamin Trial (NORVIT), used patients immediately *after* a myocardial infarction. Both studies were challenging what many retrospective and observational studies have reported for the past twenty-five years—mild elevation in homocysteine carries an increased risk of heart disease.

The actual population studied was elderly with very serious established disease, so they're trying to assess what's called *tertiary* prevention—basically preventing a second or third heart attack. There's no mention the levels of homocysteine, folic acid, or B_{12} were initially or finally measured. It would make sense to only replace those found initially deficient and had high levels of homocysteine. But did the researchers do this? John Bulushi in *Saturday Night Live* would've exclaimed, "But no!" Ironically enough, this same *Family Practice News*'s cover page article boasted "FP Residency Takes a Holistic View." They applauded the nonmedical approaches now being offered at the Maine Medical Center in Portland for medical residents. This journal, like many others, had a four-page ad for Effexor, a prescription antidepressant with many side effects, some even lethal.

Mind you also, these are published scientists and authors reporting to educated professionals. There's no mention of the dropout rate—those patients that didn't complete the study or dismissed due to various reasons. The end points, what's specifically designed to be measured at the end of the experiment, were cardiovascular death, nonfatal heart attack, or acute stroke in the HOPE-2 trial. It was the combined rate of sudden coronary death, fatal and nonfatal heart attack, and fatal and nonfatal stroke in the NORVIT trial. Since these patients were elderly and had multiple serious comorbidities, how many could complete this three- to five-year study and have the appropriate follow-up? Maybe the ones that survived longer due to the supplementation were then able to suffer another event later. Or the ones not supplemented who did have events later, were healthier or did other measures. Maybe the supplementation helped *all cause mortality or morbidity,* an

---

16   It's based upon the research article from Bonaa et al., *New England Journal of Medicine* 354, 15 (2006).

even more important end point. For example, we also know that high homocys-teine is also a risk factor for osteoporosis. The related fractures carry a 30 percent mortality rate the first year!

It would only be proper to conclude from these two studies that oral supplemen-tation with B vitamins and folic acid may not prevent the second or third heart attack or stroke in this elderly, very sick subpopulation whose vitamin levels weren't initially checked or followed to ensure compliancy and effectiveness. It's common knowledge that getting pharmaceutical grade supplementation is difficult. As will be covered later, the elderly often suffers from chronic gastritis or may be on pills blocking the absorption of many nutrients. Maybe many in this study didn't even get the actual supplementation they thought they were getting. Regardless, what the one author promoted in this article didn't match up with what was actually researched and concluded. As alluded, it may be that such supplementation may help *prevent* cardiac disease from happening in the first place—which would be a more credible and important finding—while possibly making acute or severe vessel disease worse. But that wasn't the population studied, so the issue of such supplementation in *preventing* coronary artery disease is, in fact, *not* a dead issue.

After that brief course in interpreting scientific literature, let's get back to the future. A cryonics outfit in Boca Raton was featured recently in the *Palm Beach Post*. The owners claim that since 1967 about one thousand people have signed up to be frozen after death at a cost of about $200,000 (similar to the baseball great Ted Williams' fiasco). To see how this theory pans out, let's review one of the earliest suc-cesses in gene cloning—the famous sheep Dolly. Despite making world news a few years back, Dolly only survived to six years old, a rather premature death. Why? It's really quite simple once explained. Dolly's cloned genes were from a sheep already middle-aged, about four years old. Therefore, those genes had suffered some age-related decline and mutations before being cloned. So it's no wonder, those "aged" genes survived only another six years. Well, good-bye, Dolly![17]

I believe it's safe to extrapolate this to humans as far as the following is con-cerned: If we are to use stem cells or to harvest our own stem cells (as in our bone marrow cells), we should do it at the earliest, disease-free state as possible. I am encouraged by umbilical cord blood harvesting in newborns and would suggest any early middle-aged person should look into harvesting their own bone mar-

---

17 Dolly was named after Dolly Parton because she came from a cloned mammary cell. When I googled Dolly, believe it or not, Dolly the sheep came up before Ms. Parton. Maybe country music still has a way to go or maybe sheep is more popular.

row for future use. This would come in handy if they come down with a cancer, or if a sibling or close relative needed bone marrow replacement. Further, at the rate stem cell research is going, I do believe doing this would be prudent to help reverse future bouts with Parkinson's, dementia, congestive heart failure, cancers, and many other degenerative conditions. If you plan to use stem cells, it would make better sense to use the youngest, most disease-free cells that you could produce. The major question I have is how long stem cells can be stored without becoming damaged?

Some colleagues believe today's middle-aged persons, if healthy and proactive, will often live to 120! I know what you're thinking; this is totally ridiculous! But let's look at the past and embrace such hope for the future. Today, it's not that uncommon to see patients over one hundred years old. These centenarians were born at the turn of the century, when the average life span was only 47.6 years. These *survivors* have more than *doubled* their expected life span. Many respected scientists and philosophers believe that with the technologies available within the next twenty-five years, humans may have the capacity to live hundreds of years! Who knows if that is indeed a reality? However, being proactive in the simplest terms, i.e., the proper diet and exercise, antioxidants, and proper age-management medicine, will at least optimize any health span you can conceivably enjoy now. This proven approach will only help you be in the best form, no matter what the future holds. Lastly, if future generations are going to live longer, we will have to personally and socially address the many economic ramifications. Hopefully, we may live to pay off the national debts we made during our lifetime and not pass them on to our kids!

Chapter 2. MAG feels better capable of reviewing news and research. He now knows which questions to ask his doctor and how to interpret the answers.

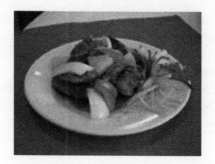

III.

Diet Basics: You Are What and How Much You Eat!

Given the facts, I want to officially decree today's Standard American Diet as SAD.

A. Introduction and Antiaging Basics. The number of overweight Americans continues to rise sharply. Even more upsetting is the news that the fastest-growing group is the very obese. From 1986 to 2000, *severely* obese Americans, those at least one hundred pounds overweight, quadrupled in number. They're on the fast track, all right—almost twice as many as the *milder* obese. Over 65 percent of Americans are now considered overweight, with reports showing increased obesity rates in teenagers, highest among minority females. This shouldn't be surprising given that children tend to follow more what their parents do, not so much what they say. This is a wake-up call, America! This lard-laden landscape unfortunately sets the stage for our young teens to experience severe old-age diseases such as adult-onset diabetes, hypertension, hypercholesterolemia, and much more. Likewise, health-care and social costs will expand as nearly nine million American youths aged six to nineteen are now overweight. Today, pediatricians are diagnosing hypertension in one-third of their overweight patients. Some as young as five are showing early signs of heart disease, prompting some to recommend routine cholesterol and diabetic screenings for obese children starting at age two![18] To this I say, "Shots happen!"

According to research done by the World Health Organization using *body mass index* (BMI), the United States had the highest prevalence of obese teens among

---

18   Blood pressure screenings should begin at age three, according to recent National Institute of Health's recommendations.

developed nations in the late 1990s.[19] Despite being generally more affluent, American students were less likely to eat a healthy, balanced diet than those from other less-privileged countries like Lithuania. "SAD" but true, American kids ranked among the top three for consuming sweets, chocolate, and soft drinks daily and were also more likely to eat potato chips or french fries. Dads, it's not good for our kids to be first in everything they do.

Ironically, it seems the poorest states with the poorest populations have the biggest weight problem. Another increase in thirty-one states in 2005 kept the gravy train of obesity chugging along.[20] Obesity now exceeds 25 percent in thirteen states. Leading the way on this train track to tragedy are most southeastern states like Mississippi. According to the report released by the advocacy group, Trust for America's Health, over $5 billion annually could be saved from only heart disease prevention if only one out of ten began walking more. I suggest the government should take a much more proactive approach in promoting a healthier lifestyle, even if it means paying for those on social programs to attend regular dieting and exercise programs. Most rising public health problems should warrant such a call to action and examine any underlying social barriers. These must be realistically addressed in order to affect any real improved public health. We must plot a course away from Tubby Town. Do we really want our toddlers to become chronically ill and be on drugs?

America is headed for "the perfect storm" in a way. Overweight-related health-care costs have been soaring, yet the government and insurance firms haven't adequately responded to promote a more preventative, proactive approach. It's hard to add up the drastically increased health-care spending on such morbidly obese-related conditions, but it's estimated at well over $75 billion annually. About half of this is paid by tax-payers through government programs such as Medicare and Medicaid. Ridiculously enough, these programs don't reimburse for the preventative counseling needed for those overweight despite the fact obesity is now considered the second biggest killer.

Yet, I consider obesity and all its related conditions to be *totally preventable*. If mild and early in onset, these are very treatable without any medications. For many reasons, only about a quarter of the 30 percent of men *trying* to lose weight are

19 Body mass index, BMI, is a measure of obesity and is covered in the weight loss chapter (I. Lissau, 2004). Body mass index and overweight in adolescents in thirteen European countries, Israel, and the United States. *Archives of Pediatric and Adolescent Medicine* 158: 27–33.

20 [22] H. M. Blanck, "State-specific prevalence of obesity among adults—United States," *JAMA* 296, no. 16 (2005):19–59. Also data compiled from *Trust for America's Health 2005* report with their recommendations.

serious enough to significantly change their lifestyle. Overall, Americans expend about $33 billion annually on weight-loss methods, some are genuine but most probably aren't. So it appears as a whole that we guys know we're overweight and may want to diet, but only a small portion of us are willing to realistically do something about it. Ah … the spirit is willing but the flesh is not. We may always be looking for a fast fix. Corporate America will always be right there, trying to make a quick buck off it. Recently, the Federal Trade Commission (FTC) fined the marketers of OTC weight-loss pills $25 million but allowed them to stay on the shelves and make their $1.6 billion in sales for 2006!

With all the above as an introduction, let's now focus on what I call the *double squeeze* on us midlife men. Although I'm hammering about the unhealthy lifestyle most *kids* have, this is pertinent for us for many reasons. First, if you were an overweight child, odds are you're still having trouble maintaining a healthier weight. As a parent, it's never too late to teach our kids to be responsible for their own health. We can do this simply by setting a proper example. It's well known our children copy more of what they *see* than what they *hear* from us. Second, these kids will turn out to be sicker than previous generations. This in turn will only cause you more heartache, downtime, and expenses later on. Also, midlife is a time when paradoxically your parents will probably be getting quite old and suffer multiple disabilities. Most of these problems will be related to being overweight and being out of shape too. You'll have a high likelihood of potentially being squeezed from both ends—dependent, sickly parents on one side and unhealthy, demanding children on the other! At the very least, a healthier lifestyle will help you fare better with all these stressors going on. It may improve your marriage even. This *window of opportunity* I affectionately refer to as midlife is the perfect time to undo some earlier damage and prevent the early occurrence of age-related disease. The (big) butt stops here!

> Unfortunately, America's youth and middle-aged are becoming increasingly at risk of getting diabetes, hypertension, and many other conditions related to being overweight. As a middle-aged man, we may feel squeezed from many directions—wife, children, job, and aging parents. Leading an example by consuming a healthy diet is a great way to prevent many of these complications.

Dieting is the most frequently discussed topic when we're trying to improve our health. It's also the most unpopular to *carry out* and then *carry on* throughout life. If overweight and out of shape, we all know we should diet. Yet, almost all have a heck of a time doing it. First, I would like to happily emphasize that most of what our parents said, or should have said, about nutrition is true. When you think about it, if these sayings didn't hold any merit, they wouldn't have been passed down throughout the ages, right? Generations before, whether they knew it or not, had preached these healthy principles based on their own *observational studies*. They directly *observed* that doing certain things, and avoiding other things, resulted in less sickness. After all, our forefathers had to be more responsible for their own health. This was a time before health insurance and many government programs existed. There were only a handful of drugs available then. Today, there are drugstores on almost every corner. It seems there's a pill and medical specialist willing to prescribe it for every conceivable symptom you could have. Maybe your parents were right; maybe everything supposedly *new* about staying healthy *is* old again.

I must stress that all the behavioral changes or modalities I present in this book work *synergistically* together. Remember, I don't believe in any magic bullets. Diet *with exercise* will work much better than just diet alone. When the two are used together, there is an additive benefit, as in 1 + 1 = 3! This should make intuitive sense. In this example, your eating the proper diet gives you more energy and results in less weight to have to carry around. This allows more enjoyable physical activity, resulting in less pain and an improved mood. Additionally, the proper rest, fluid intake, and more will help you synergistically feel better. This will be presented in subsequent chapters.

Whenever I interview a patient about dieting, I like to find out first what *had worked* for him to maintain a healthier weight in the past. I also inquire about what *hasn't* worked. That's usually just as relevant. Then, we probe further to find out *why* some things worked and *why* some didn't. This enables us to identify the barriers he must overcome to ensure long-term success. I believe any fad diet or craze is doomed to failure if it's not a lifestyle change that he can live with his whole life. This is what you must ask yourself, "Is this a diet I can't realistically stay on my whole life?" I hope this makes common sense. For example, if you went on the so-called cabbage diet for a few days and lost weight, you would simply regain the weight once you fell off the cabbage wagon. You certainly aren't going to eat cabbages the rest of your life. That would be quite silly, boring, and basically impossible. You would also suffer nutritional deficiencies and eventually suffer many side effects because of these imbalances

Eating right and in the right amounts can be tough to achieve all the time. Hey, I'm not asking you to do anything I don't do myself. I'm human too. There are indeed many personal, familial, ethnic, artistic, and social aspects when it comes to cooking and eating. Plus, food can, well … taste so good! Don't worry though, it's not true in *all* cases that "the better the food tastes, the worse it is for your health." (I'll get into that later.) We must take a cold, hard look at what we and society have created. When you were young and your heart was an open book…. No no no! That's the title of the song by Paul McCartney for James Bond's *Live and Let Die*. Anyway, when we were younger, our social activities were mostly *physical* ones. We used to meet on the neighborhood lot and play football, tag, and other sports. We had recess and PE every day at school and then continued to play long after school and on weekends. Remember the fun and camaraderie we had? Now as older midlifers, it seems most of our social activities are consumed with, well … the consumption of food and drink. We need to change this way of thinking.

Do we regret any of those times we played with our friends around the old 'hood? Of course, we don't. We lived for it! The time just flew by as if it was timeless, right? We couldn't wait to do it again and again and again. Recall how you felt when you woke up on a crisp, cool Saturday morning. No school, just playing around all day. It was more of what I call a *fun-out*, not a workout by any means. Anyway, we'll have more on exercise later; we're talking diet here. The main point is for us not to base the majority of our social activities around just eating. Instead of always driving the Harleys to get some drinks, grab some dessert, or down some dinner, let's more often join for a walk on the beach, play some tennis, or go for a swim. Let's instead have a fun-out.

Now we have to review Nutrition 101. A lot of descriptions and advice follow. There are some nice guidelines in the appendix too.

Food Group	Description/Notes	Examples
Carbohydrates	Carbon- and hydrogen-based compounds. Energy. Absorbed quite quickly. About 4 kcal/gram.	Complex: vegetables and fruits contain fiber—better. 50–60% of diet. Simple: sugars, breads, fructose, corn syrup, rice, candy are "empty" sugars—avoid!
Proteins	As above, but has amine, NH3 groups. Comprised of amino acids. Absorbed slower. About 4 kcal/gram.	Meats, dairy and nuts (have some fat, too) beans and soy. About 30% of diet. (0.8–1 gram per kg of your weight daily)

	Glycerol connected to three fatty acids. Absorbed slowly. About 9 kcal/gram.	Meats, dairy, oils, and junk foods. Fats from plant or fish are fine. Under 30% of diet or 30 grams daily. Cholesterol < 300 mg/day.
Fats		

Fig. 3.1. Nutrition 101—carbs, proteins, and fats. Other tidbits: Keep sodium under 2 g per day. Total calories you need can be roughly figured by multiplying your weight in pounds by 15, i.e., if 150 lbs, then 2250 cal daily—less if you're inactive or wanting to lose weight, more if active lifestyle.(©C. Rao, MD, 2006)

There are basically just the three food groups listed above. Any fad diet can only manipulate so much. It can basically be categorized as low carb, low fat, or low protein. Of course, it also helps to have a celebrity endorsement to be newsworthy and to get on the radar screen of the talk show or book circuit. In the end, it's no wonder people are very confused about what really makes up a proper diet. As a recent example, some researchers involved with the Women's Health Initiative proclaimed a low-fat diet may not be good for you.[21] The Atkins© low-carb diet, while helping some lose weight and improving many other aspects of health, may cause other metabolic disturbances.[22] Added to this is the confusion caused by the many fad diets and supplements' ads we daily get bombarded by and want so desperately to be true. Finally, you can lose weight while eating all you want and just lying on the couch all day—the fat just burns away. Tempting, aren't they?

Unfortunately, the reality is these gimmicks may result in some temporary weight loss at best. When you stop these shenanigans, the weight only comes back. Your fat cells may have shrunk somewhat. But they'll only come back later—bigger than ever. This is called the *ratcheting effect*. Stretching the truth even further are the tricky TV ads with wafer-thin sexy models or athletic studs with their six packs, shoveling mass quantities of beer and junky snacks into their pearly-white smiles. Most figure this has got to be healthy, right? I mean, just look at the shape they're in? Ironically, despite pushing all this junk food, the media usually promotes many unjust attitudes society has toward those overweight.

When you compare the new food pyramid with the old one, you will see the latter was more upside-down than the USS *Poseidon*. Why did this happen? Basically, the FDA decided it would be too confusing to teach the public about good versus bad fats, proteins, and carbs. Well, look where that got the once very slim Shelly Winters.

---

21   B. V. Howard, L. Van Horn, J. Hsia, et al., "Low-fat dietary pattern and risk of cardiovascular disease: the Women's Health Initiative Randomized Controlled Dietary Modification Trial," *JAMA* 295 (2006):655–66.

22   T. Y. Chen, "A life-threatening complication of Atkins diet," *Lancet* 367, no. 9514 (2006): 958.

At any rate, if you go to the FDA Web site, you will now find the new, improved food pyramid and recipes for about every ethnic group out there, Italian, Mexican, Asian and more. The new food pyramid is below. That's healthy food for thought!

Out with the old …

And in with the new! (Adapted Zone from FDA, USDA)

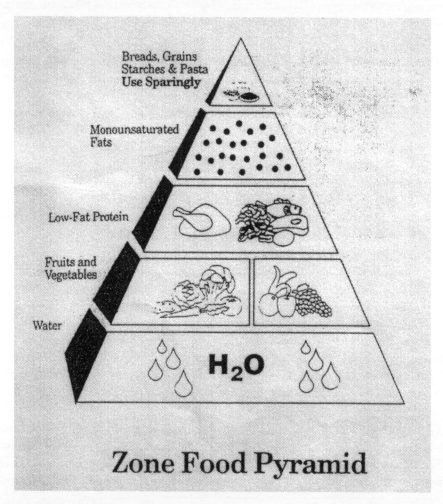

Figure 3.2. Old and new food pyramids. Notwithstanding the ratios above, there are good and bad in all the food groups. Below are some tips from the Cenegenics© diet. It parallels many of the healthy diet tips mentioned in this chapter. Use this list when making a list for shopping.

Daily Meal Guidelines

(Or the Under-Ten Commandments for a Healthy Diet)

1. **Never skip meals:** This will force your body into starvation mode and cause your metabolism to slow down, basically hoarding whatever calories you eat. Rather, eat smaller meals more frequently, based on the following suggestions. Think of food as fuel for your body. Don't put in more than you burn.

2. **Based each meal around a lean protein source:** Fish, chicken, turkey, lean beef (occasionally), yogurt (plain, unsweetened), cottage cheese, and legumes (beans, including soy). The serving size of protein should be about the size of the palm of your hand and the height of a deck of cards.

3. **Cut out high glycemic carbohydrates:** Breads, pasta, rice, cereals, candy, baked goods, pretzels, sweets, etc. This is especially important to achieve the full benefit of your hormone replacement program. **See the appendix for "Healthy Choices Based on Glycemic Index."**

4. **Eat at least three to five servings of fresh vegetables and one to two servings of fresh fruit each day:** Vegetables are an excellent source of phytonutrients and fiber. Choose whole fruits instead of fruit juice because juicing removes the fiber and increases the glycemic index. Avoid corn, potatoes, bananas, dried fruit, and tropical fruits (pineapple, mangoes, papayas, etc.)

5. **Add healthy fats to your diet:** Essential omega-3 and omega-9 fatty acids are crucial for the prevention of heart disease, arthritis, joint problems, and immune system weakness. Good sources include salmon, sardines, almonds, walnuts, avocados, flax seeds in the oil, olive oil, canola oil, and fish oil supplements.

6. **Drink lots of water:** Drinks six to eight 8-ounce glasses of pure (distilled or reverse osmosis) filtered water per day. Drink one extra glass for every caffeinated beverage and more when exercising.

7. **Keep alcohol intake to a minimum:** While 4–8 ounces of red wine daily provides health benefits, more than that can increase your health risk! Dry red wine is the best choice. Hard alcohols are also low glycemic. Everything in moderation!

8. **Choose natural products:** Avoid refined foods, hydrogenated oils, artificial colors, flavors, sweeteners, and preservatives. Avoid fat-free products, which usually make up for a lack of taste by adding artificial ingredients and sugar. Shop the perimeter of your grocery store!

9. **Take your supplements daily!** Studies show reduced caloric diets without supplementation lower metabolism, but with supplementation, the metabolism is unchanged.

Figure 3.3. Daily meal guidelines to really live by. (Adapted from Cenegenics©)

Personal Notes:

With what you've just learned, you can go to the appendix and fill out a diet log. One page is your "healthiest day." The other may be your "not-so-healthy day." It may help to note what else was happening on that not-so-healthy day. Were you rushed or stressed? Did you forget to bring your food from home? These circumstances can undermine your dietary habits and should be addressed. It's not just about the food; it's how you *think* about food when it comes to eating. (Why? How much? When? What else was going on?) Then, you can compare this to the corrected copy of an unhealthy day's diet I put in the appendix.

B. Carbohydrates, a.k.a. Carbs. Let's expand on how to manipulate insulin and cortisol, the aging hormones, to your advantage. To understand how diet affects your hormones and metabolism on a large scale, you must first appreciate what happens at the microscopic cellular level. Pretend you're like one of those scientists in that classic sci-fi movie, *Fantastic Voyage*. When you ingest food, your gastrointestinal system breaks it down to mostly carbohydrates. There are also some small protein and fat molecules. When these compounds enter the bloodstream, they then cause a relative spike in glucose levels (see the diagram below). If this is a simple carbohydrate that has a high *glycemic index*, there's a quicker, higher spike that results in you feeling that *sugar high*. This gives the betcha'-can't-eat-just-one phenomenon and fuels the cravings to sweets many can't seem to resist. A list of the glycemic index of many foods is in the appendix.[23]

---

23   We owe a lot of debt to the understanding of the glycemic index and the effects of insulin and cortisol in causing the metabolic syndrome to Gerald Reaven and his predecessors.

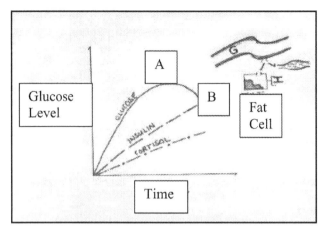

Figure 3.4. Undesired high glycemic index curves. At point A, undesired high glycemic index foods cause an exaggerated "sugar spike" in the bloodstream. Insulin then overshoots to stabilize these glucose levels. In order to keep your brain happy, a cortisol spike follows. You're hungry and tired at point B, yet the fat cell is locked tight by such high insulin levels.

Now glucose (G) causes the pancreas to release insulin (I) into the bloodstream in order to maintain an appropriate level and move this fuel elsewhere. G can either be burned up by active muscle and brain or stored in the fat cells and liver. Basically, fat cells act as the fuel tank for the body. When you don't immediately utilize this fuel, it enters the fat cells to be stored for later use. In women, these fuel tanks, or fat cells, usually accumulate in the butt and thighs resulting in the *pear-shaped* figure. This is *peripheral* fat. In men, however, this fat collects in the abdominal cavity, creating that disease-causing *visceral* fat we spoke about earlier. This results in the *apple-shaped* figure. (By the way, women possessing this apple-shaped fat distribution are at about the same risks for metabolic syndrome and vessel disease as men.)

Normally a few hours after a meal, represented above by point B, glucose dips some as insulin has steadily rising to compensate. At that point, you usually feel tired, lazy, and in a slump. Do you feel like this every afternoon after that *high glycemic* lunch? You may have the urge to put on a moo moo and take a nap, or quickly down a double espresso in order to wake up. Regardless, that *sugar high* you had an hour ago is now long gone. And now with insulin being higher, you feel tired and may even feel the urge to snack again. This is because insulin, acting like a *key in the lock of the fat cell*, is now keeping all the stored fat *locked in*. As M. C. Hammer would rap, "Can't touch this!" Glucose levels then drop. Your mind, basically running on sugar, starts to feel less sharp, maybe to the point of you feeling sad or confused. In your blood, cortisol levels start to increase in order to balance these declining sugar levels. What do you do, now? Usually, you have to resort to eating more to regain that sugar high you've become addicted.

And as you can see from above, when these high and low episodes occur time and time again, your day then becomes a virtual roller-coaster filled with many such *crash-and-burn* episodes. Maybe your coworkers note you're becoming overly anxious, *hyper,* or even maniclike during those sugar peaks, especially if you added the espresso-strength caffeine. At other times, when the glucose is in the trough, you may appear to your spouse or friends as acting distant, fatigued, or even depressed. If you're a child, these symptoms may warrant you becoming labeled as having ADHD and encouraged to then pop mind-altering drugs. If older, this erratic behavior may be mistaken for mood disorders such as bipolar, anxiety, depression, or even adult ADHD.[24]

It's much better to practice a diet that will keep your energy more constant throughout the day. By regularly consuming lower glycemic index foods during the day, not skipping meals, and having appropriate snacks, your energy is less erratic. You'll feel much livelier as you keep the aging hormones, insulin and cortisol, in healthier ranges.

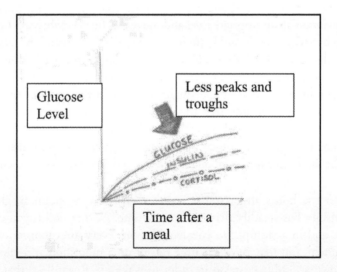

Figure 3.5. Desired lower glycemic index foods are better. With more complex carbs, there isn't such a spike in glucose and levels remain more constant. As a result, insulin and cortisol levels have a healthier profile. You won't crash and burn throughout the day.

---

24 ADHD (attention deficit hyperactivity disorder)—a syndrome typified by short attention span and uncontrollable excited behavior that can affect children as well as adults.

The importance this glycemic index of foods play in age and disease was somewhat popularized in the early 1970s James Bond flick, *Never Say Never Again*. If you recall, Sean Connery's character is now middle-aged, out of shape, and lost some of his edge. In the opening scene, one of the senior scientists scolds James for his unhealthy lifestyle and alcohol consumption. The researcher then proceeds to explain how simple sugars advance the aging process and how free radicals speed this up. "We have to beat those free radicals, James!" Although these new *radicals* aren't exactly the larger-than-life villains Bond easily wiped out in the past, he does attempt to follow the advice, albeit in his own debonair manner.

> By avoiding foods that possess a high glycemic index, we can prevent unhealthy derangements in insulin and cortisol levels. Additionally, widely fluctuating sugar levels are limited, thereby limiting crash-and-burn phenomena throughout the day.

You may wonder how these higher sugar levels cause premature aging and its many related diseases? Let me explain this in as simple a fashion as possible and give some particular examples. First, you must understand that the many protein-based messengers throughout the body rely on what's called *random collision* in order to bind with its *receptor site*. In fact, this is how insulin (key) binds to its receptor site (lock) on the fat cell illustrated above. Once bound together, these form a *receptor complex* (lock and key together) that initiates the numerous, ubiquitous reactions in the body. These mechanisms must be very specific to operate properly. Both the lock and the key must possess the right 3-D configurations in order to function correctly (open). Any deviation may cause an alarming result.

For example, many pesticides behave as a *xenohormone*. Acting as an artificial hormone, they variably bind to the testosterone receptor sites on prostate tissue. Because of an unnatural fit, the resulting action of the receptor complex is abnormal. Instead, there may be the inhibition of cell death (apoptosis) and overstimulation of cellular replication, which may result in uncontrolled growth. This could theoretically result in an enlarged prostate or even cancer.

Second, when your blood sugar remains high, it *sugarcoats* the many proteins in the body, making them abnormally sticky—a process called *glycosylation*. Instead of becoming gummy bear-like, these microscopic messengers should be very fluidlike and soft. This allows them to form the proper 3-D conformation, or the proper shape, to optimally function in the millions of complicated, cascading reactions that occur millions of times per second throughout your body. Once glycosylation occurs, there is the abnormal cross-linking of many of their molecules, which alters their conformation and binding properties. It's like the buildup of sludge inside your car's engine.

This glycosylation is what puts diabetics at a dramatically increased risk for heart attack and stroke. Besides the increased inflammation from higher insulin levels and other metabolic derangements, there are also the glycosylated lipoproteins. Carrying the cholesterol molecules in the blood, these become more gumlike and adhere to the vessel wall. This starts the initial cascade of events that eventually result in the infamous fibrofatty plaques of vessel disease. With time, this plaque slowly grows in the vessel wall until it forms a local blockage, much as a clogged pipe. Alternately, the plaque may become inflamed and unroofed. In this case, it travels further down the vessel and causes symptoms.

The level of this glycosylation on the red blood cell can be measured by a blood test called hemoglobin A1c. Doctors use this to help diabetics maintain optimal blood sugar levels or stratify their many disease risks. By keeping this low, the patient's likelihood of illness is less. The HbA1c, as it turns out, is actually the *best* predictor for disease risks in diabetics. As I put it earlier, getting diagnosed with diabetes is like you suffering from *premature aging* of your body. Accordingly, I aim to keep this marker in a much lower, optimal range than most traditionally trained doctors do for patients. This has been born out in both the monumental United Kingdom Prospective Diabetes Study (UKPDS) and the European Prospective Investigation into Cancer—Norfolk (EPIC- Norfolk) trial. In the latter trial, every 1 percent rise in glycosylation above 5 brought on a 27 percent increase in cardiac events in even the *normal* population.[25] We generally shoot for HbA1c under 4.6 percent based on the disease risk reduction shown in the scientific literature. (Most doctors inaccurately believe anything below 7 is great.)

Glycosylation is also a big player in *microvascular* disease—the kidney, eye, and nerve problems in diabetics. This is believed to be caused by the sticky situation mentioned above but is worsened by the increased thickness of the vessel wall caused by such sugarcoating. As a dirty, greasy AC filter, this impairs the diffusion of oxygen across the vessel wall, which ultimately results in poor perfusion and immune function. Usually, this leads to amputation because of poor circulation and impaired wound healing—a not so sweet of a deal in the end.

---

25   K. T. Khaw, N. Wareham, R. Luben, et al., "Glycated haemoglobin, diabetes, and mortality in men in Norfolk cohort of European prospective investigation of cancer and nutrition (EPIC-Norfolk)," *BMJ* 322 (2001): 15–18.

Third, there is also the production of *advanced glycation end products* (AGEs). For you guys so biochemically inclined, these AGEs are formed through the nonenzymatic reaction of reducing sugars with the free amino groups of proteins, lipids, and nucleic acids through the initial formation to a Schiff base and eventually to an Amadori product. When the concentration of glucose is high, as in diabetes, it causes these usually reversible reactions to be driven more toward the increased formation of such AGEs. As mentioned, these are very important because they subsequently cross-link with many proteins, altering their intended structure and functioning. This would occur in the cytoplasm of all cells, including membranes, and other vessel wall components. These further interact with cell membrane receptors, leading to them getting engulfed. This alters cellular metabolism and ultimately leads to many inflammatory events and free radical formation, a.k.a. aging.

Newer research suggests AGEs are the most significant pathogenic mediators of all diabetic complications, namely, the root cause to *micro-* and *macrovascular disease*.[26] These apparently ramp up all stages of inflammation, decrease nitrous oxide production, oxidizes LDL, and stiffen the vessel wall. Recently, many of the steps involved in the macrovascular disease process, the inflammation and blockage of the larger vessels to the heart and brain, have been better understood. However, I was curious in the past as to what causes microvascular disease.

As if not bad enough, these AGEs can also be generated from sources *outside* the body and be exponentially toxic. An example would be from cigarette smoke, which we know is unhealthy anyway. This is just another proverbial nail in the coffin for diabetics who also smoke. You may not know that many forms of food processing, even some cooking methods, can increase these disease-causing compounds. Food manufacturers know well our addiction for that great outdoor flavor, you know … *charred or blackened*. Our penchant for what is essentially burnt carbon has added many synthetic AGEs to our SAD diet. It has been shown that less AGE intake does slow the progression of diabetic-related complications in animals. Other studies have concluded that when AGE intake is lowered, other diseases such as hypertension and CHF (congestive heart failure) are improved, also. This can be easily accomplished by eating more fresh foods, avoiding those overcooked or processed, and cooking with ample water. As you can see, it's not just *what* foods we eat from the new, improved food pyramid, but *how* to best prepare them.

---

26 M. Peppa, "Glucose, advanced glycation and products, and diabetes complications: What is new and what works," *Clinical Diabetes* 21 (2003): 186–87.

Remember, this deleterious process is ubiquitous in your body. The cells that line your joints will become more stiff and painful—the hallmark of arthritis. Neurons in your brain become inflamed with gooey deposits, which result in dementia and many other neurological abnormalities. From head to toe, you're only aging *normally* according to contemporary medicine. If diabetic, or close to it, you will age even earlier and faster. Midlife is the time to prevent all this. Improve your diet and exercise regimen now. Or else, life can become quite *sticky* for you

So in the end, it may be true, *you are what you eat!* Food does play a big role in how you feel now and later in life. The big push here is for you to make healthier choices daily. Eat natural carbs that are high in fiber and antioxidants. By choosing ones with a lower glycemic index, you avoid getting diabetes, inflammation, and many other age-related conditions.

C. Good vs. Bad Fats.

If we are going to learn to fight the enteric enemy, we first need to identify it, As we will learn, it can wear some well-planned disguises, so let's not get fooled again. In 2006, the FDA finally mandated the nutrition facts label list *trans-fat* grams—the first change since the label was established in 1993. These trans fats are inexpensively produced by *hydrogenation*, the bubbling of unsaturated vegetable oil with hydrogen gas. This makes them more solidlike at room temperature, thereby increasing shelf life—a good thing for processed foods but not so good for us. Many food manufacturers switched to using these relatively unknown trans fats when saturated fats became widely unpopular. (Saturated fats are mostly animal derived.)

We now know that these trans fats are more harmful than the saturated fats they replaced. These unfavorably increase LDL, the lousy cholesterol, and lower HDL, the healthy cholesterol. Elevation of a specific trans fat was associated with an increased incidence of localized prostate cancer.[27] Many products touting themselves to be healthy and boasting "Low-Fat" and "Saturated Fat-Free" may be hiding this infamous, *invisible fat.* According to the FDA, more than 40 percent products on the shelves, including 95 percent of cookies, 80 percent of frozen breakfast foods, 75 percent of salty snacks and chips, 70 percent of all cake mixes, and almost half of all cold cereals contain trans fats. Do you know anyone who eats these? Probably most U.S. fast-food restaurants use trans fats, but there may be a recent shift to some limitation. That's welcomed news.

---

27   As suggested by Dr. J Chavarro at the 2005 Annual Meeting of the American Association for Cancer Research, this is based on data from the Physician's Health Study.

Shamefully, in our modern SAD diet, most kids only consume one to two vegetable servings per day, mostly as—you guessed it—french fries. Besides coming from a white potato, one of the high glycemic vegetables out there, fries are also processed. They typically contain other unhealthy ingredients of which you may not even be aware. A recent example is the gluten that was found in McDonald's french fries that were supposedly gluten-free. Add to this the fact that in America, these are then deep-fried in used trans fat. Some manufacturers even hide these trans fats and list them as better nutritionally sounding yet confusing terms such as *hydrogenated* or *partially hydrogenated vegetable oil, fractionated,* or *vegetable shortening.* In many countries like Holland, the use of unhealthy trans fats is considered a national health threat and has been virtually banned. McDonald's restaurants there cannot use any trans fats. Yet, they still are able to make a profit and prosper there. Why is it okay to give such addicting trans fats to America's increasingly unhealthy, overweight kids? Is it because of the free *Pirates of the Caribbean* toy that comes with the kid's meal?

How did America get this far off? Well, remember when the *low-fat craze* hit a few decades ago? Prompted by the USDA (United States Department of Agriculture) food pyramid in 1992, food manufacturers responded by making a plethora of well-marketed processed foods and snacks labeled as "low-fat." To satisfy our fat craving—that simultaneous sweet yet salty taste—they simply added more sugar and salt. When combined with our modern, increasingly sedentary lifestyle, we sort of got *sweet-talked* into today's obesity epidemic. So believe the heads of the Harvard School of Public Health and the American Society of Bariatric Physicians. For years, I preached to people the food pyramid was upside down. The USDA's position then was that it would be too difficult to educate the public about the subtleties of the various types and sources of fats, carbohydrates, and proteins and opted for a clearer simple message instead. Fast forward fifteen years of sugar and salt replacing fat and you may see part of the cause for the pandemic of diabetes in society, especially in our young.

As we age, the many membranes of our nerves, joints, and vessels harden up and become more inflamed. According to the August 2006 *American Journal of Clinical Nutrition*, obese patients having elevated free fatty acid levels are more likely to have congestive heart failure. An impaired immune system increases one's risks for infections and many cancers. Eating the right fats has an anti-inflammatory effect on the entire body. Some research suggests we should eat a handful of walnuts nuts daily. Apparently, indicators of vessel constriction and inflammation diminished after just one serving. I guess it's okay to go nuts when it comes to your health!

In the case of good versus bad fats, the ramifications are quite important. It's simple to remember: Fats from either a plant or fish are healthy when eaten in the right amounts. Fats should be less than thirty grams per day. Plant-based fats are either mono- or polyunsaturated fats and help keep you more limber as you age. Fish contain the omegas and help maintain your brain function and lower inflammation. This is so important; a section devoted to just fish oil follows. As eating these healthier fats prevent vessel disease and erectile dysfunction of older men, they help keep you both young at heart and young at hard! Use sparingly, especially fats from animal products. If you're unsure if the fat or oil in question is beneficial, a good rule of thumb is to check if it's still liquid when refrigerated. Fats should at least be liquid at room temperature. There are more tips about fats in the *Nutritional Facts Label* and *Fish Oil to the Rescue* sections that follow.

> Fats are complex, energy-rich compounds consisting of triglycerides and free fatty acids. There are two essential dietary fats, omega-3 and -6. Though important for proper neurological and immune function, fats should still be limited to less than thirty grams daily, or under 30 percent of your total diet. Get from plant or fish sources.

D. Proteins. You should avoid any processed or prepackaged meats. Proteins are comprised of chains of amino acids and in animal sources, always contain some saturated fat. So try to choose a more natural protein source as leaner organic fish, turkey, or chicken. The recommended meal portion is about four ounces—the size of a deck of cards or your fist (sorry, not the whole outstretched hand). Eating too much red meat (beef, lamb, or pork) is associated with increased colorectal cancer risks. Blackened or charred meats are even worse. According to my research, this may be due in part to the increase of bile acids being presented to the colon because of the accompanying saturated fats. This eventually leads to an increase in the production of malicious metabolites.[28] If you go to the American Institute for Cancer Research's Web site at http://www.aicr.org there are plenty of ideas and recipes to accomplish a very tasty, healthier diet containing less red meat.

So is eating fish even safe today? As I will incessantly insist, fish is proven good for your heart, brain, and lots more. But what about the mercury, polychlorinated biphenyls (PCBs), or other toxins we hear in the news? It seems again, the media has sensationalized both sides of the story so much; you don't know what to think. To make matters worse, the FDA doesn't even have published results from their

---

28 N-nitroso compounds and their metabolites.

own mercury testing of various types of seafood. Probably being a government agency, it has to be politically sensitive before recommending exactly *which* seafood and from *where* should childbearing-age women and children avoid. But before you go back to picking those blackened fatty ribs clean, let me give you some practical information and tips.

It appears oysters and Pacific salmon are safer; preferably avoid farm-raised ones though.[29] Mercury accumulates in older, larger fish such as mackerel and swordfish. So try to avoid these. Albacore tuna is probably okay, but try to buy smaller, nonartificially colored fish. I would also avoid processed or canned fish that may have fats, preservatives, and more. On a personal note, my whole family eats fish at least three times per week, so I'm not that overly concerned. We usually trim off the excess fat and skin, although mercury does accumulate in the meaty parts. Finally, it's best to cook in a way that allows the fat to drain off. Besides observing these precautions, I undergo a short course or oral *chelation*[30] twice per year to rid any heavy metal accumulation. Not just because of my preference of fish as a protein source, but because of the many other potential heavy metal and toxins out there. Overall, fish is quite safe for the middle-aged guy and offers many health benefits. Let's not throw out the caviar with the bath water!

I also recommend only *GMP-certified, pharmaceutical-grade fish oil* supplements as the best way to ensure you're getting the omegas you need.[31] This quality means a third nonbiased party has examined it for purity and pollutants and found it to be safe. Ask for this information before you buy this or any supplement. It has often been suggested that daily intake of such high-grade fish oil supplements may be safer than dietary fish consumption. Concerning dietary fish though, I believe *how* it's prepared and what it's being served *with* is more important. Lastly, I would spend more time worrying about what my child is doing on the Internet, who she's hanging out with, or how much TV she's watching. It's hard enough just to get them to eat their seven servings of vegetables or fruits a day. Life is a balance, after all. You can't be afraid of every little thing you may read.

---

29 Compiled from Institute for Agriculture and Trade Policy, Consumers Union, and Dr. W Harris of the American Heart Association.
30 The process of taking a compound that can help rid your body of toxins and heavy metals.
31 Good Manufacturing Practice (GMP) guidelines are set by the FDA (see http://www.FDA.gov).

> Proteins are the building blocks for the body but are also important for gene expression and metabolism. Giving about 4 kcal per gram of energy, there are nine daily essential amino acids. Try to eat fish, chicken, and beans. Proteins should comprise about 30 percent of your total diet. You need roughly 0.8–1.0 gram of protein daily per kilogram of your body weight.[32]

E. What about Fiber? As a preface, let me say that if you consume the higher percentage of complex carbohydrates I recommend—as in more vegetables and fruits—you probably consume enough dietary fiber. Besides their high-fiber content, unprocessed complex carbs are rich in all the antioxidants and nutrients you need to help prevent free radical damage to your body. Additionally, these are needed to construct *proteoglycans*, or *aminoglycans*.[33][35] These chemical messengers and complex structural components act much as a liaison between many genes' expression and protein function. They bridge the gap and are used for a wide array of joint, immunity, and fertility functions. There has been some recent controversy in the press about how a high-fiber diet may *not* be as healthy as previously believed, and may *not* prevent colon cancer in high-risk patients. If you're confused today about fiber intake, you're certainly not alone. But you should wonder if this represents the true convergence of evidence or just science by press?

Colon cancer is overall the second biggest cancer killer of Americans. (Lung cancer claims the top spot.) This is totally senseless, as routine preventative care including appropriate colonoscopy as indicated would drastically reduce the incidence of gastrointestinal cancers. Interestingly, immigrants from native countries that have much lower risks of colon cancer will usually match our higher rates once they've lived here awhile. This indicates a strong environmental, or acquired, risk for colon cancer. Americans may be better off in many regards; but in the end, they may have to take it up the rear more than their foreign neighbors. Get scoped! Some research facts on fiber follows.

According to recent research, men consuming a high-fiber diet significantly reduced their risk for recurrent colorectal polyps.[34] This conclusion was made by pooling data

---

32 To obtain your weight in kilograms, divide your weight in pounds by 2.2. One hundred fifty pounds equals 70 kg. The amount of protein you need can vary, depending on your individual situation.

33 Aminoglycans are essentially the same as proteoglycans (see index).

34 E. Jacobs, "Fiber may benefit men more than one and in terms of colon cancer protection," *American Journal of Clinical Nutrition* 83 (2006):343–9.

from over thirty-two hundred subjects from the Wheat Bran Fiber Study and the Polyp Prevention Trial. It's important to note that the former studied the benefits of just *cereal* fiber, while the latter utilized a reduced-fat diet with increased *fiber, fruits, and vegetables.* (The authors suggested that in postmenopausal women, increased fiber intake may block some of the protective effects of hormonal replacements.)

A recent VA (Veteran Affairs) study involving more than three thousand veterans suggests cereal fiber helps reduce your risk of getting serious colon polyps. Having been published in *JAMA*, it also found moderate to heavy alcohol consumption, tobacco use, and family history are the top risk factors. A sedentary lifestyle and obesity were also risk factors for colon cancer. So men, eat your fiber and keep moving.

Cereal fiber may reduce your risk for peripheral artery disease (PAD).[35] This refers to symptomatic blockages of (peripheral) vessels, not the ones in the (central) heart. If you get blockages in your carotid artery, then you're at risk for stroke, dementia, and mood disorders. If in the renal artery, this puts you at risk of eventually being on dialysis. If in the legs, these blockages can lead to neuropathy, nonhealing wounds, or even amputation. As if that's not bad enough, this can also lead you to not getting an erection. So, guys, eat your Wheaties© for good old Woody's sake.

Fiber intake favorably influences all lipid parameter by lowering triglycerides and LDL and improving cholesterol/HDL ratios.[36][38] Numerous other studies probably indicate that increased dietary fiber intake lowers risks of coronary artery disease (CAD). This risk may be decreased by as much as 30 percent for every ten grams of daily fiber.[37] Increased intake of fiber has favorable effects on abnormal insulin and glucose metabolism, inflammation, hypertension, high cholesterol levels, and poor clotting factors—all risk factors for CAD and PAD.[38] Insulin resistance in patients at risk for developing type 2 diabetes was improved just after

35   A. T. Merchant, "Dietary fiber reduces peripheral arterial disease risk in men," *Journal of Nutrition* 133, no. 11 (2003): 3658–66.

36   M. N. Ballesteros, "Dietary fiber and lifestyle influence serum lipids in free living adult men," *Journal of American College of Nutrition* 20, no. 6 (2001): 649–55.

37   M. A.Pereira, "Dietary fiber and risk of coronary heart disease: A pooled analysis of cohort studies," *Archives of Internal Medicine* 164 (2004):370–76.

38   Y. Ma, "Association between dietary fiber and serum C-reactive protein," *American Journal of Clinical Nutrition.* 83 (2006): 760–66.

three days of a diet high in soluble fiber.[39] Still waiting to take in more fiber? Start now. As Cat Stevens sang, get "thick as a brick."

The American Gastroenterological Association recommends about 30–35 grams of dietary fiber from a variety of sources daily. Such a high-fiber diet should begin before middle age because it may take decades to make a substantial difference. The American Dietetic Association reflects my recommendations for a diet naturally rich in fiber, originating from a variety of complex carbohydrates such as vegetables, fruits, beans, and multigrain sources. Naturally, both insoluble and soluble fiber beat processed sources.

We should appreciate that research conclusions are quite specific for a specific question and population. The widespread application of the conclusion to the real world can be quite challenging. For example, do all ethnic groups benefit from increased soluble fiber intake? I would suspect that various ethnic groups would benefit most from mimicking the more natural, culture-based diet their ancestors consumed. Most immigrants become sicker once on the SAD diet and lifestyle. The majority of our genes, and thus our metabolic machinery, would have optimally evolved through natural selection over time to thrive on such. This is certainly not meant to denigrate any particular group. On the contrary, focusing more on our unique culinary heritage may also enrich family traditions and togetherness. It's all about embracing our individuality and not falsely assuming what's good for one group is good for all. One man's meat, in fact, may be another man's poison. Homegrown food probably tastes a whole lot better too!

Currently, there may be some conflicting data when it comes to fruit and vegetable fiber intake preventing colon cancer. Over all, we should appreciate that fiber is beneficial in preventing many metabolic, vessel, and inflammatory conditions. Try to consume 30-40 grams of fiber daily. It's part of a totally healthy lifestyle. Succinctly put, "Fiber … to Uranus and beyond!"

F. Nutrition Facts Label—Just the Facts, Ma'am! Here, you will learn to become a nutrition detective. First, I recommend avoiding any processed foods, those found in a can, jar, or box. You shouldn't eat anything that has a food nutrition label in the first place. But if you must, you must. It's the real world, after all. Second, you should now be able to differentiate what's a good or bad fat, carb, or

---

39 M. O. Weickert, "Cereal fiber improves whole-body insulin sensitivity in overweight and obese women," *Diabetes Care* 29 (2006): 775–80.

protein. Lastly, and probably most important, you *must* limit your portion sizes. Now, I realize there are times when you can't avoid the tremendous urge or convenience. Without sounding like Jimmy Swaggart, I admit it; I have sinned and am guilty at times. Yet very sparingly, I might add. After all, it's what we do 95 percent of the time that matters most, not the other 5 percent. You have to become good at understanding exactly what the nutrition facts labels do and don't tell you.

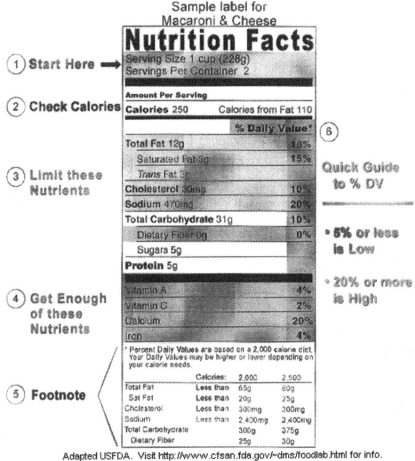

Figure 3.6. Nutrition facts label. Become a food detective. Get the kids involved too.

Initially, look at the *number of servings* and *serving size*. This is because the rest of the data is specifically based on this. Most people are misled right from the get-go on this, so don't feel bad. For example, the label lists two servings per container, but you may think it's only one serving and then proceed to eat the whole box. You may think you're eating quite healthily. *Wrong, bucko!* You've been duped … but by no small mistake of the manufacturer. To avoid this from happening, buy smaller packages, not the super-duper size. The temptation is to just graze all nightlong on the whole huge bag while being hypnotized by reality shows like *The Big Loser*, or while watching the cooking channel.

Next, look at the *amounts or percentages of fats, proteins, and carbohydrates.* Ideally, it should consist of 50–60 percent carbs, 20–30 percent protein, and 10–20 percent fat. Of course, this depends on the particular food and your overall diet. If there's no readable label, you can look at the *list of ingredients*. These are usually listed starting with the *largest* ingredient going down to the smallest. It's important to remember the idea of a balanced diet and how to combine food groups to accomplish that. For example, you may want a quick healthy snack. You could have a prepackaged snack with the right percentages listed above. Or you may have some walnuts or almonds handy. Most nuts consist of about 50 percent *unsaturated* fat, 25 percent protein, and 25 percent complex carbs. In order to balance this, you could add an apple for more carbs and some skim milk for protein. You could do this at the same time, or make it up later during the day. So a small midafternoon snack of low-fat cheese, some fruit, and roasted nuts is fine.

Next, look at *carbohydrates* and zoom in immediately on sugar. If twelve grams are listed as total carbohydrates and ten grams listed as sugar, then about 80 percent is simple sugar—not good. You want most carbs to be from *complex* carbohydrates, not from fructose, sweeteners, or syrups. Remember, avoid foods with a high glycemic index in order to prevent those unhealthy sugar and insulin spikes you read about earlier. Many foods, like juices, are all natural yet very high in sugar. So be careful; it all adds up. In the above label, only five of the 31 grams are from sugar—not bad.

As far as *fat* is concerned, keep less than thirty grams daily and limit the saturated type. Also the unhealthier trans fats should be listed. The difference between these and the *total* fat should equal up to the healthier mono- and polyunsaturated fats. Remember, the right fats in the right amounts are actually *good* for you. These would be the fats derived from fish or plant sources.

Some good news though. Because of the justifiable bad rap that trans fats are receiving, some snack makers like Kraft and Frito-Lay have responded—even to the point of some foods being labeled as trans fat free. New Yorkers are considering a ban on these trans fats. Many other countries have already beaten them to this. Hopefully, the elimination of trans fats will make common financial sense to the manufacturer. An important fact to note: If there are a less than 0.5 g of trans fats, the manufacturer can list this as being zero, or trans fat free. Well, this eventually adds up. Unknowingly, you may be eating four or five snacks a day with 0.5 g of trans fats per serving—adding up to a few grams daily of the *baddest* fat in town. If we didn't consume such junky foods in mass quantities and demanded healthier ones, there wouldn't be the vast supply we have out there today. It's basically the principle of demand and supply. We all must affect this change. Come on, baby boomers! Are you with me?

Currently, there's a somewhat haphazard movement of manufacturers to make healthier foods. As a glimmer of hope, organic foods are now more in demand than ever, prompting most grocery store chains to stock more natural foods. I find it more convenient than ever to purchase organic or soy dairy items. There are omega-enriched eggs from cage-free chickens. From pesticide-free produce to natural meat, food shelves are being filled with more options for the health conscious. Even I'm confused at the various, or dare I say, tricky labels being used for some products. Don't be fooled. Did you know the terms *all natural* or *natural* has no standard definition; it's really a meaningless marketing ploy. The USDA Web site has details on exactly what these various *organic* labels mean. Most important, remember it's a must to wash your vegetables and fruits with soap, as most pesticides aren't water soluble. We don't want to eat more *E. coli*-tainted spinach, do we?[40]

On the grocery shelves, there are protein- and omega-enriched pasta noodles like Berillo Plus© that have a healthier, lower glycemic index. Their texture is somewhat different though, when prepared al dente. I also recommend substituting white rice with those Asian bean-based noodles whenever possible. They're those yellowish clear-looking ones, and they taste fine. You'll probably need to visit the local Asian grocery store to get them. Some beans or other homemade sauce can be added for a healthier casserole, or they can be added to stir-fried food. Even for me, having salads every meal would quickly get boring. You have to have variety. Be inventive.

> Being human, you simply can't avoid eating some amount of prepackaged, processed food daily. You must learn to read between the lines and separate the fiction from the nutrition facts label.

---

40 *Escherichia coli*, a common bacteria residing in the colon, can have more aggressive subtypes and cause a number of varied, sometimes serious disease.

To get up-to-date tips on nutrition, cancer prevention, and even exercise, you should check out the American Institute for Cancer Research (AICR). They publish numerous free pamphlets that are chock-full of practical information. I feel it's far better to prevent carcinogenesis in the first place, don't you? Remember, an ounce of prevention is worth a pound of cure. I especially like *Homemade for Health: Cooking for Lower Cancer Risk*. It contains many suggestions for healthy quick-prep meals. They have a wealth of other easy-to-read pamphlets on a wide array of helpful topics: *Getting Active, Staying Active*; *How to Enjoy a More Physically Active Life*; *Nutrition and the Cancer Survivor*; *The New American Plate*; and more. You can even call their toll-free nutrition hotline at 1-800-843-8114 and speak with a registered dietitian. Being nonprofit, AICR does accept a tax-deductible donation. It's put to great use, as you can see.

G. Diet Summary. After reviewing many volumes written from various disciplines and authors, I have come to the following conclusion: Be it the Zone, South Beach, Sugar Busters, Paleolithic or Bible, Pan-Asian, or Mediterranean Diet, it really doesn't matter that much. These all have the same basic composition of a high-carb, low-calorie diet. There is usually just a different twist. In all these cases, carbs aren't bad; they just have to be the right ones. Usually, two-thirds of the plate is comprised of the lower glycemic "complex" vegetables and fruits presented earlier. Eat more vegetables than fruit, because of the sugar. The remaining one-third consists of a lean protein source, preferably fish, chicken, soy or bean based. The specific recipes depend on the ethnic, historical, or whatever shtick or theme the author emphasized. Add to that a gram of fish oil and a good multivitamin per day, then bam, you're 98 percent of the way there.

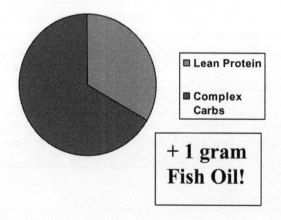

A prospective study on obese young adults concluded a diet high in carbohydrates with a low glycemic index is best for cardiovascular risk reduction.[41] The author suggests it's time to incorporate these concepts of glycemic index and glycemic load into clinical practice which, in turn, may help avoid the confusion generated by many popular diets. After all I stated above, this really shouldn't come as any groundbreaking news. Yet, it's nothing more than what your parents preached. Eat your seven to nine servings of vegetables and fruits per day. Fish is brain food. Avoid eating sugar, you'll get diabetes. Everything old may be new again when it comes to eating the proper diet! I've shown how plain logic and the scientific literature back this up.

As Grandpa Rao used to say, "Always leave the table feeling a little bit hungry." This is something I can't stress enough. If the diet is really going to work, it simply *has* to involve consuming fewer calories, or some form of portion control. *Most people don't know this, but it takes the stomach about a half hour to inform the brain it's full.* Don't wait until then to stop eating! Many seem to eat each meal as if it's their last. They feel the need to shovel food in until they feel stuffed, or even overstuffed. We have all been there; even I am no exception on Christmas, Thanksgiving, or Super Bowl Sunday! When grazing until our brain tells us we're stuffed, we invariably feel quite miserable and fatigued afterward. This is due to many reasons: one, that insulin spike I referred to earlier, as well as serotonin surges, abnormal leptin levels, and more.[42] I guarantee, if you leave the table *not* feeling completely full, you'll later feel comfortably full and still have lots of energy. You won't have to carry and metabolize all that extra food.

---

41 J. McMillan-Price, "Comparison of four diets of varying glycemic load on weight loss and cardiovascular risk reduction in overweight and obese young adults: A randomized controlled trial," *Archives in Internal Medicine* 166, no. 14 (2006): 1466–75.

42 Serotonin is a type of a neurotransmitter, a chemical message between nerves in the brain, that typically surge after a meal, maybe more so after ingesting turkey. Leptin is one of the so-called satiety hormones that indicate you're already full.

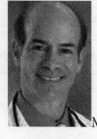More practical advice includes the following:

- Fix the proper portions of food on a small plate, then close all the pots and pans (get them out of your sight, smell, and touch) and put them *in the back* of the refrigerator.
- *Slowly* chew your food and drink plenty of water.
- Enjoy your company; converse some.
- If you are still hungry after finishing your plate, resist the temptation. As mentioned above, this will pass. Instead, get involved with another activity for the next half hour. Walk the dog after a meal, but *get away* from the table. If you're still hungry at that time, then snack on a little healthy something. (Chances are, you're not hungry any longer and feel quite good about it. Remember what I said about that postprandial glucose surge. If you rest after eating, a fat cell will get it and store it—making you literally fatter in the end. If you're active, a muscle cell will use it—a much leaner option.)
- It's better to have smaller meals throughout the day. Don't skip meals!

To summarize this in some plain lingo, put less junk in the trunk. I encourage patients on this healthier road—that's unfortunately less traveled—to look at it this way: It took a while to get things off; it didn't happen overnight. Likewise, it'll take a while to get them right again, but it'll happen. This lifelong trip starts with a few steps in the right direction. But what a fantastic destination! As the famous director Spike Lee would add, "Do the right thing!" I'll repeat more preaching from our parents, "You are what you eat." Let's prevent getting diabetes and age-related complications by practicing a healthier lifestyle—the earlier, the better.

H. Fish Oil to the Rescue

Fish is brain food. Take your cod liver oil each day!

Fish oil has long been believed to help ward off inflammation. Researchers theorize that the ideal bad fat/good fat ratio in our diets should be about 4:1. Worldwide, Asians and Japanese come closest, with a ratio around 6:1. Most nutritionists suspect this is due to their higher consumption of healthier monounsaturated and polyunsaturated fats from plant and fish sources. They generally eat less junky fat from fast food and enjoy a more active lifestyle. The SAD diet we have approximates a whopper of a figure, 20:1 or higher! When these hardened fats are assimilated into the many cellular components throughout our body, we become less nimble to play dodgeball with Father Time. This is of no small consequence. Americans have much higher rates of inflammatory mediated diseases such as cancers, arthritis, and neurological disorders.

We should regularly consume plant-based foods rich in *alpha linoleic acid*, such as canola and soybean oils, nuts, and flaxseed. The essential omega-3 fatty acids, DHA (docosahexaenoic acid), and EPA (eicosapentaenoic acid) are the most important anti-inflammatory ones and are found in fatty fish. Omega-6, present in other meats and vegetable oils, promote inflammation and therefore should be limited. It's the higher ratio of the omega-3 to omega-6 that helps limit inflammation and degeneration. Indeed, the inflammatory mediators in the body are derived from fats though the arachidonic acid pathway (please see the figure below). Most anti-inflammatory drugs as aspirin and NSAIDs (nonsteroidal anti-inflammatory drugs) work by inhibiting the cyclooxygenase (COX) system. Celebrex and Vioxx are popular examples of the more selective COX-2 inhibitors. (Currently, no drugs work on the lipoxygenase (LPO) system, although there's a lot of related research going on.) It's quite complicated to explain; but for all intents and purposes, let's say it's the *balance* of these various end products and their subtypes that either promotes or limits inflammation. The inflammation can lead to diseases in the nerves, joints, blood vessels, and basically anywhere and everywhere. These inflammatory mediators are represented below by leukotrienes, thromoxanes, and the prostaglandins. Fish oil, which contains EPA and DHA fatty acids, help inhibit these.

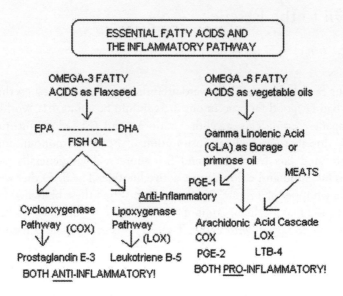

Figure 3.7. Fatty acid metabolism. More intake of omega-3 and less of trans, saturated, and omega-6 fats will help tip the scales to less inflammation. PGE-Prostaglandins-the inflammatory mediators.

Because of possible toxicities, including mercury and other environmental pollutants, found in dietary fish, younger women and children should use some caution.[43] For midlife men, any theoretical downside to fish consumption is mostly outweighed by the benefits; so relax. You can help limit this toxicity by buying only *GMP-certified* fish oil supplements. There are many books and scientific articles that focus on only one aspect of fish oil. You could read Dr. Barry Sears' book, *The Omega Rx Zone: The Miracle of the New High-Dose Fish Oil*, for more information, or visit him at http://www.drsears.com. Here's my quick lowdown:

Like David Letterman, I will amuse you with my *top ten list* of reasons to take extra fish oil.

1. You won't have to "sleep with the fishes." One gram daily of fish significantly decreases your risk for sudden cardiac death by up to 45 percent and helps pre-

---

43   Stacy Foran Melanson, MD, PhD, from the Brigham and Women's Hospital and Harvard Medical School in Boston, Massachusetts; *Archives of Pathology and Laboratory Medicine* 129 (2005):74–77.

vent *arrhythmias such* as atrial fibrillation.[44] I believe *all* cardiac deaths are rather sudden, especially if you're the one having it! It's not like you'd say, "Hey, I was just waiting for this myocardial infarction to happen. Glad it finally happened!" Amazingly, this benefit beats out practically any prescription drug. Better yet, there are virtually no appreciable side effects or risks associated with fish oil.

The very idea that fish oil may be beneficial in cardiac disease was first described by a landmark study in Greenland published way back in 1980. Twenty-two years later, guidelines published in *Circulation* recommended persons with established coronary heart disease should consume about one gram of omega-3 fatty acid daily to help prevent the incidence of new coronary events. Even the conservative American Heart Association has jumped on the bandwagon and began recommending that all patients at risk for heart disease should be taking fish oil, or at least increase their dietary fish intake. To me, this population would include anybody over fifty with or without established or suspected heart disease. Did your cardiologist accordingly recommend this the last time you visited her? If not, why? These beneficial effects are probably due to fish oil's anti-inflammatory action on vessel plaque.

Adding niacin (vitamin B$_3$) will work synergistically with fish oil supplementation to improve cholesterol levels.[45] Seeing more benefits with fewer side effects such as flushing and liver enzyme elevation, I can then recommend a more tolerable, lower dose than the usual two to three grams of niacin needed per day. I personally take one gram of fish oil with my breakfast and then one gram of niacin before bedtime. Some recent research shows this combination improves cholesterol parameters better than moderate doses of most statin drugs. Typically, statin drugs are expensive and require routine office visits and blood work to monitor their many potential side effects. Not so with fish oil.

2. It straightens out *the good, the bad, and the ugly* better than Clint Eastwood.
You'll get lower triglycerides (TG), the *ugly* cholesterol, and a higher HDL, the *good* cholesterol. These two cholesterol components, while mainly being overlooked in the past, have finally been gaining some well-deserved notoriety. For a while, most doctors and pharmacists have screamed, "Cholesterol! Cholesterol!

---

44 Arrhythmias include all irregular rhythms of the heart. Specifically, atrial fibrillation increases your risks for heart attack, heart failure, and stroke. With this disease, you need to be on risky blood thinners. D. Mozaffrian, *Circulation* 110 (2004): 368–73.

45 R. Oh, "Practical applications of fish oil (omega-3 fatty acids) in primary care," *J Am Board Fam Pract.* 18, no. 1 (2005): 28–36.

Cholesterol!" Then followed, "LDL! It's bad, bad, bad!" I feel a lot of this one-sided view was promoted by the large drug firms. At about three dollars a pop, these pills have turned out to be a real cash cow. These big corporation sponsors would have a big say in what the research would *and wouldn't* conclude. Be that as it may, lowering triglycerides help lower risks for coronary disease and many other serious maladies. These include the metabolic syndrome, pancreatitis, and much more. (Other ways to lower TG and LDL will be presented throughout the book.)

According to the large VA-HIT (Veterans Affairs High-Density Lipoprotein Intervention Trial), raising HDL by *as little as 6 percent* has been shown to reduce your risk for coronary disease by up to 35 percent! Why hasn't this been publicly promoted as much as the need to lower LDL? Well, connect the dots from the paragraph above and figure it out for yourself. There is currently *no* patented drug, and therefore no real profit, that significantly raises HDL. For the most part, it's left to good old-fashioned exercise. Luckily, this is much more affordable, has no ill side effects, and possesses many other healthy effects. How slick is that?

As mentioned above, I use these natural modalities. My total cholesterol (TC) used to be 285. HDL was unhealthily low at 45, and my triglycerides were okay, about 100. After maximizing the recommended diet, exercising, and taking one gram of fish oil with 1000 milligrams of niacin daily, my TC slid way down to 205. HDL jumped to a boastful 85! Triglycerides dove to a healthier 80. I have great blood pressure to boot. This is quite remarkable; I have a strong family history of hypertension and early heart disease. My father died suddenly at fifty-nine of a massive heart attack. According to established protocols, I should be on aggressive drug therapy. I could get my hands on all the free statin drugs I wanted from the drug representatives who visit me. Yet, I choose the more natural approach. Why? Of course, to be a role model for my patients by practicing what I preach. But wouldn't it would be ironic and quite idiotic if I didn't follow these safe, proven modalities myself?

You may wonder, with what's shared above, if I ever recommend *any* cholesterol-lowering drugs. Of course, I do, for those appropriate patients at risk when diet, natural methods, and exercise don't get them to the proper goal. The statin drugs are proven to save lives; it's hard to argue against that. Yet, there's no one magic pill for everyone. The vast majority of patients *do* tolerate these quite well. Some statin drugs I consider safer than others include Pravachol, which isn't metabolized through the liver's cytochrome p450 system.[46] Next, would be Zocor. I must reemphasize that an *integrative approach* uses a combination of proven medical *and* nonmedical methods. In treating high cholesterol for example, I may first suggest you try a low dose of a statin drug, but with fish oil and niacin. This, with certain lifestyle changes, would get you to goal, with fewer problems.

3. Your life won't end up as a total wreck! As we age, the associated increased inflammation only causes most age-related diseases to accelerate. Today, most scientists realize vessel disease has a large inflammatory component. The degree is measured by a mediator in the blood called *CRP-hs.*[47] Because of my focus on prevention, I have routinely checked these levels in patients over the past five years. This practice is just beginning to dawn in the rest of the medical community though. As a matter of fact, I have yet to get copies of any lab work done by another doctor, or even a cardiologist, that measured these CRP-hs levels. Yet, it's long been known to be much better predictor of vessel disease than LDL![48] The truth is that at least half of those having a heart attack have quite acceptable cholesterol levels. In their typical reactive approach, most insurances including Medicare only pay for this blood test if you *already have* coronary artery disease. Well, wouldn't you and your doctor want to know before it's too late? Increased inflammation causes plaque instability, thereby increasing the risk of vessel occlusion. This may erupt into a sudden heart attack or slowly evolve into other peripheral vascular conditions such as erectile dysfunction.

Discussing the pathology of vessel disease would take many volumes, but I will give you some a few analogies. I basically envision plaques, the abnormal blockages occurring in diseased arteries, as falling into two categories.

One is the stable, large plaque that builds up over decades. This eventually results in a gradual decrease in blood flow to the organ involved, i.e., brain, kidney, heart,

---

46 The liver metabolizes many drugs, many through the cytochrome p450 pathway. If this becomes overwhelmed, then the level of drugs and other toxins may be increased.

47 C-Reactive Protein (highly specific), CRP-hs, selectively measures the amount of inflammation in the coronary vessels. It can be artificially elevated in the aged or those with arthritis.

48 P. M. Ridker, M. Cushman, M. J. Stampfer, et al., "Inflammation, aspirin, and the risk of cardiovascular disease in apparently healthy men," *N Engl J Med* 336 (1997):973–79; P. M. Ridker, N. Rifai, L. Rose, et al., "Comparison of C-reactive protein and low-density lipoprotein cholesterol levels in the prediction of first cardiovascular events," *N Engl J Med:* 347 (2002):1557–65.

or legs. If you're lucky, you may get a warning before disaster strikes. It's like the dummy light on your car's dashboard telling you to check the engine right before there's pending irreversible damage. In your body, this may be a transient ischemic attack *(TIA)*, the warning of an impending stroke; or *angina,* the preclude to a heart attack.[49] To avoid getting dumped into that big junkyard in the sky, please seek immediate diagnosis and treatment if you get the symptoms.

Generally, these warnings occur in older people. They survived because the slow yet steady growth of the plaques in the vessels allowed enough time for *collateral circulation* to develop. Their vessels' blood flow may be analogous to you traveling along an old, two-lane highway with many potholes. At times, some lanes are closed down for repair. There's also the lower speed limit, occasional traffic jam, and many bottlenecks that often divert flow to an alternate back road. Fortunately, in these cases, there's enough time for the doctor to react with medications or a bypass to keep you rolling along.

The other type is the unstable, moderately sized plaque. This too often results in sudden cardiac death in the relatively overweight, middle-aged guy. He may be a smoker or have other underappreciated risks. These include *borderline* cholesterol or hypertension, a positive family history, or mild glucose intolerance. A little of bit of all these risks add up though. This nice guy will be at work or play, and suffer a massive heart attack out of the proverbial clear blue sky. Too often, we've known someone in the prime of his life knocked down like this. No one saw it coming. His wife and kids left behind may wonder how could this happen. Well, if we don't know what to look for, we'll never see it coming.

Like detectives in the popular TV show *CSI*, let's look closer and ask some serious questions. Could this have been prevented? Were there any warning signs? Microscopically, one of those silent, medium-sized plaques probably became quickly inflamed and enlarged. This results in an acute blockage. Now unstable, it could also shower smaller clots further down the vessel and damage more heart muscle. A clot only the size of a pinhead can travel further and cause a stroke. Using the analogy above, this is like you, cavalierly speeding along a curve on the wide, open highway. All of a sudden, there's a thunderstorm. A slow-moving tractor-trailer suddenly pulls

---

49   Angina is the temporary chest pain resulting from blockage of blood flow to the heart. If not treated, it may result in permanent heart damage, a myocardial infarction (MI), TIA (transient ischemic attack), the varying neurological symptoms that result from temporary insufficient blood flow to the brain. A stroke, like an MI, results in permanent loss of function of a part of the brain due to the lack of blood flow.

out in front of the cars ahead. As a normal reflex, you quickly slam on the brakes, oversteer the wheels, and start to skid out of control. Things happen fast. You're all over the road. The last sound you hear is coming from an ambulance. In this case, your vessels have not had time to develop collateral circulation. Your chances for survival are lessened as a result. Yet, a more proactive approach by you and your doctor might have prevented this tragic ending. By keeping your vehicle in top running shape, you may have been able to steer clear of this deadly pileup.

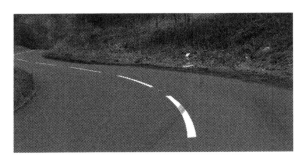

4. It'll keep you more loose than Courtney Love in her younger days. As introdu Your life won't end up as a total wrec ced earlier, aging also increases your risk of acquiring *rheumatologic and arthritic conditions.* These, of course, include rheumatoid arthritis and osteoarthritis; but you can add the whole gambit including lupus, mixed connective tissue disease, polymyalgia rheumatica, gout, and many others. These disorders not only cause disabling pain, but they also affect other parts of the body and can eventually lead to depression, fatigue, and even increase the risk for many cancers. Some can cause permanent blindness, as in the case of temporal arteritis.[50]

Do all these have to happen as we age? This should be no big surprise once you think about it; this is how many of us envision old geezers. It's just that, as we reach midlife, many accept the early, milder symptoms of aging. Ask any child to imitate her old great-grandpa. She will stoop over, shuffle, and move slowly. Asking the same questions again and again, she may also incessantly complain about her declining health. These actions amount to the *normal* aging syndrome as many have come to know: Osteoporosis and Parkinson's disease with frailty syndrome, dementia, depression, urinary incontinence, and so on. Does getting

---

50   There are many rheumatological conditions including the ones mentioned above. They all represent an exaggerated inflammatory response against various tissues throughout the body. The various names depend on which parts of the body are affected.

old always *have* to have such bad outcomes? No, but you shouldn't *let* yourself *get* old in the first place. George Burns also quipped, "You can't help getting older, but you don't have to get old."

Fish oil has long been known to effectively lower arthritic symptoms without the undesired side effects to the liver and kidneys that NSAIDs possess.[51] By the way, all the hoopla that lawyers are making about the increased hypertension and risk of heart attack is a *class effect* of almost all NSAIDs, not just Vioxx or Celebrex. This holds true for Advil and Aleve, both available OTC. Probably, the most dangerous risk is acute gastrointestinal bleeding. This can be caused from gastritis or a more serious ulcer, and can occur whether you have been taking NSAIDs for a few days or many years. Half the time, there are no warning signs. Most of these victims are the elderly or alcohol users. About half as many Americans die from NSAIDs' side effects per year as do from bullets! The lesson is that drugs can kill too, even the ones available without a prescription. Fish oil can help improve arthritic conditions safely.

5. Taking fish oil will make you happier than David Spade the week he dated Heather Locklear. Age-related inflammation probably helps explain our increased incidence of dysphoria, or feeling blue and stressed out in middle age. As published in the medical journal *Primary Psychiatry*, one daily gram of fish oil improved 83 percent the conditions of those suffering from clinical depression.[52] The severity of depression improved over 50 percent. (Interestingly, those taking over a gram had less improvement, although were still significantly better.) There were basically no adverse effects, unlike most prescription remedies. This work was not funded by any pharmaceutical firm.

Most prescribed antidepressants don't approximate this success rate and possess many potentially serious side effects. These commonly may include weight gain and sexual dysfunction and worsening psychiatric symptoms. Extra caution should be used in youths. I generally find that the EPA (eicosapentaenoic acid) component in fish oil helps inflammation, whereas the DHA (docosahexaenoic

---

51   NSAIDs are nonsteroidal anti-inflammatory drugs that can cause many serious effects on the liver and kidneys. Supposedly, about eighteen thousand Americans die annually from NSAID-induced gastrointestinal bleeding. These can be prescription medicine or available OTC as Aleve or Advil.

52   [54] EJR, "Omega-3 fatty acid DHA shows efficacy for treatment of depression," *Primary Psychiatry* 11, no. 7 (2004): 15. Based on research by Mischoulon, M from Harvard Medical School (*APA* 2004).

acid) may better benefit mind and mood. Reflecting this, I may push up the dose of DHA to help treat neurological conditions such as dementia, Parkinson's, multiple sclerosis, or ADHD. (For rheumatoid arthritis or related inflammatory conditions, I usually titrate up the EPA dose.) The specific amounts I recommend are highly individualized, being based on the clinical picture. The benefits probably result from lowering the ratio of bad to good fats. Currently, there are blood tests available that can measure the various levels of fatty acids. These may help in the initial evaluation of a patient, but I tend to use them to find out just how high I need to push up the dose. After all, taking a few grams of good fish oil a day isn't exactly cheap. All this shouldn't be a big revelation,. Historically elders have pushed kids to take their cod liver oil each day. Fish is brain food, right?!

6. Momma will have her *squeeze box* playin' all night long. Patients suffering with *asthma* or *emphysema* can be helped by omega-3 supplementation.[53] Improvements were noted in their six-minute walk test, dyspnea scores, and arterial oxygenation. Levels of many inflammatory mediators were also noted to decrease. Lastly, hyperinflammation, mucus production, tissue destruction, and bronchospasm were lessened. The multiple chronic obstructive pulmonary disease (COPD) medications prescribed today are, at best, minimally effective in controlling symptoms and offer no real cure. They have multiple serious side effects among them such as immunosuppression, osteoporosis, diabetes, acute gastrointestinal bleeding, and more. Significant side effects of fish oil—zero. The benefits—priceless!

7. You won't get confused with Rush Limbaugh. *Chronic back pain* has an inflammatory component, which is improved by adding omega-3 fatty acid intake.[54] The body's pain mediators, like substance P, are theoretically inhibited. There are also volumes of research suggesting the improvement of many other inflammatory and autoimmune contributors to back pain. These conditions are associated with increased levels of interleukin-1 and leukotriene LTB4, which are derived from pro-inflammatory prostaglandins. As you can see in figure 3.7, these modulate the *yin and yang* of the inflammatory mediators in the body. By consuming more monounsaturated fatty acids (MUFA) and polyunsaturated fatty acids (PUFA), you can tip the scales to less overall inflammation.

---

53 Matsuyama, "Effects of omega-3 polyunsaturated fatty acids on inflammatory markers in COPD," *Chest* 128, no. 6 (2005). Many major inflammatory players as leukotriene B-4, interleukin-8, and tumor necrosis factor significantly decreased.

54 J.C. Maroon, "Omega-3 fatty acids (fish oil) as an anti-inflammatory: An alternative to nonsteroidal anti-inflammatory drugs for discogenic pain," *Surg Neurol* 65, no. 4 (2006):326–31.

8. You won't have to melodramatically cry out, "Doctor, ... my eyes!" Higher intake of omega-3 long-chain polyunsaturated fatty acid and fish was associated with decreased risk of getting neovascular *age-related macular degeneration*(AMD).[55] This is based on the results from the large AREDS (Age-Related Eye Disease Study) that looked at over forty-five hundred patients aged sixty to eighty years. I find this very relevant because most fear getting blind as they age. AMD is the most common cause of blindness in the United States. Along with taking a good multivitamin with zinc, you can help prevent this.

10. You may finally live to outsmart Alex Trebeck on *Jeopardy.* Data analyzed from the large Framingham Heart Study revealed people who took an average of 180 mg or more of DHA from fish oil daily exhibited *40–50 percent less Alzheimer's* and other dementias.[56] This intake matches the equivalent of consuming fish about three or more times per week. Your brain mostly consists of fat, and about 50 percent is DHA; so it's very important to eat the right fats. More than going blind or even dying, older people fear losing their cognitive and mental abilities. As reiterated by many generations, fish is brain food and you should take cod liver oil each day. Think about it, fish are in schools their whole lives!

Lastly, how about the other sources of omega-3 and -9, such as *flaxseed, borage, or primrose oil?* Obviously, I can't present a lengthy discussion on all these. My one-minute take is that fish oil supplementation has the most scientific evidence concerning safety and benefit. These other omegas are precursors and rely on your body for conversion to the preferred, anti-inflammatory DHA and EPA. (Figure 3.7 illustrates these pathways.) As a matter of fact, some older people don't metabolize these very efficiently. They may also be on multiple medications that often inhibit these needed conversions. In the end, there may not be the expected benefit. On the otherhand, for some that's allergic to fish, or simply refuse to take fish oil for whatever reasons, these other sources may be a necessity. When practical, these should be an adjunct, not a replacement, for fish oil—the real deal. Lastly, no matter which you choose, remember to buy GMP-certified, pharmaceutical-grade products. Like using the best motor oil in your vehicle, it'll keep you well lubed and will more than pay off in the long run. Your body will thank you for it.

55 J. Seddon, *Archives of Ophthalmology* 124 (2006): 995–1001; B. Chua, *Archives of Ophthalmology* 124 (2006): 981–86; J. P. SanGiovanni et al., in 2004, from the National Eye Institute in Bethesda, Maryland.

56 Dr. E. Schaefer, director of the Lipid Metabolism Laboratory in the Human Nutrition Research Center on Aging at Tufts University, as presented to the American Heart Association, 2004.

As you age, the many diseases resulting from the usual rise in inflammation has been further accelerated by today's SAD diet. Heart disease, dementia, arthritis, and many other metabolic disorders are worsened by your body's pro-inflammatory milieu. By taking a daily gram of fish oil, you help keep these to a healthier, younger minimum.

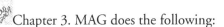

Chapter 3. MAG does the following:

- Starts following a diet that's 2/3 complex carbs (vegetables and fruit with a low glycemic index) and 1/3 lean meat. He cuts out all bread, rice, and pasta for now. It's now just one glass of wine per day, max.
- He starts one gram of fish oil per day.
- Drinks more filtered water.
- Avoids anything that has a nutrition facts label.
- Doesn't skip breakfast anymore and avoids eating late at night.

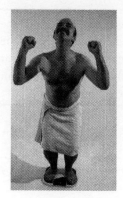

IV.

Weight Loss: This Time, You Will Lose Weight

If you don't change direction, you'll probably end up where you're headed.

A. How Do You Know You're Overweight? Much was introduced in the prior diet chapter or will be complemented by subsequent chapters, but I wanted to specifically address *weight loss*.[57] Obesity is the root of all evil. I can never stress enough that *weight loss* is not as important as *weight control*. Obtaining and then maintaining the proper *body composition* should be the main goal. It's where the weight is that's really important.If you achieve this, you needn't worry about all the other outcomes of being overweight. All else will fall in place. Let me explain by giving you an example. If you were to lie in bed all week, you may be surprised to find you would actually *lose* weight. But before you get any bright ideas, you would actually lose muscle mass—not a good thing. Furthermore, you would gain some disease-causing fat mass—again, not good. This is referred to as *sarcopenic obesity* and is common in immobilized, sickly patients. This is not your ideal role model.

---

57 The most difficult part of writing this book has been trying to organize, or separate, the knowledge into specific topics as diet, hormones, exercise, sleep, etc. The body doesn't act as individual parts though; it's all interrelated. For example, it is impossible to write about how the proper diet lowers insulin and cortisol, and not mention the important relationships with proper exercise and hormonal balance.

The same argument can be made for fad diets or pills that cause a loss in *water* weight. That's not the root problem, either. Too much fat, especially visceral fat, *is* the problem. Too little muscle is the other concern. Even weight or mere fat loss, as a sole indicator, doesn't tell us the whole story. I'd say a successful program results in you obtaining an optimal weight, improving lean body mass, and boosting your energy level.

> It's not merely losing weight but obtaining an optimal body composition that will prevent you from becoming inflamed, fat, and frail before your time.

First, how would you even know if you are overweight? The simple answer is, "Come on, you know." Historically, you know what your basic body type was when you were younger, say in your twenties. Were you the muscular type? Or were you the skinny guy or somewhere in-between? How was your stomach size in proportion? If you forgot, take a look at some old pictures and compare them to the man in the mirror. No, I don't mean Michael Jackson—that's not exactly the visual I meant. What has changed though? Then, contemplate some about what your overall life style consisted of then, including diet and activity. Compare this list to what you do, and don't do, nowadays.[58] Are you still on the right track? Where would you like to be in five to ten years?

I present this here because we are dealing with the *total* you. In the normally intelligent individual, improper weight may be a symptom of some deeper physiological or emotional concern or both including addictions, abuse history, rivalry, guilt, control or self-esteem issues, and so forth. Therefore, in order to obtain effective long-term weight control, you must learn how to deal with these potential barriers, with some degree of success. The mind and body has to be in sync, as we are ultimately attempting to optimize *total* health, right? A healthy mind is a healthy body and vice versa. Both the brain and body fat are interactive organs in our body. Proper weight is only one means, albeit an important one, to achieve proper health. The mind and spirit has to go along for the ride too.

---

58 Contemplate about the time and effort you spend doing various things each day. Are they in line with your earlier priorities and goals? How are your relationships at home and elsewhere? What effect may they be having? Being overweight is often a symptom of a life out of balance.

Conversely, being overweight may be the consequence of other conditions that should be identified and treated. I find that in most *mild to moderate cases of being overweight*, it's usually due to the following:

- Lacking willpower or commitment, for many reasons.
- Not knowing enough about the right diet and exercise regimen.
- Being out of balance with life's more profound priorities.

In more *severe cases of obesity*, these self-defeating cycles have just been going on for a longer time, unchecked, and usually since early childhood. You've only been chugging along the wrong road for a longer time. Getting overweight begets getting more overweight—the body just gets spins more out of control. This makes it more difficult to effectively change direction to a healthier path, *but it can be done.* Are there any other better options? As Carlos Santana sang, "You've got to change your (not so) evil ways!"

To effectively change the outer self, you must first start with what's going on with your inner self.

Basically, you're overweight if you can no longer button that top button on the pants you bought five years ago. Or, if you're a normally built man and your waist size has become over 35 inches. Looking in the mirror at your basic shape also helps. If you're *apple shaped* like most middle-aged men, you have that increased unhealthy visceral fat we've often mentioned. You may not be able to pinch much of this peripheral fat because it's actually *inside* the muscular wall. If you bang on your stomach in a King Kong manner, you'll believe it's hard as a rock. Well, you may have had a six-pack underneath there at one time. Now, the only problem is that a *keg* is hiding it. You may be pumping lots of iron at the gym, yet still sporting this big *beer gut*, or *breadbasket*.[59] If we attempted to use fat calipers that pinch only peripheral fat to estimate this inner fat, it would be grossly underestimated. Those handheld gizmos or weight scales that supposedly measure fat aren't that reliable either. I usually recommend you get a percent fat composition at the same time as a dual energy x-ray absorptiometry (DEXA) bone density scan. You'll quickly get

---

59 It seems our ancestors inherently knew that both bread and alcohol causes a big gut. We now know it's due to the high glycemic index of these foods and the resulting higher glucose, insulin, and inflammation factor.

an accurate picture of your lean body mass as well as risks for osteoporosis, both important biomarkers of physiological aging. With minimal radiation, we'll be able to monitor your disease risk reduction as you improve on these parameters.

HEIGHT (In shoes)	WOMEN FRAME Small	Moderate	Large	HEIGHT (In shoes)	MEN FRAME Small	Moderate	Large
4'10"	92-98	96-101	104-119	5'2"	112-120	118-129	126-141
4'11"	94-101	98-110	106-122	5'3"	115-123	121-133	129-144
5'	96-104	101-113	109-125	5'4"	118-126	124-136	132-148
5'1"	99-107	104-116	112-128	5'5"	121-129	127-139	135-152
5'2"	102-110	107-119	115-131	5'6"	124-133	130-143	138-156
5'3"	105-113	110-122	118-134	5'7"	128-137	134-147	142-161
5'4"	108-116	113-126	121-138	5'8"	132-141	138-152	147-166
5'5"	111-119	116-130	125-142	5'9"	136-145	142-156	151-170
5'6"	114-123	120-135	129-146	5'10"	140-150	146-160	155-174
5'7"	118-127	124-139	133-150	5'11"	144-154	150-165	159-179
5'8"	122-131	128-143	137-154	6'	148-158	154-170	164-184
5'9"	126-135	132-147	141-158	6'1"	152-162	158-175	168-189
5'10"	130-140	136-151	145-163	6'2"	156-167	162-180	173-194
5'11"	134-144	140-155	149-168	6'3"	160-171	167-185	178-199
6'	138-148	144-159	153-173	6'4"	164-175	172-190	182-204

One reference for weight in men and women. Note, no one graph tells the whole story.

Figure 4.1. Height-Weight Chart. One chart doesn't give all the answers we need. (Adapted USDA, FDA)

Also, to see if you're pulling extra poundage, you can measure your *body mass index* (BMI) and get a numerical estimate by using the equation below. It's much easier to use the chart in the appendix though:

$$BMI = weight\ in\ kg/height\ in\ m^2$$

- If the result is 25 to 30, you're in the yellow zone and mildly overweight. It's time to get happening on diet and exercise.

- If over 30, you're in the red zone and obese now. Losing weight should be job 1. You're now pathologically overweight to the point of adversely affecting your health, resulting in glucose intolerance, back pain, shortness of breath, etc. Drugs may be warranted, but I prefer hormonal balance first. (This will be covered.)

- If close to 40, it's time to think more seriously about weight-loss drugs or even surgery. You're on track for a forced early retirement from life.

Note that BMI doesn't differentiate between excess muscle or fat weight, so lean bodybuilders may get an incorrect result of being unhealthily overweight. A frail, older woman with low muscle and bone mass, yet a high fat percentage may wind up with a good value. Again, measuring only one feature while blindfolded, you can't adequately describe the whole animal.

Likewise, the rule of thumb we were taught in medical school—adding 6 to 106 pounds for every inch over 5 feet—may also be off. As you can see, it can be quite challenging and even frustrating to know what you should weigh. All the above measurements have their use and their limitations. For the doctor and the patient, this only adds to confusion and can undermine early efforts. Concerning your optimal weight, it seems like a plot from the start to even determine where you are now and what your proper destination should be—two essential yet complex points to plot on the treasure map to a healthier weight.

Add to that the age-related hormonal and metabolic changes introduced earlier, and it's no wonder this has truly become a lifelong *Battle of the Bulge*. Sad but true, the natural progression of things as we age is to *lose* one percent of muscle and bone mass and to *gain* one percent of fat mass per year—unless we fire back. By learning Mother Nature's war strategies, we can launch a successful, preemptive strike on her many metabolic missiles. We'll be in far better mental and physical shape to deal with her accomplices—Father Time and ultimately, the Grim Reaper. Remember our defense plan, comrade—health span? It's all about that *morbidity compression* introduced earlier. Live life to it's fullest, or at least die trying.

In getting to the proper body composition, there's unfortunately no shortcut around exercise and diet. Both are needed. Concerning exercise, no matter what shape you're in, there are many exercises you can do to improve your physique. A safe yet effective exercise program mostly helps those in the worst physical shape. Sorry, no excuses here. Get a prescription from your doctor, as insurance usually pays for physical therapy if you have orthopedic or other limitations, and mutually decide on a safe routine. I see people with no legs or a bad back in the gym doing exercise with just their arms! Remember, a personal trainer can help you a lot. As far as diet is concerned, do what is going to work for you long-term, no fads; but try to approximate what we recommend.

If you don't seem to be losing weight, the following four things are usually going on:

1. You're not really trying. There's still too much junk food, alcohol or soda, and late-night binging. The more you eat out, the more you lose control over exactly what's in your diet. A daily soda can pile on fifteen extra pounds in a single year. No breakfast still? How's your daily one-hour exercise routine going? Are you stretching the truth a bit?

2. Hormonal testing and replacement probably needs to be done. If not, you're fighting even more of an uphill battle. You're at risk for losing motivation and giving up. Mother Nature is winning the battle. Don't let her win the war.

3. There may be underlying food allergies that should be tested and treated appropriately. Clues include associated bowel disorder, allergy, rashes, or unexplained fatigue and aches. One man's meat is another man's poison! I will expound on this throughout the book.

4. There may be underlying emotional concerns. Depressed? Stressed? Addicted? There are effective treatments out there; not all are drug-based. Don't be ashamed; get help. More on this follows in the men's special topics chapter.

B. Why Lose Weight? According to the 2001 Canadian Community Health Survey, boys are three times more likely to be grossly overweight if at least one of their parents is obese. For girls, it's even worse—about six times. Like their southern neighbors, Canadian adults are generally more sedentary and eating poorly compared to their earlier generations. It's only natural that our *children imitate more what we do, not what we say.* As midlifers with kids, it's important to set an example for future generations. It seems as though with industrialized nations worldwide, kids are being raised in an *obesogenic* society. According to research by the University of Minnesota published in the December 2003 *JAMA*, it's healthier for our young to be more physically active, or *fit,* than *thin.* This makes some sense; a *skinnier* person can have less muscle mass yet have relatively higher fat. More active muscle burns more stored fat, thereby lowering insulin levels and the subsequent risk for diabetes. Despite the current paradoxical energy crisis, the World Health Organization estimates that by 2025, the number of diabetics worldwide will double to three hundred million. Not very sweet news, is it? As incredulous as this seems, walking only thirty minutes a few times per week and losing 10 percent of your weight can cut your risk by about 60 percent! Your whole family can sing that song, "I like to move it, move it!" as they jog along.

There's no denying that weight loss by proper dieting beats any magic pill and costs much less. The *Diabetes Prevention Program* revealed that by three years the incidence of type 2 diabetes was reduced by *60 percent* using intensive lifestyle interventions compared to drug therapy (metformin) at *30 percent*.[60] The lifestyle interventions cost half the amount of drugs at $15,000 versus $31,000 per case of diabetes delayed or prevented. It was further estimated that the lifestyle intervention used would decrease direct costs by over 70 percent. In the real world, insurances don't believe in reimbursing physicians for such intense counseling. (Most do it anyway, gratis.) At the risk of sounding cynical, I find most of the time my advice falls on the insured's deaf ears because they're seeking today's magic pill. They are also unaware or may be denying that a more expensive and sicker life is just around the corner. There it is, right by the doughnut shop. Because of the nearsightedness on all these levels, society will eventually get stuck with the higher price tag. Ultimately though, the only one that has a vested interest in keeping your mind and body healthy will be you.

Another interesting study along these lines was published in *JAMA*, which concluded that a low-fat vegetarian diet including soy, eggplant, and almonds can reduce cholesterol levels about as much as the widely used statin drugs. Involving men and women with high cholesterol, the one month study showed the *vegetarian* group's LDL dropped by 29 percent, which was equal to the reduction seen in ones on a low-fat diet plus 20 mg daily of Mevacor.[61] Just as important, CRP-hs, the inflammation marker, decreased the same 10 percent in both groups. Another study found using margarine that-contained plant stanols along with a lipid-

---

60 The lifestyle intervention achieved and maintained a reasonable 7 percent reduction in initial body weight through behavioral counseling, diet, and moderate physical activity. Additionally, the lifestyle intervention costs about $31,000 versus about $100,000 for medical intervention per Quality Adjusted Life Year (QALY) gained. The Diabetes Prevention Program Group, "Within-trial cost effectiveness of lifestyle intervention or meformin for the primary prevention of type 2 diabetes," *Diabetes Care* 26 (2003): 2518–23; J. A. David," *JAMA* 290, no. 4 (2003): 502–10.

61 J.A. David, "Effects of dietary portfolio of cholesterol-lowering foods vs. lovastatin on serum lipids and c-reactive protein," *JAMA* 290, no. 4 (2003): 502–10.

lowering diet further lowered LDL in patients already receiving optimal doses of statin drugs.[62] So there's no denying the cholesterol-lowering benefits of a healthy diet. Just say no to drugs.

As preached earlier, diabetes is about the worst disease that you can get. To put it succinctly, it's premature aging of the body. Basically, all age-related diseases you wouldn't get until sixty-five or older occur decades earlier. This covers the gambit of medical problems such as heart attack, stroke, cancers, kidney failure with resulting anemia, and related complications such as neuropathy, blindness, loss of limb, etc. As if not enough, there is also increased risk of depression and dementia such as *Alzheimer's*.[63] As alluded before, glucose intolerance and insulin resistance are not black-and-white conditions like pregnancy or HIV. It's more of a reversible, subclinical progression of multiple abnormalities. The appreciation of this latter point has prompted the modern diagnosis of *prediabetes*, which is much like you receiving a D grade at midterm in school. Likewise, in middle age, there's still time to improve things and wind up getting an A in life!

Insulin resistance and the metabolic syndrome increase risks of both depression and Alzheimer's disease (AD). Persistent glucose intolerance among patients with depression leads to the typical nerve degeneration, beta-amyloid plaques, and neurofibrillary tangles seen in AD. In fact, brain scans show deranged glucose metabolism in specific areas in patients at risk even years before symptoms start. This is especially prominent in patients with a single copy of the apolipoprotein E-4 gene, an inherited AD risk. The link between insulin resistance and depression goes back to 1985 when it was discovered that successful treatment of depressed patients improved insulin resistance. These findings should encourage aggressive lifestyle changes and interventions to help prevent dementia in these depressed patients with various degrees of glucose intolerance.

---

62 M. C. Cabezas, "Effects of a stanol-enriched diet on plasma cholesterol and triglycerides in patients treated with statins," *J Am Diet Assoc.* 106, no. 10 (2006):1564–69. Subjects on the standard low-fat diet saw only an 8 percent drop.

63 N. L. Rasgon, "Insulin resistance in depressive disorders and Alzheimer's disease: revisiting the missing link hypothesis," *Neurobiogy of Aging* (26 Suppl) (2005): 103–7. Dr. Rasgon presented similar conclusions at a meeting of the International Psychogeriatric Association in 2003.

Completing the enigma of living past your time, it's been shown that having the metabolic syndrome also makes you twice as likely to become *frail*.[64] This association is quite profound because of its subsequent compounding conditions. Complications such as hip fracture, dehydration, malnutrition, or immune system compromise can buy you a one-way ticket to the nursing home. Don't worry; as these gradually worsen you may get a discount at the local funeral home because of pulmonary embolism, pneumonia, serious urinary infections, and much more. As you can see, diabetes puts the early nail in the coffin by advancing all age-related conditions. But which occurs first: the inactivity, then diabetes, and then frailty or the inactivity, frailty, and then diabetes? At any rate, despite modern medical advances, proper lifestyle intervention is still the most economical preventative measure.

> Let's teach future generations how to be responsible for their health. This will help keep health-care costs low for all of us. The proper lifestyle can help reduce cholesterol and sugar as effectively as most drugs. This, in turn, lowers risks for the most debilitating diseases that send us to nursing homes.

C. Weight-Loss Diets. Preliminary results from one of the largest, most current studies on overweight diabetics found subjects are less likely to lose weight if they believe this inability is due to an endocrine disorder or their own eating and exercise behavior.[65] Although these conclusions were quite unexpected by researchers and nutritionists alike, I' m not so shocked, frankly. Health professionals must understand the real facts and learn ways to deal with them in order to find out why weight-loss diets often fail. Why *do* diabetics have these inexplicable attitudes?

---

64 *A* study presented at the Third World Congress on Insulin Resistance Syndrome by Dr. Barzilay followed about twenty-four hundred nonfrail sixty-nine- to seventy-four-year-olds for about nine years. The roughly twelve hundred that developed frailty or prefrailty had significantly higher fasting insulin levels, higher white blood cell counts, higher CRP levels and higher factor 8 levels. They were also more likely to have metabolic syndrome at baseline.

65 Preliminary report from the SHIELD Study, a five-year observational-type study. This disheartening news was presented by Dr. A. Green at the Thirty-third Annual Meeting and Exhibition of the American Association of Diabetic Educators held in August 2006.

I'll try to explain my rationale. First of all, for someone to become a type 2 diabetic would mean he has been practicing a self-defeating lifestyle for decades. This would include a lack of self-control and acting irresponsibly for his health by putting proper dieting and exercising last. To his defense, there are many genetic predispositions and hormonal imbalances compounding his likelihood of becoming so obese and diabetic. With his increasing age, these only worsened and made his losing weight more of an uphill battle. Earlier on though, by practicing the proper lifestyle, he could have helped suppress these factors. Being more proactive on his part would have prevented this. The conclusions above make perfect sense to me, for if it truly weren't for his hormonal imbalances and improper lifestyle, he probably wouldn't have diabetes.

It all boils down to this: Diet alone isn't going to *make* you lose weight. Rather, it's what I've said all along. You have to take a commitment to change your behavior—the way you think and then act toward all food and exercise. These are bidirectional and quite individualized. There is no one diet that works for everyone out there. Everyone out there isn't looking for the same diet either. This is infinitely more variable than the car we choose to drive or the clothes we wear. After this bittersweet dose of reality, here's my take on the most popular diets out there. Pick and choose as you see fit. Then, try one on *for size*!

There is a lot of good data on the benefits of the **CRAN** (calorie restriction with adequate nutrition) diet. Proportion-wise, this is the same diet that we recommend; however, it probably has about 35 percent less calories than the normal healthy person consumes. The CRAN Diet has been shown to cause a healthy rise in human growth hormone (HGH) and to lower many of the body's inflammatory mediators such as insulin and cortisol—the so-called *aging hormones*. An interesting article I found in a recent *Science* magazine suggests that it's never *too* late to benefit.[66] Here, a British team analyzed life and death patterns among seventy-five hundred fruit flies. They found the ones that started dieting in middle age had a reduction in death comparable to those that had been dieting their *entire adult* lives. Conversely, flies that switched from the restricted diet to a full diet experienced the same corresponding death rate. Bottom line: It's probably never too late to eat right and reap some benefits, even for us midlifers just buzzing around.

There has been much animal- and human-based research on this diet's effect, starting back in the 1930s. There is strong evidence the CRAN diet can add

---

66 *Science* 301 (5640): 1731–33.

healthy decades to one's life.[67] As mentioned above, the *calorie-restricted* intake has shown to help subjects obtain healthier levels of HGH, DHEA, insulin, and cortisol. These levels reflect a healthier body composition, lower risk for metabolic diseases, and possibly improved DNA repair. Less food intake means less free radical production. The *adequate nutrition* component lowers inflammation, increases fiber and antioxidants, and further boosts the immune system. Decreased insulin resistance means less deleterious AGEs and glycosylation. More information on the CRAN diet, including recipes, can be found in the nonprofit Calorie Restriction Society's Web site, http://www.crsociety.org.

You could just follow the dietary advice of the Okinawans by eating until you're *80 percent* full. They enjoy having one of the highest life expectancies in the world with many healthy centenarians—about thirty-five per one hundred thousand compared to about ten in industrialized nations like the United States. Or you could listen to your parents' advice, "Eat to live; don't live to eat!" Notwithstanding that general advice, there are probably just a small minority of people who are able to follow the rigors of the CRAN throughout life. Usually this diet consists of 250 to 350 calories *less* than the current recommendations of 1600 calories daily for a small, inactive woman and up to 2800 for a large, active man.

Caution! Your spouse and entire household must be willing to tolerate your extremism, as well. You may want to review the pros and cons with them before you get any more bright ideas. It's remarkable to note that the CRAN diet *is* one of the longest-studied, proven-safe, and beneficial regimen. Good luck. You're a better man than I am if you can do this long term. As I said before, though, there isn't *one* diet that works for *all* people out there.

Some people *can* be completely complacent consuming the CRAN diet. However, this gets back to the importance of finding the individual's balance to the *quality* versus *quantity* of life. Why not have some of both? This involves achieving a personal compromise between realistic goals and what you're willing to routinely give up. By just cutting calories 10 only percent, you'll still enjoy significant health benefits, though maybe not as dramatic as mentioned with the CRAN diet. Eat less; live more.

---

67 L. Heilbronn, The Journal of the American Medical Association, vol. 295 (April 5, 2006): 1539–48. Eric Ravussin, PhD, professor, Pennington Biomedical Research Center, Louisiana State University, Baton Rouge, La. Fontana, L. The Journal of the American Medical Association, vol 295 (April 5, 2006): 1577–78. WebMD Medical News, "Low-Cal Diet May Slow Heart's Aging," news release, *JAMA/Archives*.

In most cases, the CRAN diet may be useful during the *induction* phase of dieting, when substantial *weight loss* is desired. Behavioral modification and willpower, nutritional education, and the so-called shrinking of the stomach may be other needed benefits. Once proper weight has been accomplished, then *weight control* may be all that's needed. During such *remission*, a more practical yet less restrictive diet may be more realistic in the long term. Occasionally, when falling off the proverbial wagon—say, during holidays or vacation—and gaining some unwanted poundage, you may have to go back to a CRAN-like diet a little while. Alternately, you could trim off calories *before* an event. For example, lose a few pounds before going aboard a cruise ship. I'm not recommending a yo-yo approach though. This would be quite counterproductive in the long term, of course. Though, you could finally inform your cabinmate, "Honey, I shrunk the beer gut. Now, shiver me timber!"

How about the **DASH diet**? There's good news for those desiring a more natural approach to controlling hypertension. According to a study done by Kaiser Permanente, lifestyle changes for those overweight with *pre*hypertension normalizes blood pressure as effectively as common drug therapies.[68]The *control* group received behavioral intervention including exercise and dieting advice and follow-up. The *interventional* group received the same support but followed by the DASH diet. Accordingly, these participants significantly increased their intake of complex carbohydrates, fiber, dairy products, folate, and other minerals. (These have many other health benefits.)

In the end, rates of those obtaining normal blood pressure were 18–24 percent in all three groups—comparable to the blood-pressure-lowering effects of drugs. As expected, overall physical fitness improved in all groups. However, there was the usual trend toward a partial regaining of the initial weight loss between six to eighteen months. Again, this emphasizes the importance of committing to *long-term weight control* as opposed to *short-term weight loss*. This is a common dilemma with any dieting program. As I say, any diet to be successful long term

---

68 Even the obese and those with only what's considered pre-high blood pressure (early or mild hypertension) benefited. The study was funded by the National Heart, Lung, and Blood Institute and followed 810 subjects for eighteen months with systolic blood pressures of 120 to 159 mmHg. Published in the *Annals of Internal Medicine*, 2006: 144. Also, information is from the Dietary Approaches to Stop Hypertension study. For a review, you can go to the "Sixth report of the Joint National Committee on Detection, Evaluation, and Treatment of High Blood Pressure," *Archives of Internal Medicine*, 157 (1997): 2413–46.

has to be one you're willing and able to stay on throughout life. More information on the DASH diet can be found at the Web site, http://www.nhlbi.nih.gov/health/public/heart/hbp/dash.

An interesting article entitled "Lifestyle Changes May Prevent or Reverse Prostate Cancer" relates to the DASH diet. A research by the well-known Dr. Dean Ornish suggested the diet's beneficial effects on men with biopsy-proven prostate cancer. PSA levels ranged from 4–10 ng/dl.[69] The interventional group ate an entirely plant-based, low-fat diet that emphasized unprocessed whole foods. Virtually identical to the anti-inflammatory diet I recommend, this consists of 70 percent complex carbohydrates and 20 percent protein—mostly soy based. All the subjects had declined medical treatment methods yet engaged in moderate aerobic exercise, stress management, and psychosocial group support. They also took fish oil and vitamins. This mirrors my integrative, mind-body-based approach to staying well. The PSA levels *decreased* 5 percent after just three months. It *increased* 1 percent in the control group. After one year, PSA levels decreased by 3 percent, but increased 17 percent in the control group. Although challenged that lifestyle changes may have affected PSA levels without truly affecting the underlying prostate cancer, a more specific prostate tumor marker LNCaP argued against that.

I find the above research important on many levels. First, prostate cancer is worsened by the extent of inflammation in the body. This is based on the fact that many prostate cancers become antihormonal *nonresponders* after a year into treatment. This means the standard therapies used, such as Lupron and Casodex, may become ineffective.[70] No one is exactly sure why this occurs, but it's theorized the tumor has now mutated and is more stimulated by inflammatory mediators. Second, this same diet recommended decades ago by Dean Ornish had helped lower inflammation and the resulting cardiovascular disease. In the earlier section on fats, it was mentioned some trans fats are associated with increased prostate cancer risk. All these benefits are achieved only with a healthy lifestyle. That shouldn't surprise you.

---

69   PSA stands for prostate specific antigen. It is a blood test that helps in screening and monitoring prostate cancer. PSA can also be elevated in benign prostate conditions (see the men's special topics chapter). D. Ornish, 2003. AUA 98th Annual Meeting: Abstract 105681. *Journal of Urology*, news release, September 2005, University of California, San Francisco.

70   Antihormonal treatments block the production of testosterone thereby slowing the growth of the prostate cancer. More on this in the Special Topics chapter.

Lastly, *microscopic* prostate cancer is hard to detect early and has about the same incidence worldwide. However, in societies with the predominately SAD diet, like those with a high intake of pro-inflammatory animal fat and protein, there are more clinically apparent, aggressive prostate cancers. Another sad fact to consider is that immigrants originating from countries with lower rates of breast and prostate cancers gradually reach our rates. For example, the native Japanese women have about ten to twenty times *less* breast cancer than Americans. Once they've lived here awhile, their rates increase to approximate those of the general American population.

How about Hollywood's **Macrobiotic diet?** If you glossed through your significant other's glamour, trash magazines, you've probably come across some celebrities boasting about this diet. *Macrobiotic* in Greek means "long life." Having a catchy name, it boils down to about the same as the Paleolithic Diet, Mediterranean Diet, and the diet I recommend too. Again, it focuses on complex carbohydrates, i.e., vegetables and fruits being about two-thirds of the diet and lean protein sources mostly from fish and seafood. There's also the push for healthy fats and the avoidance of refined or processed foods. These suggestions are really nothing new, right?

According to Columbia University research, people that enjoy a **Mediterranean-like diet** can significantly reduce their Alzheimer's disease risk by up to 68 percent.[71] A previous study in June 2006 noted a decreased risk for other degenerative neurological diseases. This diet has been earlier associated with lower risks for several forms of cancer, obesity, dyslipidemia, hypertension, abnormal glucose metabolism, and coronary disease. In studies that followed those aged seventy to ninety for ten years, the Mediterranean diet and lifestyle resulted in a *50 percent lower death rate* from these causes.[72] This diet reflects the typical southern Italian diet, rich and fruits, vegetables, beans, cereals, and fish. It's low in saturated fats from meat and dairy products. It makes you wonder why we're spending so much research money on drugs that will never reach that effectiveness. A healthy lifestyle, as described above, doesn't need extreme sacrifices, nor does it cost any more. Certainly, it's not one to die for!

---

71 Columbia University research published in the October 9, 2006, *Archives of Neurology* by Dr. N. Scarmeas. A previous study in the June 2006 *Annals of Neurology* also reflected these findings.

72 Taken from the HALE, SENECA and FINE studies, as reviewed, 2004. K. Knoops, *JAMA*, 292 (2004):1433–39, 1490–92. Also, A. Trichopoulou and colleagues from the European Prospective Investigation into Cancer and nutrition study (EPIC) studied about seventy five thousand healthy people aged sixty and above, April 8, 2005, online first issue of the *BMJ*.

There may be seasonal variances to the Macrobiotic diet, though nothing I find deviates from most cultural practices. For example, this diet recommends lighter, cooler foods during the summer and somewhat heavier foods, i.e., stews and such, during the winter. The shtick here is the supposed "Eastern influence" and suggestion of balancing the assigned *yin* and *yang* properties of different foods. Well, some may say the Californians, and especially those living in Hollywood, are more eccentric than most and may set the trend as far as fads or extremism is concerned. It has to be packaged differently to sell in Beverly Hills, right? In the end though, I find that this diet amounts to a somewhat different trip that arrives to the same healthy destination—namely a balanced, nonprocessed diet.

> I feel the Mediterranean, Pan-Asian, Biblical, Paleolithic, Zone, Sugar Buster's, and Macrobiotic diets amount basically to the same thing your parents promoted. There is nothing different from the dietary suggestions made throughout this book. However, these may represent a slightly different path to the same goal—a healthier, longer life. Although there may be individual preferences to the specific type of foods and spices, *you* need to adjust to the proper lifestyle, not vice versa.

The **Atkins diet,** in my *opinion,* is half right—which means it's also half wrong. The right parts promote calorie restriction and the avoidance of *simple* carbohydrates—that much we know does wonders. The *wrong* parts push the increased intake of basically any and all fats—including saturated and those horrible trans fats—and limit disease-fighting, complex carbohydrates. These fats would theoretically promote inflammation, something we clearly don't want. There would also be less fiber, vitamins, and antioxidants. Most of the research I've reviewed showed Atkins probably *does* result in loss of visceral fat because of healthier, lower insulin and cortisol levels through the avoidance of *simple* carbohydrates. This in turn would result in the proven benefits we see in people on Atkins—improved weight, blood pressure, glucose and cholesterol levels, and many other benefits. However, because of a theoretical rise in inflammation, I wouldn't be surprised if some long-term clinical effects aren't as good.

The Atkins diet does result in weight loss and improvement in many disease risks or their severity. However, in my opinion, it does this at the expense of an increased intake of pro-inflammatory fats and obviously less nutritious foods. Some people wind up doing what's called a *modified* Atkins, which *may* be better on many levels.. Others are simply trying on a diet and may just accessorize with whatever fits their lifestyle. Instead, it should be the other way around. It should be the *person* that conforms to the change. It's all about behavior modification, remember? Others may find it too hard to stick to Atkins throughout life. Once they modify it to include some healthier veggies and fruits, and cut back the bad fats, it more closely resembles the diet we recommend, after all. Even Atkins gurus agree with this view.[73] Lastly, the Atkins diet may be quite useful for some people during the initial weight loss portion of a new diet regimen. Its results would provide important, needed motivation.

> There are no long-term published, controlled studies to verify any diet's effects, except maybe CRAN. On the other hand, there's no one diet that works for all people out there. There has to be flexibility when it comes to something so personally and socially intertwined. So, if a particular diet works for *you* and is complemented with other lifestyle changes, it's probably okay. It should include nonprocessed protein and fats, more veggies and fruits, and a good daily multivitamin.

The following further explains the rationale of my diet suggestions. Harvard School of Public Health found that low-carb dieters can consume an *extra* 300 calories a day and still lose just as much as those on the standard low-fat American Heart Association Diet.[74] According to contemporary nutritional beliefs, the Atkins dieters should've ended up with an additional seven pounds. Just the opposite of what researchers feared, cholesterol levels didn't go up either. These results baffled most all the professionals and nutritionists at the conference; they found all this, well, quite hard to swallow. Their long-held, revered belief is, "A calorie is a calorie is a calorie, no matter where it comes from … it all goes to the waistline the same way." Many others expressed disbelief, shaking their hands while leaving, stating, "It just doesn't make sense, does it? It must be wrong!" I opine it's actually them who are wrong; the facts are true.

To me, it all makes perfect sense. The professors must have forgotten what they were taught in biochemistry and endocrinology classes. We physicians aren't adequately trained in nutrition, anyway. This fuels our traditional medicinal approach

---

73   In January 2004, the director of research and education for Atkins Nutritionals advised people on the diet should limit the amount of red meat and saturated fat. Atkins officials are now recommending limiting saturated fat intake to 20 percent, mostly from vegetables and fish sources, rather than beef and dairy. They recommend more fish and chicken, and again emphasize eating until you're satisfied, not stuffed.

74   Penelope Greene as presented to the American Association for the Study of Obesity,

when it comes to the prevention and treatment of disease. I don't know what the excuses for the nutritionists are, as they should know better. I will make these results quite clear to you though and hope in the end that *you* can teach *them*. We doctors should remember a vital lesson we're taught in medical school—we learn more from listening to our patients, not from reading textbooks.

Yes, it's true that a calorie is a calorie, but we must look at the true definition of a calorie and how that's determined. It's basically the amount of heat energy expended when a fixed amount of a food is burned in a Petri dish in a controlled laboratory environment. That's not what actually happens in our body now, is it? That's indeed one of the errors made; they ignore the complex machine—us—who are *using* this fuel. How does this interact? We must appreciate a calorie as only *one* quality of many that a particular food possesses. It does help you compare apples to apples, but there's more to it than that. Does a gallon of gas get the same mileage in all cars? Even in the same automobile, the mileage depends on many factors. Are you going uphill or accelerating? Is the car older? Has it been recently tuned up, oil changed, and are the tires properly inflated? You get the picture, guys.

Let's start to put this together by remembering what I said earlier about the glycemic index of foods. This is an indication of how fast they enter the bloodstream as glucose. As a quick review, the more simple the sugar, the faster and higher this sugar spike occurs. The higher the sugar spike, the higher the resulting insulin and cortisol levels. This, in turn, promotes glucose intolerance, diabetes, visceral fat, and the many other metabolic disturbances we older guys can get.[75]

If we replaced the typical high-glycemic carbs in our diets with more slowly absorbed fats and proteins, there would be less sugar spikes. This results in more favorable glucose levels throughout the day. Thus, in lower-carb diets like Atkins, the insulin and cortisol levels are improved. So besides just the inherent calories, or potential energy, the particular food possesses, it's important just how quickly it's *absorbed* into your body.

> The Atkins diet teaches us that there are many other important qualities of food we should consider besides just calories. We need to also factor in the glycemic index—how fast that food is absorbed into the body.

---

75   Review the diet chapter if needed. *Also, there is another quality, the *Glycemic Load*. This is the glycemic index times the amount of food. Suffice to say, eat the right-sized portions.

Next, think about what happens *after* the food is in the bloodstream. In our analogy, we noted all automobiles don't use the same amount of gas per day. Of course, it depends on the fuel used; but it depends on what the car is doing too. Your body burns more calories when running, or going uphill. On the other hand, it conserves fuel when turned off, coasting, or going downhill. Likewise, if you're physically active after a meal, the glucose is used by active muscle cells. However, if you rest after eating, it's stored inside fat cells. As alluded to many times, this breadbasket creates risks for many future metabolic disturbances. Instead of just lying around after eating, go for a walk.

It's also important to learn the body can be fooled into believing it's going downhill. This is basically what happens when this increase visceral fat tricks the liver into believing the body is in a starvation state. Much like a fattened bear during hibernation, the couch potato watches TV for nights on end, but does this throughout the year. This stored fat releases many substances that cause the liver to release glucose. This starts the ball rolling for many age-related metabolic disturbances and rise in inflammation—all undesired effects.

This also occurs when you skip a meal, though to a smaller degree. Your metabolism drops and you then feel more lethargic, or sluggish. These result in *less* energy consumption and less calories burned. Subsequently, your body will want to *store* more fuel when the next meal comes. You're eating less and gaining more weight, quite a paradox. At any rate, it's always good news to those overweight to hear it's bad to skip meals. Wasn't it your parents that said not to skip your breakfast; it's your most important meal. It literally means to *break* your *fast* from the prior night.

Also remember, past generations didn't have all the abundant foods we now enjoy. There were no twenty-four-hour supermarkets, fast food joints everywhere, instant junky snacks, and so on. Instead, there were droughts and famines, many epidemics, and parasites—many environmental pressures we never even heard of. These naturally selected for us to possess the genes that most effectively metabolized and stored food. It's simply a matter of *survival of the fittest.* They survived, and their offspring—again us—inherited these traits. These predispositions are great, but only for those bygone, very different times. What happened …? Somebody switched the whole game board of life while no one was really watching. The rules have changed much too quickly. We humans haven't had enough time to adapt to this new plentiful, less manually laborious lifestyle. Given our long life span, evolution takes time for us humans. Maybe, nature is now trying to correct this improper lifestyle and metabolism machinery gone awry. At any rate, don't blame your parents; they mostly preached and led a good example.

Next, it matters what *you* do after the food is ingested. If you're active, the food is taken up by muscle. If not, it's stored by a fat cell. This soon adds up to more severe, age-related diseases.

Last but not least, it also depends on *when* the food is absorbed. Let's learn how this ties in with some of the other hormones affecting weight and metabolism, not just insulin and cortisol. Remember what was mentioned earlier about the few but important HGH spikes? These occur during the deep stages of sleep in the early morning. HGH, among its many other effects you'll read in later chapters, helps keep you lean. It just so happens that the higher insulin and cortisol get, the less frequent and intense these HGH spikes become. This relationship again reinforces the important, delicate, and natural, optimal balancing of all the hormones—the *yin* and *yang* of them.

Let's see what happens if you eat a late dinner, just before going to bed. (This also occurs in those who may stick on a feed bag or graze all night while watching TV.) This causes blood sugar levels to rise. As usual, insulin and cortisol are then secreted to stabilize such levels. Unfortunately, this all occurs while you're fast asleep. This, in turn, decreases the number and quality of HGH spikes.[76] Less HGH can lead to increased visceral fat, decreased muscle mass, lowered energy, and many other symptoms listed in the appendix. It's almost like you're sleeping with the enemy! Some with deaf ears may have been told it's not good to eat before going to bed; they'll get fat.

To simply look at foods from merely caloric perspective is like you being blindfolded, feeling one part of an elephant, and then trying to describe the whole beast. Calories are only one angle to a multifaceted statue. It's not just about the single *type* of food; it's about the *combination* of foods. It's *when* it's absorbed into the body and *where* it goes. It's also *how* the body then interacts with it. We do become *what* and *how much* we eat. (I should accordingly add, *when we eat* too. It just was too much for a chapter title.)

---

76   HGH (human growth hormone). Its importance was introduced earlier and will be covered later in the human growth hormone chapter. Suffice to say, HGH spikes are integral to one's physical and emotional and mental balance.

Getting back to the researchers' confusion on the Atkins diet, I'm not at all surprised when less simple carb intake resulted in weight loss and improved many metabolic parameters in those studied. Given what you've now read—you should expect this outcome too. I'm still concerned about the lack of complex carbs and increase in fats and protein. I hope your level of understanding get to this next level—one that most doctors and learned nutritionists don't grasp yet. Indeed, the facts presented bring things full circle. These connect common sense and many generations of observational studies with cutting-edge nutritional, biochemical, and endocrinological science. As promised, I presented both the convergence of evidence and what your parents already knew. What more could you Atkins groupies want, perhaps some ice cream and whipped topping?

> *When you eat* is also important. Skipping meals just makes you feel tired and doesn't result in weight loss. Eating too late will raise your insulin levels, which then lower HGH production. Unknowingly, these hormonal imbalances can undermine your otherwise healthy lifestyle and can lead to difficulties.

Along those lines then comes the obvious reality. Basically, there is no *one* diet that works for *all* people out there. It has to be individualized. To be successful, it must incorporate lifelong lifestyle changes the person is willing to maintain— mainly eating less. Quick gimmicks or fads don't work long term. In 2001, the USDA invited the late Dr. Robert Atkins and Dr. Dean Ornish, as well as other diet gurus, to battle it out in what was termed "The Great Nutrition Debate."[77] Various studies were compared and evaluated, as well as an entertaining live shoot-out—I mean, debate and discussion. I wouldn't be surprised if this took place at high noon. That *would* be lunchtime. The bottom line is that all the diets studied—Atkins, Weight Watchers, The Zone, and Ornish—produced about the same amount of weight loss *but* with some minimal, variable health benefits.

There were higher dropout rates in the most extreme diets, those two being Ornish and Atkins. Some in the Ornish group complained they ate so many vegetables and such little fat, they felt like a rabbit or a cow. Some in the Atkins group, eating mostly meat and dairy, got tired of the lack of variety. It's important to mention though, the Ornish group did not do the full recommended program, which emphasizes stress management. The Weight Watchers group didn't go to any of the usual support

---

77 M. Dansinger, AHA 2003 Scientific Sessions: Abstract 3535. Presented Nov 12, 2003. Since then, the National Institutes of Health has funded further studies comparing popular diets.

group meetings. This was done in order to keep all four diets on the same level of intervention, but leaves out unique important aspects of their therapies.

The results weren't that predictable. Subjects on the Ornish diet initially experienced a small rise in insulin levels. In the end, they actually wound up with lower levels than those on Atkins. (The carbs are more complex carbs.) Their LDL was lowered the most at about 17 percent. Despite eating a higher fat content, the Atkins' group had lowered their LDL by 8 percent and raised HDL by 15 percent. Rounding out things, Weight Watchers' followers won when it came to raising their HDL by almost 19 percent. That rivals most drugs! As you can see, all these diets have their good points and unique challenges. Ultimately, when all the dust at the diet showdown was settled, less total caloric intake mostly determined the amount of weight loss. Losing twenty pounds resulted in a 30 percent reduction in heart risk score.

Additional research in 2006 compared variations of the DASH diet.[78] Patients were randomized into four groups, but given the same amount of calories. One was on a strict DASH diet, which is mostly fiber and complex carbs as described above. The second substituted 10 percent of carbs with nonmeat-based protein. The third substituted 10 percent with monounsaturated plant-based fat. The fourth ate the standard American diet. As expected, all three specialty diets significantly improved blood pressure and LDL cholesterol. The higher soy protein diet was the best overall. Triglycerides *improved* in both the higher unsaturated fat and protein versions. HDL *decreased* in those with less saturated fat and cholesterol intake; the high-protein diet lowered it the most. This reinforces the points made earlier. Depending on personal preference and goals, the DASH diet can be realistically modified without sacrificing its benefits to LDL and blood pressure.

A *balanced*, natural diet consisting of complex carbohydrates, plant-based fats, and nonmeaty protein is probably the best, over all.[79] There's no one specific diet that appeals to everyone, but it has to be nutritionally sound and simple to maintain in order to work.

78 W. Karmally, "Can altering carbohydrate, protein and unsaturated fat intake improve patients' blood pressure and lipid profile?" *Nat Clin Pract Cardiovasc Med* 3, no. 5 (2006): 254–55.

79 M. Schabath, *The Journal of the American Medical Association*, vol 294 (Sept. 28, 2005): 1493–1504; L. Dacey, *The Journal of the American Medical Association*, vol 294 (Sept. 28, 2005): 1550–51; *Arch Intern Med.* 166 (2006):79–87; Paul Elliott,

D. Weight-Loss Supplements and Drugs.

It seems we're bombarded daily by tons of cheesy TV and radio ads touting the latest magic cure for fat. Annually, we dump enormous amounts of money on pills that supposedly help us lose weight, block fat or sugar absorption, or simply melt the fat away. Some sprays may falsely claim to help boost HGH levels. Remember, since all supplements aren't FDA regulated, it's like Forrest Gump's mom would advise, "They're like a box of chocolates … you never know what cha gonna get." As presented earlier, dietary supplements may contain toxins, dangerous prescription drugs, caffeine, ephedra, diuretics, animal hormones, heavy metals, or other hidden compounds.[80] Don't risk it. There's really no secret pill that's going to do the work for you. Your behavior must change. At most, taking these may complement all the needed modalities presented in this book by about 5 percent. Of course, any help is welcomed as obesity is the number two killer *with a bullet*. Here's my take on a few worthy ones:

- **Chromium.** Diabetics have been shown to be low in chromium, but there is minimal if any valid research showing that supplementing with such appreciably improves glucose metabolism.[81] Clinically, I've not found it to be much effective by itself. However, many good supplements include a little chromium, so what the heck. It's usually quite safe. I would avoid any megadosing, of course. It may work synergistically with other options as L-carnitine.

- **L-carnitine.** I find this more effective in helping some people gain muscle mass and lose fat mass. As presented in the supplement chapter, some research shows it to be as effective as testosterone replacement but without any appreciable side effects or risks.[82] Most supplements containing L-carnitine have way too little to have any real effect though. I would recommend 750 to 1000 mg per day. L-carnitine helps with fat metabolism inside the mitochondria within the cell.

MB, PhD, from Imperial College London in England, and colleagues from the INTERMAP Cooperative Research Group; *Arch Intern Med.* 166 (2006):79–87; D. Jenkens, *JAMA* 290 (2003):502–510, 531–33.

80 R. Saper "Heavy metal content of Ayurvedic herbal medicine products," *JAMA* 292 (2004): 2868–73; *MMWR* 53 (2004): 582–84; Y. Waknine, "Brazilian dietary supplements contain prescription drugs, FDA warns," *Medscape/WebMD* Jan. 13, 2006, article 521545. You can find or report such instances by calling 1-800-FDA-1088 or visit online at http://www.FDA.gov/medwatch.

81 *Diabetes* 46 (1997):1786–91.

82 According to Italian reproductive researchers who studied 120 symptomatic healthy men with a mean at age of sixty-six for six months. *Urology,* April 2005.

- **Various OTC Carbohydrate or Fat Blockers.** Again, you never know what you're really getting inside the bottle, so why not just eat a little less fat or carbohydrate in the first place? Do you really plan to take these the rest of your life? If not, once you stop, you'll simply regain the fat and ratchet up even more fat cells. What's the use in the long run? If you aren't committed to substantially changing your lifestyle, things won't work. Besides, the OTC so-called *blockers* lack any scientific proof. Recently, the FTC fined the marketers of OTC weight-loss pills $25 million because of false claims they cause weight loss. These included Xenadrine EFX, CortiSlim, One-A-Day WeightSmart (Bayer), and TrimSpa. Amazingly enough, the FTC and FDA will still allow these potentially dangerous, fraudulent pills to stay on the shelves and make their $2 billion annually. Even the prescription fat blocker Orlistat© has minimal long-term effects compared to diet and exercise alone.[83] A milder dose may become OTC soon.

  All the fat blockers have appreciable gastrointestinal side effects such as nausea, cramps, bloating, and socially unacceptable flatulence. The more effective the drug and the more fats you consume, the more undesired the side effects. It can be so bad; it would make the campfire scene from *Blazing Saddles* seem like a formal tea party in a library! Lastly, they're nonspecific, which means they may block the bad as well as the good carbohydrates or fats your body need. The absorption of certain pills and vitamins may also be affected negatively. To compensate, I would recommend adding a good multivitamin at an opposite time of day.

- **Phentermine** or similar **Meridia©.** These category 4 prescription drugs basically belong to the "appetite suppressant" or anorectic category and are modern, somewhat safer version of the *speedlike pills* that were popular in the 1950s and '60s before these were appropriately outlawed. You also may remember the highly publicized fen-phen scare of the 1990s. It consisted of combining two of such class pills, fenfluramine and phentermine. Although never scientifically proven to directly cause heart problems, its mere *association* in twenty-four people studied by the Mayo Clinic resulted in it being pulled off the market. Their publication in 1997 eventually resulted in many millions of dollars being handed out. Phentermine, *by itself,* has long been proven safe and effective when used correctly, although most studies were only for a year or less. There are still substantial, potentially life-threatening side effects such as primary pul-

---

83 Obesity. *Prescriber's Letter,* January (2004): 4.

monary hypertension that warrants ongoing, lengthy dialogue with your physician.[84] Meridia is considerably more expensive; and most insurance plans don't reimburse for this one either. Yet, I may consider Meridia somewhat safer, overall. Side effects for these may also include worsening of hypertension, palpitations, nervousness, or any mood disturbance, including insomnia. You can google to find out more, but talking to your doctor is best.

I may—and I emphasize *may*—prescribe it to the right individual during the so-called *induction* phase of weight loss as part of a comprehensive program. The ideal candidate would be mostly healthy yet historically suffer from considerable food cravings that would undermine our recommendations and early success. Despite the obvious food addiction, the person would have to be free of other addictions, psychiatric illness, and should possess proper insight. Its use may also be appropriate for a prn, or *as needed basis*, for those who can't help but frequently overindulge at riskier times; for example, from Thanksgiving to New Year's Day. This regimen may help keep them from *falling off the food wagon* and may be safer in the long run.

- Rimonabant works by being a cannabinoid-receptor inhibitor. Drugmaker Sanofi-Aventis is on an all out blitz to educate doctors about this new class of weight-loss drug. Yes, you're right! Cannabinoids are the active ingredients found in marijuana that gives you the munchies and also get you high. According to their research, it was quite effective in weight loss, decrease in waist size, and metabolic parameters. I'm not so convinced yet. Who knows, though? Maybe they'll try to get you hooked by having celebrity spokesmen as Cheech and Chong!

- Miscellaneous: Most other supplements have suspect, or minimal if any, established substantially remarkable research on proven weight loss. (I can't describe all these in this one book; but remember, there's no one magic herb.) These include Panax ginseng, cinnamon, ginger, etc. Alone, I don't believe they appreciably add much, but recommend them *ad libertum* in their *natural* forms to crank your diet up a notch. BLAMM!

---

84 Primary pulmonary hypertension is basically high blood pressure in the lungs' vessels. This can be life-threatening. Common symptoms include sudden shortness of breath, edema, or chest pain.

E. Liposuction. This is a *cosmetic* procedure that doesn't remove what's really bad to the bone in most men—that *visceral* fat. Liposuction simply sculpts out what pear-shaped women usually sport—that *peripheral* fat. According to the *New England Journal of Medicine*, there were no beneficial medical effects in women who underwent this.[85] The author stated, "Had these patients lost this much fact by dieting, they would have expected to see marked improvements in insulin sensitivity and other risk factors for heart disease." I am mildly surprised at this, as well. Although predicting losing visceral fat would have more substantial health advantages, I would assume even losing peripheral fat would have some measurable benefits. There should be less production of adipokines. These are the by-products of fat cells that amplify the many metabolic disturbances of being overweight. It's been previously emphasized how the visceral fat distribution, *android* shape, increases multiple risk factors for serious age-related diseases more so than peripheral fat, the *gynecoid* shape, does. Apple shape is worse than pear.

Besides the usual risks of outpatient surgery, there are other concerns. Obviously, there should be a complete consultation with the plastic surgeon to review goals and expectations. It is, after all, body *sculpting* and is considered a permanent procedure. Therefore, you should possess your realistic body composition so that the sculpting fits you long-term. For example, you wouldn't want to undergo body sculpting when you're rather heavy and then lose or gain a substantial amount of weight. This could result in some undesirable, uneven contours later.

However, liposuction does have many appropriate applications. Some midlife guys may have lost about all the visceral and peripheral fat they reasonably can, but still have a wee bit of a pouch hiding that six-pack. In the right surgeon's hands, lipo offers a quick and relatively safe option to that *cut* look. Remember, imbalanced hormones can also limit the desired loss in fat, so you need to get those back in sync too. That healthy look starts from the inside out. In more extreme cases of weight loss, as after successful bariatric surgery, there's probably a substantial need for abdominoplasty *and* liposuction, as there's usually an appreciable amount of unattractive, redundant tissue left hanging around.

F. Bariatric Surgery. This may be a last ditch option for morbidly obese patients, i.e., those sporting a BMI over forty. I must admit,to having mostly bad feelings toward this procedure. Everything I have written thus far explained the true underlying pathophysiology of many age-related diseases brought on or

---

85 S. Klein, *New England Journal of Medicine,* June 17, 2004. Even removing about 20 percent of body fat from obese women, there were no beneficial medical effects.

worsened by your being overweight. Then, based on these, I went on to express the mostly natural, proven long-term modalities to combat them. I challenge any surgeon to show me the research indicating that in chronically obese patients with subsequent metabolic and hormonal disorders, the inciting abnormality is an enlarged stomach or any underlying gastrointestinal pathology for that matter.

To take this a little further, I opine bariatric surgery brings medicine back to *the dark ages* of improper rationale; preys on the unmotivated, uneducated patient; negates over fifty years of progress in nutritional and hormonal knowledge; and may even contribute to society's apathetic attitude toward losing weight. Keep in mind, it should really be improved *body composition* that's the goal, not just arbitrary weight loss. We need to combat that age-related loss in muscle and bone mass and the added fat to best prevent disease. Research has shown it's better to be fit and overweight that just less overweight. Where has it ever been proven that being overweight is caused by some form of stomach pathophysiology whose only corrective option would be surgical? Rather, I say practically everything else *but* the stomach plays a role in proper weight control! Bariatric surgery reflects today's typical reactive, cost-shifting approach as opposed to a better proactive, preventative, holistic one. The profound individual emotional and mental contributors are often discounted which would limit overall success.

The best analogy I can make is the incredulous time, not too long ago, when surgeons performed frontal lobotomies on the mentally ill. This is a similar adage of what other medically trained physicians would refer to as the typical surgeon's mentality: "If it's bad, cut it out! Forget all that medical mumbo jumbo." Modern research has elucidated it's actually the brain's neurochemical imbalances that cause most forms of psychiatric illness. This then lead to the many effective medical cures we have today. We don't cut the brain out any more, do we? I ask you to ponder, didn't these organs evolve or were specifically designed for a reason? It's not the stomach that causes obesity. Certainly, the two-thirds of Americans now overweight were born with a perfect functioning gastrointestinal system.

To add to my disfavor, I believe bariatric surgery has only gained popularity because of the change in the economic picture. Surprise! Once insurances and Medicare were medicolegally forced to pay for this, hospitals and surgeons sprung up overnight like Starbucks Coffee shops. Glamorous ads followed. In the end, though, we all pay for these operations that costs tens of thousands of dollars each. Yet, are there any incentives for physicians to do the more feasable outpatient counseling in order to prevent or even treat weight loss? Heavens, no! Even today, if I were to list *obesity* or *weight-loss counseling* as a diagnosis code, the payment for that visit would invariably be denied by Medicare and all insurance carriers I know. It's estimated that over one hundred fifty thousand bariatric operations were performed in 2005. Maybe one day, the hospitals can start putting up the golden arches like McDonald's and boast the numbers carved to date.

Again, the health-care system is quite upside down. Given what I said about modern society's epidemic of obesity, especially in our kids, shouldn't we make preventing and treating obesity job 1? It's shameful; but as usual, society is waiting for us to get clinically sick before we get any help. Basically, we have to "fall off a cliff" before a rescue attempt is made. Meanwhile, open-heart units and drugstores are sprouting up on every corner, profiting everywhere. Guess who pays for all this? This modern-day reactive attitude was recently expressed in my office by an overweight teenage girl who was accompanied by her mother. I've been seeing them for years for only acute problems, yet I've always been throwing in some counseling for her to lose weight. After I finished my most recent pro bono spiel about dieting, she kept looking at her polished nails and cavalierly remarked that she will just wait and eventually just get bariatric surgery. The mom kept silent as I looked at them both in amazement and at a lost for words, myself.

It's important to realize bariatric surgery is a far cry from a benign procedure. It's a major life-threatening intra-abdominal surgery. The most commonly performed is the *Roux-en-Y procedure,* which basically converts the stomach to a 30 mL pouch and then bypasses the first two parts of the small intestine, connecting directly to the ileum. Thirty milliliters is the volume of six teasoons. I think it's important to recall this operation was historically performed only as a palliative measure for those suffering from end-stage pancreatic, stomach, or intestinal cancers. Understandably, these unfortunate patients had no other options available. The associated high risks of life-threatening infection, respiratory failure, and pulmonary emboli were usually accepted. The risk of all these serious complications is estimated at about 10 percent. About 50 percent get gallbladder stones. That's more good news for surgeons. Wound infections will occur in up to 20 percent.[86] Research that reviewed insurance claims found nearly 40 percent of bariatric surgery patients experienced a complication within six months after discharge, while

---

86 These statistics are from references stated in the American Family Physician, April 15, 2006. Then, in October 1, 2006, *Family Practice News* ran a story entitled "Six-Month Bariatric Complication Rate Worrisome," which stated complications six months after bariatric surgery may be higher than what previous research suggested.

22 percent of patients had a complication *prior* to discharge.[87] Overall, this represented over an 80 percent increase in complications six months after surgery. This is much more than the 10–20 percent ranges usually found in the literature. Men may even be at higher risk.

Morbidly obese patients usually have accompanying diseases that put them at increased risks for a while. Recently, a review by Medicare estimated as high as one in twenty of their younger beneficiaries died the first year from related complications.[88] That's a whopping 5 percent first-year mortality rate! Hello, is anybody listening? Granted, this specific population was high risk, but geez, that's exactly who usually gets this procedure. Also, many long-term risks are yet unknown. These can include risks for stomach ulcers and stenosis. Studies show about a 40 percent overall morbidity rate, including early and late complications.

As this is a permanent procedure, there are other *lifetime* consequences of malabsorption and nutritional disturbances. You would have to follow up throughout life with a medical physician specially trained in the long-term maintenance of such special needs. Make sure this is addressed *before* the surgery. Lastly, there are many emotional and psychiatric issues you may also have to deal with. The surgery itself is also known to sometimes worsen other addictions such as gambling. Therefore, the necessity of lifetime emotional support exists. For some, being obese offered a good excuse for not becoming more in life. Others may have had other secondary gains not even recognizable on a conscious level.

I expressed these things to a very competent general surgeon that began doing this only a few months ago at our local small-town hospital (which by the way, was on an all-out ad blitz). In a defensive manner, he asked me what's *my* long-term success rate and proof concerning my weight-loss methods. I replied, "It's not *my* weight-loss method, rather, it's nature's. Show me anyone who has maintained the proper lifestyle, with no hormonal abnormalities, who is overweight? And then show me the biopsies from your surgical specimens that reveal *any* gastrointestinal pathophysiology? Weren't these people born with the same normal guts we all have?" I believe it borders on malpractice to remove healthy tissue from younger, mostly healthier individuals that still have the full gambit of options

---

87   William E. Encinosa, PhD, from the Agency for Healthcare Research and Quality (AHRQ) in Rockville, Maryland, and colleagues. *Medical Care* 44 (2006):706–12.

88   D. R. Flum, Early mortality among Medicare beneficiaries undergoing bariatric surgical procedures. *JAMA* 294, no. 15 (2005):1903–8. This study involved over 16,000 Medicare patients who underwent obesity surgery between 1997 and 2002.

available. As if that's not bad enough, the push now is to perform bariatric surgery on *all* ages, even teenagers. As a future trend, many patients that were left with "deformed" layers of flabby skin are now demanding that insurances pay for abdominoplasty too! It's quite unfair that the (few) healthy, proactive insured are all lumped together and have to pay the increasingly higher premiums for the others that regularly choose an unhealthy lifestyle.

Notwithstanding the above, I do believe such surgery has its proper, "noncelebretized" role. It's probably appropriate in the emotionally stable, motivated individuals who, for resolved reasons, previously ignored their health for decades and believe nothing else now is going to help. As explained previously, the comprehensive natural modalities I mention are more preventive and proactive, than reactive and curative. I prefer to safely help the person get down the cliff, not to wait to catch them once they fall. If a person has basically ignored a proper, healthy lifestyle and hormonal replacement for decades, all the resulting abnormal metabolic changes we've discussed have sent them far down the highway to early morbidity and mortality. In this instance, there is probably no other way to get back on the proper track without such drastic, riskier measures. Yet, that risk may be the only viable, realistic option left compared to the inevitable.

You would want a good life raft before jumping off a sinking ship, right? Likewise, make sure there is a good integrative team with the verifiable qualifications and experience to fully address the gambit of long-term concerns. Also, get your insurance carrier to guarantee the follow-up care. In the experienced surgical hands and with long-term support, bariatric surgery may be the only real option available for the appropriate morbidly obese candidate. Of course, assuming the surgery is a success, the patient should still commit to the necessary lifestyle changes and optimal hormonal replacement in order to ensure total health and proper body composition. I recommend routinely checking levels of iron, folate, vitamin B_{12}, vitamin D, and fatty acids in these individuals. I do follow a few patients that have undergone bariatric surgery.

Still, I don't believe bariatric surgery is the only magic bullet for the obese. Look at Jarod from the Subway's ads. I've had many patients lose substantial amounts of weight and gain proper body composition. One that comes to mind is a male I had been warning for years about being a borderline diabetic. Despite my efforts, it never sunk in. (He now claims he was in was denial.) Eventually, I recommended Metformin to help with his metabolic syndrome. Well, he didn't take this suggestion either. To make a long story short, he called one day feeling quite ill;

and I urgently worked him. He had become a frank diabetic with sugars running in the 300s! Immediately, he was put on insulin therapy. He was now listening to what I had to say and began the diet and the Metformin. Despite not exercising and only adhering to the right diet for three months, he lost fifty pounds. His complexion, mood, back pain, and irritable bowel symptoms were also much improved. Sugar and cholesterol levels normalized, so he was able to wean off his medications. Since that time, he added some exercise and lost over five inches of belly fat. Using myself as an example, I lost twenty pounds and four inches of waist. I now have more endurance and strength than when I was in my twenties!

G. Summary. I will close with yet more incentives to maintain a healthy weight:

- According to the July 2006 issue of *Archives of General Psychiatry*, fat people are, in fact, not jollier. Actually, obesity is strongly linked with depression and anxiety disorders. Furthermore, the drugs used to treat such mood disorders can compound these problems. Social expectations and prejudices may further complicate matters. Again, which came first, the mood disorder or the obesity? Maybe one day, Santa Claus and the Pillsbury Dough Boy may become spokesmen for Prozac. It can happen.

- As presented in the diet chapter, lower caloric intake means decreased fasting insulin levels, body temperature, energy expenditure, and the resulting free radical—induced DNA damage, which are all well-known biomarkers of longevity. The lower your caloric intake is, the better your chances of a longer, healthier life. As your parents said, "Eat to live; don't live to eat."

- Obesity increases your risk for almost all cancers, which are the biggest killers of people under eighty-five years old. The associated increased fatty acid levels cause an increased resistance to insulin, which, along with increasing cancer risks, is associated with development of diabetes, metabolic disorders, and heart disease. If not already, obesity will soon replace smoking as the number 1 preventable cause of most common cancers. See the above quote again for a cheap flashback.

- Obesity also increases your risks for nonalcoholic fatty liver disease, which affects up to 30 percent of Americans. This condition can be worsened with the use of alcohol and drugs, even the prescribed ones. This underappreciated form of hepatitis can progress to liver failure and even increases risk for liver cancer. The usual comorbidities such as diabetes and metabolic syndrome can complicate things further. The good news is, improvements are seen with dieting and exercise that result in a weight reduction of 10 percent or more.

- For men only: According to *JAMA*, diet and exercise that resulted in weight loss improved sexual functioning in obese men with erectile dysfunction (ED). One hundred ten "healthy" men aged thirty-five to fifty-five with a BMI of 30 or greater were followed for two years. In the intervention group, BMI decreased while erectile scores dramatically improved.[89] Even more importantly, there was also a decrease in blood vessel inflammation. This was indicated by lowered CRP and interleukin-6, which indicates improved endothelial function and lower risks for cardiovascular disease. I find that most guys tend to listen to diet and exercise advice when they find out it puts more lead in their pencil. Unlike Viagra-like drugs, there are no undesirable side effects such as possible blindness and death. Unfortunately, such natural approaches lack the little blue pill's Hollywood glamour and catch phrases. Here may be one though: Get up to exercise and exercise to get it up!

I would like to reemphasize there are no magic bullets when it comes to weight loss. What works for one person may not work for the other. Understandably, the approach needs to be individualized. The fact of the matter is that there are good and bad proteins, fats, and carbohydrates. I hope to have given you the knowledge to know the difference. Eating less amounts and selecting healthier foods are the only proven, safe dietary manipulation. Just gulping that extra can of soda a day can pile on fifteen pounds in a single year—so drink water with a lemon slice. If you look at your current diet and simply eat one-fourth less, you'll really lose weight. Don't eat three cookies, eat two—no biggie. Another way is to reduce your intake by 500 calories per day. By just doing this seven days per week, you would lose one pound of fat, or 3500 calories, per week! Not bad. This is very doable and practical in the long term, as any diet should be.

Of course, increased physical activity must be included. No excuses! Hide all remotes, or better yet, avoid TV altogether! Take the stairs. Ride the bike or walk your errands after eating. Take some advice from the International Obesity Task Force to your workplace or neighborhood and make things happen (see below). Get involved. If you can't afford a half or a full hour of exertion per day, break it up into smaller time allotments during the day. Pencil in and devote this relatively small amount of time just for you. Although you may have other commitments to family or job, you must realize the best way for you to be able to care for others is to first take care of yourself. You'll only be a better you for a longer time to come. You deserve it!

---

89   K. Esposito, *JAMA* 291 (2004): 2978–84, 3011–12.

Top Ten Recommendations from the Obesity Task Force:

1. Families should limit television and computer use to two hours a day and never at dinner. Parents should also provide healthy snack options.

2. Businesses, governments, associations, and organizations can collaborate to promote lifelong healthy nutrition.

3. Faith-based organizations, civic and service clubs, and voluntary health agencies should promote helpful nutrition opportunities.

4. Community should promote lifelong access to physical activity, including investing in bicycle and pedestrian paths.

5. Community planners should develop roadways and pathways for bicycles and pedestrians.

6. Faith-based organizations, civic and service clubs, and voluntary health organizations should include increased physical activity opportunities into current and future initiatives.

7. Health-care providers should be empowered to support healthy eating and increased physical activity.

8. Promote health-insurance effort that supports science-based eating and physical activity programs, and offer incentives to people who practice healthier lifestyles.

9. Promote weight loss and weight management in programs focused on diabetes, congestive heart failure, and hypertension.

10. The Department of Health should continue promoting lifelong physical activity.

Figure 4.2. Taken from the Obesity Task Force. Top ten weight-loss recommendations we all should follow. Sounds like old-fashioned advice.

This does take a long-term commitment on your part, but it's for your biggest asset, your optimal health. Ultimately, it's *all* about behavioral modification—the way you look at your life and improve your attitude toward your dietary and exercise regimen. As presented, there are no downsides to this proven and safe approach. No gimmicks, fads, knives, or pills. Remember what I said at the get-go, "If you don't change direction, you'll probably end up where you're headed." Fast food just gets you to the graveyard quicker! Get your life in order now and set a course to a healthier destination. Midlife presents the window of opportunity.

Chapter 4. MAG feels that the diet we recommend is fine. After all, that's exactly what his mom used to feed him when he was a kid. No more candy and soda! He drinks soy milk though, and snacks on nuts and an apple or some dried apricots. He starts to take a GMP-certified supplement that has 1000 mg of L-carnitine and 250 mcg of chromium.

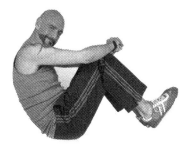

V.

Exercise: Use it or lose it!

Think of it as you when younger; have a fun out, not a workout!

A. A Pep Talk. It should come as no surprise; exercise also helps prevent age-related illnesses. There's indeed a profound mind-body connection—a healthy body promotes a healthy mind and vice versa. It seems quite ironic that on one hand, America, and the whole world for that matter, is going through another energy crisis. Meanwhile, health costs are soaring because of the obesity epidemic and its related conditions. *These are mostly brought on by the population's unwillingness to expend enough energy.* What's going on, people? If we'd start walking and riding our bikes more, fuel consumption, health care costs, and even pollution would improve. My first goal here is to provide you with the facts and then offer suggestions to help you overcome any barriers to establishing and maintaining a regular exercise regimen. But you must walk around the block, get your heart pumping, and mind jumping first.

I must emphasize again, your health is your biggest asset, or it can be your worst liability. You will only get out of your life what you put into it. Let me make an analogy. Most of us devote a lot of time per week working for *the man*, or maybe *the woman* for that matter. You give forty hours per week or more. Why? To make money, of course! So that the eagle shits and you get that paycheck. All that dedication and work in order to pay your bills and, hopefully, you'll have some leftover to save for retirement. Ah … those golden years you've heard so much about. Granted, one day having financial security and not having to work *is* a main priority we middle-aged men focus on a lot—maybe too much. But remember what I emphasize: your health, it's your most important asset. Think about it. Do things seem a little topsy-turvy in your life?

Indeed, money is very important. But your health should come first. Let's assume you're the typical middle-aged man. You've worked hard your whole life and saved some for retirement. Like most guys, you put your health on the back burner, so now you're overweight with borderline hypertension and diabetes. Your doctor has threatened to put you on more pills, besides the cholesterol pills you're on, if you don't improve. She routinely harps on you about diet and exercise, but this falls on deaf ears. You *almost* start to exercise and diet. Thanks to your wife, you're eating more salads, bought some exercise outfits and running shoes, maybe even joined a gym and went a couple of times. You may have lost a few pounds and an inch off the waistline, but not seeing the dramatic results needed to combat decades of … well, let's say, not-the-best lifestyle. Eventually, you give up. Well rest assured, you're not alone.

You probably believe or convinced yourself that you simply don't have the time to regularly exercise. You are either too busy getting ready for work or being at work or coming home from work or picking up the kids or fixing dinner or finishing up on work at home or going to bed. You basically fell into the trap of *working for the weekend*. Weekends are usually spent catching up on work at home and, granted, some well-deserved leisure time—watching a game or two and having a few brewskis. And it's tough, I know. When you come home from work, tired and frustrated, there are some choices to make. It's like those many cartoons we saw as a kid where they had the little angel on one shoulder and the minidevil on the other. One may say to get a beer, relax on the couch, or get online to read your e-mail. The other pleads for you to go outside in the heat and jog for two and a half miles. These are tough decisions. Most would, and do, choose the beer and sofa.

But as they say, you can only reap what you sow. In other words, you only get out of something what you put into it. For example, what if you only worked only a few hours or even one day per week? Would you have the money then to pay your bills? Would you have enough leftover to save for retirement? Of course, you wouldn't. Likewise, with the investment you routinely need to make toward your health—again, it's your most important asset. Eating right or exercising just one day per week isn't going to really cut it. You have to invest daily, or usually three things happen. This is sort of like what Mr. Scrooge went through with the three ghosts in Charles Dickens' classic novel *A Christmas Carol.*

The first scenario assumes you're lucky enough to live into older years. You may have some money saved, but you're also suffering some with the usual age-related decline and increase in diseases. You may still have the money to buy a boat or take a trip or get a new a car, but you're too weak or achy to really enjoy them. What's the use then? The second is that you *had* the money to buy all those things, but you now spend all your retirement on hundreds of dollars of medications per month, on multiple specialists, and on hospital bills. Remember, these are supposed to be the golden years. They can be. Unfortunately, sometimes this means you now give all your gold to the doctors and hospitals. The third scenario is that you die before you even get to enjoy any of your saved money. In this case, someone else will enjoy it for you. By the way, the same above scenarios can happen to your spouse, which may have an even worse outcome. That's why it's best to accomplish optimal health, together. There are no armored cars following a hearse. Or as they say, "You can't take it with you."

Okay, so maybe what I said above didn't click. I have two other quick analogies that may help you see things better, get motivated, and see the light. One is, imagine you were given only one car, one vehicle, to use your *entire* life. This may sound crazy, but think about it. Wouldn't you be sure to take *extra* special care of it? Well, of course! You would wax it, make sure it doesn't rust out, and keep it well tuned and oiled. It's best to prevent any problems from becoming costlier ones down the road, right? Well, when it comes down to it, your body is truly the one vehicle you have. It must last your whole life, right? It takes you around your whole life. It's the most intimate vehicle you'll ever have. So you should take extra special care of it, making sure it doesn't break down and wind up costing you a whole lot more. Unfortunately, you can't trade your body in on a new one now, can you? Well, at least that's not an option yet.

Similar to the analogy above, some people's bag may be to have a big house, a big fancy automobile, or a bigger whatever to show off to their neighbors. (By the way, why is it that the bigger the person is, the smaller the car they drive?) Think of the money that house costs each month and then total that over thirty years—that's a lot of paychecks. A house can be your biggest asset … or liability if you don't perform routine preventative maintenance. Or in four years, that fancy sports car will be worn out and will be worth a quarter on the dollar. Think of how much you've wasted on automobiles during your lifetime. If you're a jackass like me, it's way too much. At any rate, I'm just trying to put things in the proper perspective. We are blasted with ads twenty-four hours a day with silly things we don't need to buy or spend our time doing, yet very little is spent educating or promoting healthier lifestyles—a much more important prerogative.

> To summarize, you probably give forty-plus hours plus a week of sweat to "da" man. Shouldn't you be able to give a measly three to five hours per week *to yourself*, to *your* health? After all, it is your most important asset, isn't it?

More so than any car or house, you should invest in your health *every day* with healthier lifestyle choices. Unfortunately, once a week simply won't cut it. If you do the right thing, you'll start having better health now and future reserves to draw from in older years. When you think about it, being in better shape is really one of the best ways to care for your loved ones too. You can leave a legacy of healthier attitudes. If not, your health will simply not be there when you need it. You will become a burden to these very same loved ones, as well. Your health account will be over drawn. Account closed, NSF! C'mon, don't be a scrooge when it comes to giving some time to your health. As they say, money isn't everything!

As greatly emphasized, diet and exercise play very important roles in your overall health. These probably make up about two-thirds of what you need to obtain optimal health. There are many other books that go into more depth than I can here. I hope to show you the facts, encourage you some, and help you overcome some common barriers and problems. The other players, proper hormonal balance and nutraceuticals, complete the rest of the health puzzle. These make the difference between you just feeling good and feeling *great* for your age. You'll be getting out and *living* life as opposed to finding excuses all the time. Getting these parameters right will provide you with the power needed to help you slow down, even reverse, many of the age-related bad cards that Mother Nature starts to deal you around middle age.

Most patients I see for age management are quite proactive about their health to begin with, or else they wouldn't be spending their extra time and money. They already realize the importance of investing some extra effort in their health. Most have read a lot and are knowledgeable about the many things we emphasize. Many have been misinformed, as well. The men we see can be grouped into three basic categories:

(1) The younger middle-aged guy, MAG1, who feels great and wants to *keep* feeling great. He knows now is the time to do it and wants to prevent pills and disease in a more natural way. It's better to keep up than to play catch-up on aging later.

(2) The middle-aged guy, MAG2, is like our MAG example throughout this book. He used to feel great, but now feels well, only *okay.* He's been to a few contemporary doctors with the many vague complaints of feeling middle-aged—which they really don't care to hear about or be reminded. On return visits, he was told the lab work was completely normal; there's nothing wrong. "Get used to getting older!" In actuality, there were probably many subacute diseases or *predisease* states going on that aren't apparent to the traditionally trained doctor. Probably, disease risk markers like CRP and insulin weren't even measured. Insurance wouldn't pay for these unless there were abnormal symptoms first. Realistically, health insurance should be called *sick* insurance, not health insurance. It kicks in when you're sick.

(3) The older middle-aged guy, MAG3, now has established, overt medical problems requiring medications, yet wants a more balanced, integrative approach in order to regain better overall functioning in the safest way. Seeing the light now, he wants to get off the old train to disability and get on a better path and final destination. Although some may unfairly consider this somewhat too late, it's always better late than never. He'll still benefit greatly from being more proactive.

Let me say that we can help all three of these people. I love the scenario of MAG1; it makes my job the easiest and most fun, as I can help prevent a lot of age-related conditions in the first place, optimizing his health and performance. This guy is on the right road; we just have to make sure he stays on it and doesn't get lost on the way. He is usually in his early to midthirties, is proactive about his lifestyle, exhibits good body composition, and enjoys overall great health. As stressed in the introduction, midlife presents the window of opportunity to prevent the premature onset of age-related conditions. The earlier you start, the better off you'll be.

MAG2 and MAG3 are similar in a lot of ways—only the additional decades on the wrong path separate them. They are both on the same *normal* aging path that Mother Nature intended, although shortened and rushed somewhat by the unhealthier lifestyle today. MAG3 is just further down that same road in distance. MAG2 is to be commended somewhat, because he may be really trying his hardest. He's doing the diet and exercises the best he can, although inconsistent. This lack of motivation may partially be due to his not seeing the results he used to when younger. I was like MAG2 about five years ago.

Typically the problem with MAG2 and 3 above is that they are fighting the same age-related uphill battle. They think about when they were younger and never had to worry about silly dieting and exercise. They were basically young studs or at least the closest that they'd ever get to being one. There lies the dilemma. What's different about them now? Why is it so hard to have that same *boing* or *schwing* they used to sport around? Aren't they the same person as before, with the same genes? Well, of course, they are. The *typical* lab work would probably show very little difference from when they were younger. They're *normal* for their age. But they know something has changed. What *has* changed is their hormones are no longer optimized the way they were when they were in their teens or early twenties. Mother Nature made sure their original warranty wore out. That new car smell has long disappeared and is being replaced with creaks, leaks, and squeaks.

Although individual needs and treatments vary widely, getting all the hormones back to their optimal physiological levels will help all things come together. The improvement in mind and mood will give you the willpower and mental edge to get and stay on that healthier track. The increase in muscle mass and strength will help you see the real results you had when younger. As visceral fat is lost, risks for all the age-related diseases mentioned previously will decrease. Immune, sexual concerns, aches, fatigue, and more improve. Getting the hormones in tune will synergistically work with diet and exercise to achieve optimal mental and physical shape. If you think you are doing all you reasonably can do to lose weight and stay fit and it just *ain't happenin'*, chances are your hormones are out of whack. If you're MAG2, you better reverse and get on the right path now to avoid becoming MAG3. When your hormones aren't optimized, you're basically fighting uphill battles against a very experienced Mother Nature. You'll quickly lose the war on aging and its many complications. Suffice to say, you have to have all cylinders firing and gun locked and loaded to win. (Hormones are covered later.) Well, after that important digression, back to exercise.

B. Exercise Benefits. Here's a few:

- **Cardiovascular Disease:** Physically fit people are eight times less likely to suffer and die from cardiovascular disease than their unfit cohorts.[90] *You gotta' have heart!*

- **Mind:** Understandably, being physically fit decreases your risk for metabolic disorders and chances for getting dementia and stroke. Exercising releases natural mood enhancers such as enkephalins and endorphins, giving you the "runner's high" and decreasing pain. "A sound mind is a sound body" was the conclusion from a very interesting study that began

---

90 S. Blair, "Physical fitness and all-cause mortality," *JAMA* Nov. 3, 1989.

in 1932 by Scottish researchers.[91] They were able to measure IQ scores of subjects eleven and seventy-nine years old and compared these to their physical fitness. According to the author, "The important result here is that fitness … contributed to later life cognition after adjusting for child-hood IQ. At the level of the general population, being fit is not only good in itself, it is also associated with better cognitive functioning … For a clinician, surely this just reinforces the message that is a good thing to be as physically fit as one can be."

- **Cholesterol**: Regular exercise helps raise HDL, the *good* cholesterol; low-ers both the LDL, *bad* cholesterol; and the *ugly* triglycerides. Lowering triglycerides prevents heart disease and progression to diabetes and the metabolic syndrome, as well as many other maladies. As mentioned before, raising HDL by only 6 percent decreases the risk of cardiac prob-lems by up to 35 percent.[92] Lowering LDL has well-known, established health benefits. All without drugs! Here's the truly natural way to go.

- **Hypertension**: Regular exercise helps reduce blood pressure—both systolic and diastolic—and helps decrease your risk for prehypertension. The latter is indicated by blood pressures that run 120/80 to 139/89. Better pressure readings mean less risk for premature death, CAD, CHF, stroke, dementia, and a whole lot more. Lower systolic blood pressure was associated with increased life expectancy to seventy-five years old for middle-aged men from the Framingham Study.[93] So, feet, don't fail me now!

- **Body Composition**: Of course, regular aerobic and resistance exercise will help maintain bone and muscle mass. This prevents the frailty syn-drome we often warn about. If you don't lose muscle mass, you won't lose bone mass. Additionally, you'll have less visceral and peripheral fat, decreasing you chances for metabolic syndrome, CAD, chronic back pain, and related conditions. Don't become a *girly man*!

- **Stress and Sleep Disturbances**: Proper exercise is the best way to reduce stress and risk of chronic pain disorders. Being in shape makes you less prone to injuries. Exerting yourself during the day helps keep normal diurnal rhythm patterns of cortisol. This helps you sleep better come nighttime. Exercise produces the "runner's high" and releases endorphins

---

91   I. Deary, "Physical fitness and lifetime cognitive change," *Neurology* 67 (2006): 1195–1200.

92   GISSI Investigators, "GISSI prevenzione trial." Lancet 354(9189) 1999: 1556-57.

93   This, according to research by the University of Massachusetts Medical School pub-lished in the *Archives of Internal Medicine,* March 1996.

and enkephalins, giving you that natural high. A normal body habitus help prevents obstructive sleep apnea and its related illnesses. Get high with nature; take a hike.

- **Cancer Prevention**: Being fit helps boost the immune system and keeps inflammation down, thereby helping prevent carcinogenesis in the first place. Cancer *is* the number one killer for people aged eighty-five years and under. Why go through all that chemo if you don't have to?

- **Optimal Sex Performance**: No surprise, older men do suffer from increased sexual dysfunction. This can be delayed or improved with a healthier lifestyle. Over thirty-one thousand men between the ages of fifty and ninety were studied by the Harvard School of Public Health in 2003. About 33 percent reported erectile dysfunction (ED). (This was similar to the large Massachusetts Male Aging study report of about 50 percent in men aged forty to seventy.) Risks for ED included watching TV and being overweight, i.e., being a couch potato. Expectedly, risks such as peripheral arterial vessel disease, diabetes, and hypertension, even antidepressant medications were also noted. Yet, those men with an active lifestyle reported a 30 percent *lower* risk of ED.[94] It's important to note one-fifth of men don't respond to Viagra—which possesses some potentially serious side effects. So again, there is no magic bullet to fall back on; the best way to keep Mr. Johnson happy is to keep your whole self in tip-top shape. Use it or lose it!

C. Exercise Tips.

Unfortunately, I can't give you personal advice, but I'll assume you're a basically well middle-aged guy, like MAG1 or MAG2 above, who was moderately fit when a teenager. Like most, you probably don't have an exercise regimen. If you do, that's great. More power to you. Still, you may pick up important tips to help you reach the next level. Some caveats before we get started.

I firmly believe a personal trainer can help out a lot. He'll be able to address any barriers or physical limitations you may have. Additionally, a lot has changed in the decades since you were a teen; he can get you up to speed. You two can establish a safe, balanced exercise regimen that will get results. Some people do need a personal trainer to help them regularly show up and stay on the ball.

---

94 C. G. Bacon, "Sexual function in men older than fifty years of age: Results from the health professionals follow-up study," *Annals of Internal Medicine.* 139, no. 3 (2003):161–8; R. C. Rosen, "Lifestyle management of erectile dysfunction: The role of cardiovascular and concomitant risk factors," *American Journal of Cardiology* 96(12B) (2005):76M–79M.

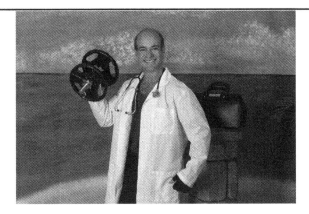

Three aspects to *generally* consider when designing an appropriate exercise regimen:

1. I recommend all guys over forty to devote **one-third of their exercise time** to stretching. As age would have it, most things you don't want stiff get stiffer. Overall, our joints, tendons, and ligaments become less flexible, which only increases risks for injury. To prevent this, I find this important step is typically underdone. Stretching should start before exercising, during the warm-up phase. You may also do your stretching during the exercise program, while taking a small break, between repetitions, or while resting to lower your heart rate. This is crucial after exercising, during the cool-off period. This is a good time to meditate. You can incorporate some yoga, tai chi, or silent prayer. Or you may just practice deep, slow breathing and get in your own zone—whatever floats your boat. Stretching warns your body that you're about to exert yourself and as a bonus, it helps relieve stress naturally. I even have some patients who pay someone else to stretch them out daily.

2. **One-third of the time should be cardiovascular (aerobic) exercise.** I generally explain there are *two* categories of aerobic exercise. Which you perform depends on your overall shape and goals:

   • If your main objective is to lose fat, then you'd be better off doing a treadmill, or similar machine, for a *longer* amount of time. For about fifty minutes or more, you want to just *moderately* raise your heart rate. If your baseline heart rate is 80, raise it to about the 110s. Basically, you're trying to *burn off* the fat. Metabolically, you have to use up the sugar in the blood and muscles first. This will cause insulin to drop, thereby unlocking stored fat from fat cells everywhere. The results are improved glucose tolerance and insulin sensitivity, all desired effects.

- If your goal is to have better cardiovascular and overall conditioning, then you may be better off safely getting your heart rate higher.[1] If your baseline heart rate is in the 70s, getting it up to the 130s may be the goal. You really don't need to do this for as long a time as stated above, twenty-five to thirty minutes are usually fine. Remember what I said about this being a *fun out*? Many people pass the time reading or listening to tunes on the iPod. Some may learn a new language or study jazz music. Get some socializing done. Network or reacquaint with old friends.

- Stop doing *dumb* exercise! What do I mean by this? More recently, I try to get patients to do more of an interval-like routine. This *"intelligent exercise"* produces a hormonal advantage to obtain better body composition. Basically, you need to get to lactic acid production—that point of metabolic and functional fatigue. But not too strenuous a level, you should be able to still speak comfortably. This approach stimulates a small spike in human growth hormone and testosterone. There is also a longer rise in your basal metabolic rate. The end result is better body composition with less caloric expenditure.[2] Think of the frailer appearing marathoner compared to the really cut sprinter and you'll start to appreciate the difference with this method. It's not just how long you exercise or calories burned, it's also about *how* you exercise. Talk to your personal trainer about this; it should be attempted safely.

---

1   At midlife, you may want to get a cardiac stress test to know exactly what is safe and what to shoot for. All increases in exercise should be gradual. Your doctor can help you. Two hundred twenty minus your age is a *general* rule for maximal heart rate; example: 220 minus 50 years old equals 170 maximum heart rate per minute. This can vary greatly though! Start off at 70 percent and slowly work your way up to maybe 90 percent. You can go to http://www.cdc.gov and look up Nutrition and Physical Activity and get more exercise tips, like the Borg Rating of Perceived Exertion Scale.

2   Thanks to a paper by Jade and Keoni Teta, ND, CSCS. King, et al. 2001. A comparison of high intensity vs. low intensity exercise on body consumption in overweight women. *Medicine and Science in Sports and Exercise* 33. Tremblay, et al. 1994. Impact of exercise intensity on body fatness and skeletal muscle metabolism. *Metabolism* 43: 814-18. Treuth, et al. 1996. Effects of exercise intensity on 24 h energy expenditure and substrate oxidation. *Medicine and Science in Sports and Exercise* 28: 1138-43.

3. ***One-third should be resistance exercise.*** I assume you're moderately out of shape, but not too bad. The biggest mistake you could do is to do too much, too soon, and too fast. Again, I strongly recommend a personal trainer or *buddying* up with somebody who knows. If that doesn't happen, make some new friends by asking someone in shape who looks like he knows what he's doing. You can usually ask the gym employees for some free advice. They usually toss this in when you join; or better yet, they may have special group classes. Most are quite glad to do it. Borrow free exercise videos from the local library. Don't be intimidated. I find most people going to the gym enjoy the camaraderie and mutual encouragement.

- I also emphasize starting off with ***strengthening the central, or core, muscles*** and then working your way to the peripheral ones. Most macho guys will incorrectly start pumping biceps, triceps, and lower legs. They'll invariably start getting back and neck problems. Think about it. You must first strengthen the core, or the foundation, then work your way out. This means getting your abdomen and back in shape first. If, instead, you start lifting weights using the extreme periphery of the body, like in the arms, you're putting a tremendous amount of torque and torsional strain on the back and neck. Don't overextend the joints, especially knees and shoulders. You then may break down, get frustrated, and maybe even give up. We don't want that to happen. Remember, while it took a while to get out of shape, it'll take a while to get back into it. Have patience, you will get there! Don't break your back trying to rebuild Romulus in one day.

- As far as the proper amount of weight to lift, use the weight that you can comfortably lift about eight times. Get to that point of muscle fatigue mentioned above. Eventually, once you can lift this amount twelve times, crank up the weight some, and repeat. Go slow. It should take twice as long a time to let the weight down as when you lift it. You can count 1-2 when contracting and 1-2-3-4 when passively relaxing a muscle.

- It must be a ***balanced*** program, alternately working on upper, mid, and lower body. While doing repetitions, try to ultimately push and then pull the particular muscle groups. Appropriate rest time is needed between workouts to allow your muscles to repair themselves. This is especially important as we age. It's okay to be a *little* stiff the next day after working out, but you shouldn't hurt. If so, you're doing something wrong. It's not, "No pain, no gain." It's better to have "No pain, no pain!" Typically, I work out an hour and a half, three days per week. The other days I may do some artwork or play my drums. With the kids, I try to do sports at the nearby park or do chores at home.

- *Change your routine every three to five weeks* so that you gain the most from the particular workout. Doing the same routine week after week results in less gain, as the neuromuscular system adjusts and becomes more efficient with time. This can be avoided by switching from using machines to free weights or using resistance bands, for example. (By the way, the bands are great to pack in a suitcase when going away on trips.) To switch things around a bit, you can lift less weight but do more reps; use a slightly different but appropriate angle.

At any rate, I do recommend to progressively, but gradually, advance the number of repetitions and the amount of weight. If you do the same routine month after month, year after year, you will only *slow down* the rate of age-related decline in strength. Not bad, but you're doing the same old routine—not improving. So instead of looking like you're thirty-five when you're actually forty-five, you'll feel twenty-five if you're regularly advancing your routine. As stressed before, this should be done appropriately and monitored so that that you don't break down. No pain, no pain, remember? Get the proper advice from a personal trainer.

Most research shows that resistance training keeps your basal metabolic rate (BMR) increased longer than after just an aerobic workout, thereby lengthening caloric expenditure. Furthermore, some suffer from mobility problems or such that prohibit them from doing adequate aerobic exercise. In this case, *progressive resistance training* (PRT) may help fill the gap.[1]

PERSONAL NOTES:

---

1   Further advice on PRT can be found at K. A. Willey, *Diabetes Care* 26 (2003): 1580–88.

Now let's assume the gym may be entirely out of the question for whatever reasons. What to do now? Well, you're going have to be more innovative and flexible. You may have to get *sporadic* exercise throughout the day instead. This may mean a brisk fifteen-minute walk first thing in the morning or a walk around the parking lot at lunch. With the energy crisis, this may mean riding a bike to work. They do this in Europe all the time. Depending on the season, it may include a half-hour of physical labor around the house each day. This may be raking, sweeping, washing the car, or even painting the house, for example. This is great when the kids are still too young to go to the gym. This allows them to learn about life and feel like part of the home team. Then on the weekends, since all the house chores are done, the whole gang can walk or ride bikes to the local park and have a good old-fashioned family *fun out*. Bring a healthy picnic lunch too! Did I mention that no TV is needed?

Indeed, even a moderate exercise program can reduce risk of cardiac-related deaths by 25 percent and all death rates by 20 percent. According to some studies, such "no sweat" exercise has substantial benefits.[95] This includes significant decreases in risk for stroke, diabetes, dementia, fractures, and breast and colon cancers. The famous long-term Framingham Heart Study showed that people who regularly exercise enjoy almost four years of additional life compared to their couch potato cohorts.

According to Duke University researchers, even overweight, *nondieting* adults can prevent further weight gain by performing the equivalent of just a half hour of brisk walking per day.[96] This may not seem much good, but we generally would gain 1 percent of fat mass per year. The more aggressive subjects *lost* weight. As will be mentioned many times throughout this book, exercise is one of the very few proven ways to safely prevent the early complications of aging. This is good news for those of us that can't seem to diet yet may enjoy getting more activity.

Unfortunately, they're two ends of the exercise spectrum—the majority that doesn't exercise enough and those few that exercise *too* much. **Overtraining** often backfires, sending athletes into a tailspin that may end their career.[97] This may

---

95 H. Simon, "Moderate exercise: No pain, big gains," *Medscape Internal Medicine*, March 28, 2006.

96 S. Klein, *Archives of Internal Medicine,* Jan. 12, 2004.

97 You can find more information from the American College of Sports Medicine. University of Indiana sports psychologist John Raglin presented this at the national meeting of ACSM in Denver, July 2006.

cause the *staleness syndrome*, which is marked by vague symptoms such as depression, illness, soreness, sleep disturbance, and loss of appetite. There is a psychological screening tool known as the Profile of Mood States (POMS) that may help identify if you're overdoing it.

Signs of Overtraining

- Decreased performance
- Increased recovery needs
- Changes to resting heart rate
- Chronic fatigue
- Sleep and eating disorders
- Menstrual disruptions
- Muscle soreness and damage
- Joint aches and pains
- Depression and apathy
- Increased illness
- Lowered self-esteem

Source: American College of Sports Medicine

Figure 5.1. Signs you may be overtraining. Symptoms can even last for months after you slow down.

D. What about Sports Drinks or Protein Bars? Here's my take on these. First of all, you shouldn't be skipping meals and eating junk anyway, right? I don't recommend exercising on an empty stomach, nor do I recommend eating or drinking *too much* before working out because of upchuck risks and cramps—very embarrassing. Do replace fluids *during* and *after* exercising. And use common sense; don't exercise in extreme heat or sun exposure. Find a shady spot or avoid midday sun.

I don't recommend sport drinks high in sugar because of the high glycemic index and because of the phenomenon of *hitting the wall.* This occurs when you *carb up* before a workout. The sugar is used up quite fast and only lasts so long. At that point, you basically run out of gas and go flat. But usually, if you eat right about an hour and a half before working out, you should do fine. Having an energy bar or a drink that has protein and is under 50 percent carbs is okay. This may even help your performance.[98] If I hadn't eaten in a while before working out, I may do such a bar and just drink bottled water. To tell the truth, most of the time I find it inconvenient to have a protein bar or drink handy. They can also vary widely in calories and contents. They're processed and not that cheap, either. Read the label. Most of the time, I just bring my bottled water from home and replenish things after the work out … I mean, fun out.

Depending on how hard I worked and when my next meal is due, I may fix my own protein drink after working out. It consists of about thirty grams of whey protein, sixteen ounces of orange juice with pulp, one teaspoon of olive oil, and one gram of creatine. (This is about the only time I have any sort of juice.) Or I may quickly have a glass of skim milk with a little chocolate syrup. That has protein to help muscle repair and helps replace the glycogen that was used up during the exercise. If I'm going to eat soon, I'll just have my regular well-balanced meal with a low-calorie drink such as tea or water.

> As Rod Serling from the *Twilight Zone* would say, "Imagine if you will … Nananana♪ … Nananana♪ … The famous theme song, remember? Maybe if none of this is sinking in, you need that flying door to hit you in the head. At any rate, imagine a pill that could do all that merely exercise achieves, with no bitter taste or side effects. Friends say you look great. You feel great. No insurance plan's hassles, copays, or deductibles. Well, this is a reality. Just add good old-fashioned exercise. If you really want to reach your *twilight* years in great health, you must get in the proper *zone* now. If not, your life can become quite frightening! (You can add Vincent Price's laugh now.)

---

98 M. Saunders, *Science and Medicine in Sports and Exercise*, July 9, 2004.

Chapter 5. MAG gets a personal trainer and finds out he was doing many things wrong. He needs to start with the core muscles, stretch more, and get a more balanced program going. He wants to burn off fat, so he does the treadmill for fifty minutes every other day. MAG is fully committed to three one-and-a-half-hour sessions per week. His wife is impressed, and now they both go. (They arranged for a neighbor to watch the kids.) They have a *fun out* three times per week now. Feeling closer than they have in a long while, they enjoy more lovemaking! Their *sleep* has improved, too.

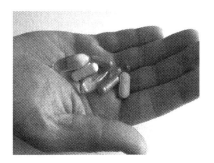

VI.

Supplements: Helpful, or Are You Just Urinating Your Money Away?

I haven't seen any "natural" pills growing on a plant yet. They're all made in a factory somewhere.

The topic of supplements could easily take up many books. Many are devoted to one supplement such as fish oil or coenzyme Q_{10}. I will try to give you some facts, background, and recommendations on a few I believe are helpful. This way, when you follow up on the further resources provided, you'll be better able to discern the *news* from the *noise*.

First, you must realize supplements aren't regulated by the FDA; they're categorized as dietary supplements, not drugs. This means you must trust the manufacturer to relay the truth about the ingredients, potential benefits, and risks. To me, this is like letting the fox watch the hen house. Ergo, I only recommend GMP-certified or pharmaceutical-grade supplements. This means an unbiased third party has approved the manufacturing process and examined the particular supplement for quantity and quality. These standards are similar for an FDA-approved drug. Don't be fooled. A product being touted as a *natural, holistic,* or safer alternative to medical therapy may not be. Many herbs will entice you with a label featuring an Asian or Indian (Eastern or Western) figurine. Any manufactured pill contained in a bottle is man-made. It's *unnatural,* be it a prescription pill or a supplement, right? When it comes down to it, the only *truly natural* methods are proper diet, regular exercise, and optimal hormonal replacement. But if you want to supplement these, you'll need the *real deal*. It's well worth it. Again, you only get what you pay for. It's not good to skimp when it comes to your health; you're only shortchanging yourself. Another *red flag* is if the particular herb claims to cure *all* ills that you, or everyone else, could possibly have.

Research has shown many Internet- and store-bought supplements carry unknown risks. What the label states on the outside is not necessarily what you get on the inside. You don't know if you're getting *any* of what you *think* you may be getting. The amount can vary widely. A good example would be the warning from a *Mayo Clinic Proceedings* 2003 review article on DHEA. After listing the many potential benefits, the authors couldn't advise routine replacement after all. This was because the actual amounts in store-bought DHEA varied from 0 to 150 percent of what was stated on the label.[99] Add to that the fact that many of the supplements or their ingredients are manufactured outside the United States. China, India, and elsewhere don't adhere to our strict manufacturing principles. I only mention those two countries because there have been many reports in the literature of serious heavy metal and other toxins found in so-called Chinese and ayurvedic supplements.[100] There were several known cases of death in recent years from heavy metal exposure from these. I'm concerned the glass containers may contain lead too.

There have been recent reports of prescription drugs being hidden in many OTC supplements. No warnings for these were listed either. These include Viagra, the drug for ED that can potentially worsen heart problems and cause blindness. Another is glyburide, a diabetic medication that can lower glucose to dangerous levels, even causing a coma. Recently, there were even amounts of Prozac, a prescription antidepressant, found in OTC weight-loss supplements originating from Brazil. Some herbs claiming to safely and naturally boost energy have been found to contain caffeine, ephedra, librium, animal thyroid extracts, even illegal stimulants that could result in you getting a positive drug test and being fired![101] All these ingredients are quite scary. If you recall, L-tryptophan was touted as

---

99 K. Ketan, "DHEA: Is there a role for replacement?" *Mayo Clinic Proceedings* 78 (2003): 1257–73.

100 R. B. Saper, "Heavy metal content of Ayurvedic herbal medicine products," *JAMA* 292 (2004): 2868–73; *MMWR* 53:582–84.

101 Y. Waknine, "Brazilian dietary supplements contain prescription drugs, FDA warns," *Medscape*, Jan. 13, 2006. According to the FDA, these were marketed over the Internet and were distributed from Miami, Florida. They warned other manufacturers and suppliers may exist.

a non-narcotic sleep aid from Japan. It became associated with many mysterious deaths in the 1990s and was eventually banned. You can find out up-to-date information by going to the FDA Web site, http://www.fda.gov/medwatch, or calling 1-800-FDA-1088.

Even ones made here in America have diverse and serious risks. Recently, PC-SPES and SPES, herbs that many took for prostate health, contained warfarin (a potentially very dangerous prescription blood thinner) and alprazolam (a prescription, short-acting, Valium-like drug). There are also warnings about kava kava supplements causing liver failure in some people, even necessitating transplants. Well known Metabolife© and Cortislim© have both had multiple issues with the FDA in the past concerning false claims or their ephedra and caffeine content.

Remember, anything OTC cannot legally claim to prevent, diagnose, treat, or cure any disease and doesn't have to undergo third-party testing and approval. You really shouldn't entrust your health to a mere cashier in a vitamin shop, or maybe worst, just any Web site administrator. Lastly, supplements can dangerously interact with medications, even with other supplements. As a simple example, it is quite common foe me to discover a patient is taking way too much vitamin A once reviewing *all* their supplements. This can result in quite serious health problems such as liver failure, despite the patient believing they were trying to do themselves some good. Similar to prescription drugs, it's not *if one is good, then three should be better*, rather it should be the view of *what's the least amount of quality supplements I need to obtain my main health goals?* It is very important for your doctor to know everything you take, OTC and prescription. I recommend you bring all your bottles to every medical visit.

Physicians rarely recommend supplements to their patients. Why is this? Well, I feel a lot has to do with what's mentioned above. Physicians want to recommend treatments that are first safe and then have scientifically proven benefits. All our decisions should be evidence based. Often with supplements, the evidence doesn't all agree. But such complex decision-making should be what separates us from the other lesser-trained *health-care providers* out there today. This, and the ethics and dedication we should possess. Other contributing factors variably include their lack of knowledge of supplements, or having to spend more time learning more about these integrative modalities. Some are into it, and some aren't. You really can't blame them, as there are exponentially increasing medical discoveries made every year that makes just keeping up with contemporary medicine quite difficult. Also, insurance reimbursements for office visits have been steadily decreasing for decades while doctors' overhead has skyrocketed. This has basically forced physicians to *see* more patients each day, limiting the time of the visit, and therefore no time to adequately address all these options. Stressing this delicate balance between time constraints and quality of care is the fact that patients are now older, sicker, more medicated, and demand more. Most docs will simply defer to the safest saying, "When in doubt, cut it out."

So why do I recommend supplements? First of all, I chose family practice as a specialty because I enjoy treating the patient as a whole. Usually, this involves a long-term personal relationship that focuses on prevention. This includes counseling and follow-up on lifestyle, such as smoking cessation, various addictions, diet, exercise, and other nonmedical means to keep one healthy. Of course, these dialogues are a two-way street; I must listen to gain his trust. In medical school, it's emphasized for us to listen to our patients—they are our best teachers, after all. I never forget that. So naturally, over the past decade or so, I increasingly had more patients that felt comfortable disclosing they took supplements to prevent or help treat a chronic disease. Many wouldn't mention this to their other doctors for fear of being ridiculed or even discharged.

Usually, these patients had hypertension, arthritis, or hypercholesterolemia. Some would claim glucosamine and chondroitin sulfate would help their joints, when nothing else would. Others praised red yeast rice, garlic, and flaxseed for lowering their cholesterol, or black cherry extract for curing their gout. Patients would ask if I had heard of these or if they're safe to take with their medications. Initially, I didn't know how to answer them, as I wasn't originally trained in this, nor were there much published medical research out there. As their family physician, I felt obligated to find out; yet as a scientist, I had to remain very skeptical. I began researching the scant, inconsistent evidence available. Keeping an open mind, I tried not to prematurely discount these new modalities. Initially, my search focused on the safety and any potential drug interactions the supplement may cause. I was referring to chiropractors and physical therapists when this was still quite taboo.

Some may be wondering that if they're doing the proper diet and exercise, why is there a need to supplement at all? That's a very good question. But it's a SAD fact, the vegetables and fruits simply don't contain the vitamin and nutrient punch they had years ago. The nutrients in the soil has been washed away and used up. In today's world, it's difficult to eat enough vegetables and fruits to *supply* your body with what's optimally needed. Add to that the multiple decades' worth of pesticides, heavy metals, and other toxins that have been accumulating on Mother Earth. You may begin to appreciate this increased *demand* to help boost the repair of all these damaging effects. Remember, in the introduction I reviewed the free radical theory and its contribution to age-related degeneration. Basically, we age when the damage done to our body outpaces its repair. Or, in other words, the *demand* for free radical scavengers and building blocks surpasses the *supply*. A better, more natural paradigm would focus on *preventing* disease. Supplements, albeit with very few exceptions, are generally considered safer than most all medications. Furthermore, they work synergistically with diet and exercise, clearly a more integrative, proactive approach.

There are many supplements that, in fact, have been proven to be beneficial and safe when used appropriately. As stressed earlier, I find most can help prevent various diseases, especially when synergistically used with a healthier lifestyle. They can potentially help limit the toxicity and side effects of some drugs by supporting the drug's metabolism or by lowering the dose needed. A few of such instances will be mentioned below. There still remain the questions presented in this book's introduction:

(1) Which supplements, if any, are best at *preventing* a particular disease?
(2) Which ones are safe and effective *during* an active disease state?
(3) Which ones are helpful after a disease is *cured or stabilized*?

An example may be the use of flaxseed in prostate cancer survivors. Is it beneficial, or harmful? Lastly, I will hopefully give some knowledge and resources for you to do some private investigating on your own that's particular to your situation and goals.

A. Omega-3.
If I were to recommend only one supplement for you to take, it would have to be—you guessed it, pharmaceutical-grade fish oil. This was covered in detail earlier. Here's a quick review. Fish oil is anti-inflammatory and helps boost the immune system, both of which help many age-related diseases such as osteoarthritis and rheumatoid arthritis. The latter significantly improved with fish oil supplementation.[102] It also has antiarrhythmic property and has been shown to decrease sudden cardiac death by up to 45 percent—basically beating out any single drug out there. It lowers triglycerides and raises HDL. Combined with niacin, fish oil can lower cholesterol better than all but the highest dosing of statin drugs without any appreciable side effects as liver failure and muscle aches. These aches

---

102 According toresearch by Joel Kremer as published in *Arthritis and Rheumatism*, June 1990

can be a sign of more severe rhabdomyolysis, or muscle breakdown, which leads to kidney failure and possible death. (These effects prompted the withdrawal of Bayer's drug to treat high cholesterol, Baychol.) For people that may get a flush when taking niacin, inositol, the pro-drug to niacin, may be a better option. Fish oil alone may minimally raise LDL levels according to scant research, but this can be reversed with moderate intake of garlic.[103]

Personally, I eat a lot of roasted garlic throughout the week and take 1000 mg of inositol before bedtime. My cholesterol went from 285 to under 200. HDL increased from 48 to 85. Triglycerides are now under 50 and my LDL under 100. I do have a positive family history—my dad had a heart attack and died at fifty-nine. Both parents have, or had, hypertension. Despite this high risk, my blood pressure is fine and, although I could get free samples of all the statin drugs I want, I much prefer the safer integrative means I recommend to my patients. I should practice what I preach, right? I'll bet my life on it!

This reinforces the evolutionary basis and subsequent recommendation of a balanced diet—as the Mediterranean Diet mentioned earlier, which includes a lot of fish, olive oil, and garlic. Back in 2002, the American Heart Association updated its recommendations to include the daily intake of the equivalent of 1 gram of fish oil. There is even some data from the Physician's Health Study and the GISSI-Prevention trial to suggest keeping your omega-3 index, the percentage of total red blood cell fatty acids comprised of EPA and DHA fatty acids, above 8 percent. This is especially true if you are at risk of sudden cardiac death. Fish oil may be a viable safe option for those *aspirin nonresponders*, or those allergic to aspirin, desiring an alternative for coronary disease prevention.

Alone or with higher doses of vitamin E and C, fish oil has been shown to help prevent all dementias by 40 percent.[104] This makes sense when you consider our brain is *two-thirds* fat. If more pro-inflammatory fats are assimilated, we're predisposed to such degenerative diseases such as dementia, Parkinson's disease, multiple sclerosis, and more. Alternately, when the fat possesses more anti-inflammatory properties, there is less free radical damage, plaque formation, and cholesterol-related pathology that typify these conditions. Important to note, the blood has

---

103 According to research by Adam Adler and published in the *American Journal of Clinical Nutrition*, 1997: 65.

104 This is according to a study on nine hundred participants in the Framingham Heart Study examined during 1986 to 1990 and presented to the American Heart Association by Dr. Schaefer.

only about *5 percent* fat. So routinely consume dietary fish or take pharmaceutical-grade fish oil supplements, especially if a child or fertile woman.

Its anti-inflammatory properties also help many other diseases such as COPD and irritable bowel syndrome, as presented earlier in the section devoted to just fish oil. One gram daily has been shown to have a 69 percent success rate in helping those suffering from clinical depression.[105] There are basically no risks or side effects, very unlike changing any dose of prescription antidepressants.

Well, all this shouldn't be mind-boggling; as it's been said many times, "Fish is brain food" and "Take your cod liver oil each day!" It's nice to finally see research that bears out what previous generations have advised. As far as interactions with other medications are concerned, they may be only a few. Fish oil naturally keeps inflammation down and thereby limits pathologically "sticky" blood components. While fish oil doesn't pathologically *thin* the blood, it may cause typical blood thinners such as aspirin, vitamin E and C, and Coumadin to have more effect. Because of this, I urge caution in patients taking these, observing for any signs of increased bruising. If the person is on Coumadin, I recommend they monitor their blood work more closely. Obviously, if you're allergic to fish, you'll probably react to fish oil too. You may need to entertain other options, as mentioned below.

B. Other Omegas such as Borage, Primrose Oil, or Flaxseed. A few caveats about this, the first being that these need to go through a few steps to convert to the most usable and beneficial forms of the omegas, namely, DHA and EPA. (Please review figure 3.7, Fatty Acid Metabolism.) As people age, get chronic diseases, and take multiple medications, their bodies may not perform the necessary conversions. Second, most valid research has been done specifically on fish oil, not these other omega-3 precursors. Not all omegas are the same, so it's improper to simply extrapolate this data to all the other omega sources. Third, flaxseed may aggravate an enlarged prostate, so I generally don't recommend that men take it. Yet, for men that are allergic to fish, or simply can't stand taking fish oil, it may be an okay option. I must add that fish oil does come in a variety of concentrations with natural fruit flavors, and in gel capsule or liquid forms. Personally, I prefer the gel capsule, but my children like the orange-flavored, refrigerated liquid variety.

---

105 This is according to research in the October 2002, *Archives of General Psychiatry by* H. Peet. Also, *Primary* Psychiatry 11, no. 7 (2004):15–16. COPD is the same as emphysema. See the diet chapter on fish oil for more detail and references.

What about the dosing of fish oil? As stressed earlier, make sure it's pharmaceutical grade or GMP certified. Still, the concentrations of EPA and DHA can vary depending on the preparations and manufacturer. The dosing depends on what you're wishing to accomplish. For routine *prevention* of heart and mind conditions, I recommend about 250 mg of DHA and 350 mg of EPA daily. I find DHA to be more important for mind, neurological, and mood concerns. In cases of dementia, neuropathy, or ADHD, I may recommend a higher DHA component. EPA tends to have more anti-inflammatory actions, so I may substantially increase this for rheumatic or arthritic conditions. How much of an increase depends on clinical factors and response. By adding SAM-E, I can usually obtain superior and a much safer results than with aspirin and NSAIDs. This may help to also lower the dose of DMARDs (disease-modifying antirheumatic drugs), the newer drugs for rheumatism, and their resulting toxicities.[106] As mentioned before, there are specific blood tests to measure various omega fat levels and ratios. These may be useful when we need to get higher concentrations of EPA or DHA in the body.

C. Vitamin C—Ascorbic Acid.

C is mostly known for its important role in collagen synthesis. Remember learning in grade school how the early sailors got scurvy? It's also a very important antioxidant and protects fatty acid degradation. Involved with the synthesis of many neurotransmitters, C also has an integral role with many important chemical reactions involving iron, copper, and a wide array of peptides. For optimal amounts, I generally recommend 1000 mg maximum daily. Together with zinc, this probably helps your immune system to a degree. Linus Pauling, recipient of two Nobel Prizes and the son of an American druggist, is usually given the credit and has the reputation for recommending much higher amounts. Adding some credence to other possible benefits, research found individuals with the highest level of vitamin C had about a 25 percent lower prevalence of *Helicobacter pylori* infections. This is the bacteria that causes many stomach ulcers and increases risks for stomach cancer.[107] Such infections with *H. pylori* or *Cytomegalovirus* may further increase your risks for stroke and coronary disease. On the other hand, I've seen a few patients that have gone through an extensive workup for vague symptoms; yet once they confessed to taking megadoses and stopped, they got better. It's not true that if you're taking one of something does good, then taking two is even mo' better. Again, because of the inherent synergy occurring in nature, I believe it is more beneficial and safer to just take one good

---

106 Sam-E (s-adenosyl methionine), a natural anti-inflammatory molecule that's OTC in America. NSAID (nonsteroidal anti-inflammatory drug) as Aleve or Advil. DMARD (disease modifying antirheumatic drug) as Embrel, Remicade, or methotrexate.

107 August 2003 issue of the *Journal of the American College of Nutrition.*

pharmaceutical-grade multivitamin daily than to gulp down a few megadoses of supposed magic bullets. Although with good intentions, excess intake of one vitamin can have detrimental effects on the absorption and excretion of others. This practice can even lead to increased oxidative damage and distinct disease states—what we're trying to prevent.

More pertinent to men's health, recent research studied a small number of infertile men aged twenty-five to thirty-five years old. After the subjects received 1000 mg of vitamin C twice per day for two months, their mean sperm count, motility, and morphology improved.[108] As concluded, such supplementation in infertile men might have a role in improving semen quality toward conception. Maybe C helps both seaman *and* semen.

D. Vitamin D. Really a provitamin that is converted to its active form by the sun's ultraviolet rays, D comes from plant and animal sources. The latter is a product of cholesterol and is the most important. Calcitriol, the active version, relies on healthy liver and kidney function. Until recently, D has mostly gone unnoticed because of the old belief routine sun exposure is enough to get all you need. Because of such, Vitamin D receives my Rodney Dangerfield's *I Get No Respect* Award.

You may be surprised vitamin D has gained more importance than calcium in preventing and treating osteoporosis—the bone loss that contributes to the frailty syndrome. You may say, "What do I care about osteoporosis. Men don't get that!" You would be wrong, bucko. In fact, men *do* get osteoporosis; but because of their initial higher bone mass compared to women's, it appears about ten years later on the average.[109] Also, women generally live longer than men, increasing their chance of becoming frail in their latter years. Understandably, if you're planning to live a long time, you want to have healthy bones to go with it. One-fifth of those suffering from osteoporosis are men, and it appears they're sicker overall. You don't want to become that frail Mr. Magoo I spoke about earlier.

Men's risk for osteoporosis is increased with history of smoking and steroid medications, including shots for conditions such as allergies, asthma, colitis, and

---

108 M. Akmal, "Improvement in human semen quality after oral supplementation of Vitamin C," *Journal of Medicinal Food,* September 2006.

109 National Osteoporosis Foundation, "Osteoporosis in men: Fast Facts on osteoporosis." More information may be available at http://www.nof.org. Accessed November 2006.

arthritis. Recently, according to the Malmo Preventative Project that prospectively studied over twenty-two thousand men for decades, the biggest risk factor for disabling fractures was diabetes. This is another reason to prevent such metabolic disorders while in midlife.

More unknown, yet more profound, vitamin D deficiency can also contribute to autoimmune diseases such as rheumatoid arthritis, and even worse, cardiovascular disease.[110] As we age, these quite common and increasingly disabling conditions usually require multiple risky medications and procedures. Low D also increases risk for many diverse cancers in men.[111] According to a recent VA study involving three thousand veterans, proper intake of vitamin D and cereal fiber helped reduce serious colon cancers. Other researchers are hopeful D may play a preventive role in prostate cancer. I recommend 1000 iU daily for routine maintenance.

Obviously, I believe it's most important to find the proper diagnosis and contributing factors, thereby affording effective and safer treatments. If you think you suffer or may be at risk for any of the above, then ask your doctor to check your 25-hydroxyvitamin D level with any other workup she may recommend. You should have a level above 35 ng/dl. If below, then aggressive replacement with vitamin D_3 is warranted. Since this information has just come to light over the past year, I have discovered and successfully treated many vitamin D deficient patients with recalcitrant fibromyalgia-like symptoms and osteoporosis.

E. Vitamin E includes the gambit of isomers known as the tocopherols and tocotrienols. The absorption of E can vary widely especially those with impaired fat absorption. This may result from bariatric surgery or from gastritis of old age. Its main function as an antioxidant is to protect intracellular liposomes and mitochondria from oxidation. You can get by with lower doses of E if you take supplemental ascorbic acid and beta-carotene because of the synergy. Yet, with increased polyunsaturated fat intake, the need may be increased. Since also being part of the glutathione peroxidase system that limits free radical damage, increased E supplementation may help people with low selenium. Although there are stronger antioxidants than E, its high concentration in so many different tissues makes it relatively more important. Its popularized role in preventing coronary disease

---

110 M. Holick, "Vitamin D: Important for Prevention of Osteoporosis, Cardiovascular Heart Disease, Type 1 Diabetes, Autoimmune Diseases, and Some Cancers," *Southern Medical Journal* 98, no. 10 (2005): 1024–27.

111 E. Giovannucci, *Journal of the National Cancer Institute.* 98 (2006):428–30, 451–59. For each 25 nmol/L lower level, the risk for cancer mortality decreased 29 percent.

is rooted in its protective role in reducing many inflammatory and atherogenic mediators.[112] Its other secondary but vitally important roles include sex hormone synthesis, fertility, and proper immune function.

Researchers collecting data from the Cache County Study, a very large population-based investigation on Alzheimer's and other dementias, found a reduction in such risk when subjects took supplements containing larger doses vitamin E and C together. As mentioned above, people who took both vitamins E and C were less likely to develop Alzheimer's disease, although varied doses were used. Vitamin C works quite synergistically with vitamin E. For *treatment* of dementia, reflecting the higher doses used in this research, the recommended vitamin E intake may be as high as two grams daily. However, I have yet to recommend that high a dose because of possible pro-inflammatory concerns and the equivocal data. I usually promote 400 to 800 units per day, tops.

Recently, there have been a lot of challenges to the long-held belief that vitamin E supplementation is beneficial. Most of this came from the HOPE-2 Trial published in 2005.[113] Basically, it surprisingly concluded *high-risk* cardiac subjects that *reported* taking 400 units daily of vitamin E had no difference in the incidence of cancer or cancer deaths. Furthermore, there were higher risks and hospitalization rates for heart failure. This definitely contradicted many previous long-term trials that used a large number of subjects, though those studied were healthier. This would include the Nurses' Health Study and earlier published research.[114]

So what's my take on all this? I eluded many times earlier, it may be that some modalities used to *prevent* a disease in an otherwise healthy individual may not necessarily be what's appropriate for a sicker, older individual with chronic disease(s). For example, I wouldn't tell a patient suffering from unstable angina to go out and start an exercise program. Naturally, that would put him at risk of suddenly dying from a heart attack. But, in fact, if he was more *proactive* with diet and exercise

---

112 Less phospholipase and lipoxygenase reactions, and reduced thromboxane production.

113 HOPE and HOPE-TOO trial investigators, "Effects of Long-Term Vitamin E Supplementation on Cardiovascular in Events and Cancer: A Randomized Controlled Trial," *JAMA* 293, no. 11 (2005): 1138–47.

114 Rimm, using about forty thousand men, published in *New England Journal of Medicine* 1993: 328 (20); and Knekt, using about five thousand healthy Finish men and women thirty to sixty-nine years old, published in the *American Journal of Epidemiology* 139, no. 12 (1994)..

years before, he probably wouldn't have severe heart disease in the first place. In addition, once his heart condition was *reactively* stabilized through pills or surgery, exercise and diet would be critical to his long-term health and survival.

Some proponents for vitamin E reply it's the quality and quantity of the varying tocopherol isomers, *alpha* to *gamma*, that's important. This plausible point wasn't addressed in the HOPE and HOPE-TOO trials. From what I have read on vitamin E, I believe doses of 400 units probably do have anti-inflammatory properties for healthy individuals. However, a higher dose may possess pro-inflammatory effects in the sickly. (This was also suggested when lung cancer patients took vitamin E and experienced a worse prognosis.) Again, I believe there are no magic bullets, and it's better to take a wide assortment of low dose vitamins with resulting synergism. Pair this with a healthy lifestyle, and you're all set. Reinforcing this is research showing beneficial effects of vitamin E, mostly alpha-tocopherol, in preventing bladder cancer.[115] This elusive, silent cause of death of about thirteen thousand Americans annually is also the fourth biggest killer cancer of men. Obviously, it's much better to prevent carcinogenesis and heart disease in the first place. That's probably the *convergence of evidence,* as it stands right now.

As a cautionary addendum, both vitamins C and E can "thin" the blood, so watch for increased risk of bleeding especially if you're on aspirin or NSAIDs such as Aleve or Advil, fish oil, or many herbs that can thin the blood such as St. John's wort or ginkgo biloba. Extreme caution should be taken if you're on blood thinners such as Coumadin or Plavix. You may be asked to stop these to help prevent excess bleeding when undergoing a surgical procedure.

F. Folate and B$_{12}$ are very important for proper nerve function and red blood cell production when low, *irreversible* neuropathy; pernicious anemia; brain dysfunction including dementia; and many more serious consequences can happen. However, mildly deficient symptoms can vary widely and can be quite vague. Most have to do with symptoms of fatigue, and nutritional and neurological complaints. Levels are heavily influenced by diet, hereditary factors, and drugs. B$_{12}$ and folate work synergistically in the varied synthesis and delicate balance of many integral proteins throughout the body.

---

115 E. Jacobs, "Vitamin C and vitamin E supplement use and bladder cancer mortality in a large cohort of U.S. men and women," *Am J Epidemiol* 156, no. 11 (2002): 1002–10.

Now in the old days, it was common for Marcus Welby-like doctors to treat elderly patients with such nonspecific complaints of fatigue with a monthly B_{12} shot. This was basically based on subjective evidence, meaning that patient's reported improved overall well-being and the shots—well, they're quite cheap and benign. At any rate, for those few needy, difficult-to-treat patients, this offered relief and an opportunity to get things off their chest and get some attention. This eventually fell out of favor though, with newer doctors' increased dependence on lab work, which would typically show only low-normal, but nonetheless *still normal,* B_{12} levels.[116] Most third-party payers, including Medicare, either severely discounted such shots (actually paying only a few cents if the deficiency is so severe it causes pernicious anemia) or stopped paying for them altogether. As ridiculous it may seem, Medicare and most insurances don't deem it medically necessary to check for this easily treatable cause of irreversible neuropathy and dementia.

More recently, there's research reinforcing the importance of maintaining optimal folate and B_{12} levels. About one-fourth of people over sixty develop significant B_{12} deficiency.[117] Because of the current folate fortification in our food, doctors may not see the enlarged red blood cell size in the blood work that typifies *pernicious anemia.* Because of this, the deficiency can be easily missed. Despite an estimated third of the population suffers from low folic acid, those with even proper levels may *mask* low B_{12} symptoms. This can lead to permanent neuropathy—the loss of proper nerve function. I recommend virtually all elderly patients should be on supplemental B complex vitamins as there is basically no downside.

Since 2004, the National Academy of Sciences has urged older people to meet their recommended daily B_{12} intake through supplements. This is based on the fact that long-standing B_{12} deficiency is associated with irreversible cognitive decline. Reinforcing this position was a small study where elderly patients low in B_{12} with cognitive impairment, receiving B_{12} supplementation, significant improved.[118] The effect was better in those with short-term cognitive impairment. Probably the

---

116 Range is from about 250 to 1000 ng/dl. If you get a value of 275, most doctors will say this is normal. It isn't, it's a D minus.

117 According to Dr. Ralph Green, speaking at the 2004 Annual Meeting of the American Association for Clinical Chemistry as presented in *Family Practice News*, January 1, 2004, by M. Zoler.

118 *Journal of American Geriatric Society* 40, no. 2 (1992):168–72. Eleven out of eighteen elderly geriatric patients low in B_{12} with cognitive impairment receiving intramuscular B_{12} supplementation had significant improvement in their cognitive scoring as presented in same *Family Practice News* (2004).

most widely known serious health risk of low folate is neural tube defects in the developing fetus. In addition, the risk for depression, worsening depression, and lack of response to antidepressant therapy have been linked to low B_{12} and folate.

Major sources of folate are leafy green vegetables and fortified bread. B_{12} is derived from meat sources; therefore, vegetarians are at risk of becoming deficient. As we age, our risk for atrophic gastritis increases. Subsequently, B_{12} and folate absorption by the stomach is compromised. If you add improper diet and heavy alcohol use, levels are compromised even further. If on an H2-blocker drug such as Zantac or Pepcid, or a proton pump inhibitor such as Prilosec or Nexium, your acid production is diminished. This further impairs the absorption of these nutrients. Iron too. A high index of suspicion should be used in those with intestinal bacterial overgrowth or possible malabsorption like in Crohn's disease. I routinely supplement all patients with any of the above risks with oral B complex vitamins. When you can't absorb oral B_{12} well because of the lack of intrinsic factor production by the stomach, pernicious anemia (literally "bad" anemia) occurs. If mild, this can still be overcome with oral B_{12} supplementation, although higher amounts are generally needed.[119] However, monthly shots may be needed.

When testing for levels, it's important to note that "normal" lab values for B_{12} and folate can vary widely. Normal B_{12} levels can range from about 250–1000 pg/mL. I have seen many patients with lab work from other physicians showing a level of 280, and who were told this was normal. I disagree and recommend an *optimal* range above 1000. I normally shoot for folate levels above 24 ng/ml. I especially suggest these higher levels for those with central or peripheral nerve disease.

Supplementation with folate, vitamin B_{12}, and vitamin B_6 helps reduce homocysteine (Hyc) levels and theoretically reduce risk for cardiovascular events. According to newer research by Schnyder published in *JAMA* 2002, supplementation produced lower rates of mortality and nonfatal myocardial infarction, as well as reduced the need for revascularization procedures in those *at risk*. This reinforced two of the earlier landmark trials back in 1997 that studied patients for about five years, and mostly confirmed this relationship.

As a background, Dr. Kilmer McCully truly faced an uphill battle back in 1969 when he first introduced in the *American Journal of Pathology* homocysteine's pos-

---

119 C. Butler, "Oral vitamin B_{12} versus intramuscular vitamin B_{12} for vitamin B_{12} deficiency: A systemic review of randomized controlled trials," *Family Practice* 23 (2006): 279–85.

sible role in heart disease. To make a long story short, much as the first doctor promoting laparoscopy or the first suggesting that an infection can cause stomach ulcers, he was discredited and basically excommunicated from the entire medical academic community. Unfortunately, such disbelief, cynicism, and ridicule are common when introducing new ideas to such large conservative groups such as the medical establishment, which is heavily influenced by political and financial supporters. Similarly, physicians and small groups promoting a more integrative approach in preventing the profound consequences of aging often face unfounded ridicule from their contemporary cohorts who profit better in today's more invasive, reactive medical atmosphere. Hey, the ERs and ORs are overcrowded. Why is that so?

As they say, to each his own. I believe it only takes a passionate few to effectively start a paradigm shift. I hope it catches on, for all our sakes. Speaking for myself as a family physician, this outlook definitely makes life more interesting and meaningful. By the way, it took until the mid-1990s for the Physicians Health and Framingham Heart studies to show a direct correlation between Hyc levels and heart disease. McCully was finally vindicated by being labeled the Father of Homocysteine! For more interesting readings on this topic, I recommend *The Heart Revolution: The Extraordinary Discovery That Finally Laid the Cholesterol Myth to Rest* by Kilmer McCully, MD.

The big push today is still Cholesterol! Cholesterol! Cholesterol! I would like to know how much money drug firms have made in the past decades on these statin drugs costing about three bucks a pop. Yet, half of those suffering myocardial infarctions have relatively *good* cholesterol levels. Common sense would say there must be more to it, right? I believe there are many modifiable risk factors—not so much just LDL cholesterol, but the amount of *inflamed* LDL cholesterol. More predictive are the ratios of triglycerides, HDL, and subfractions such as apolipoprotein(b).

Further relaying the possible deleterious effects from high homocysteine levels was research published in *JAMA* March 12, 2003. Heart-healthy patients from the Framingham Study with levels in the upper 50 percent were twice as likely to get congestive heart failure (CHF) than those in the lower half. However, being an observational study, this doesn't address if methods to lower levels—say, with folate replacement—would necessarily lower risks for CHF. The elderly, especially men, have higher Hyc levels. This may be due to the beneficial effects estrogen has in women. Hyc is a sulfur-containing amino acid that undergoes oxidation.

In theory, this produces damage to the coronary vessel wall and the nearby myo-cardial cells.

In the May 13, 2004, article in the *New England Journal of Medicine* entitled "Homocysteine Levels and the Risk of Osteoporotic Fracture," an increased level was a strong *independent* risk factor for this disabling fracture in older men, *regardless* of bone mineral density. Hyc—it's bad to the bone.

I usually recommend lowering Hyc levels to below 9 micromoles per liter or so. Artificial elevation of Hyc can occur if there are delays in processing blood work or when collected nonfasting after a protein-rich meal. Elevated levels may be an indication of kidney failure. Additionally, some drugs that may increase levels include methotrexate, trimethoprim, L-dopa, hydrochlorothiazide, and antiepileptic drugs.

G. Coenzyme Q_{10} (CoQ_{10}).

Also known as ubiquinone, this fat-soluble vitamin is quite popular as it accounted for over $200 million in sales back in 2002. Isolated in the late 1950s by Dr. Folkers at Merck, it is vital to many intracellular metabolic activities directly related to energy production. Additionally possessing antioxidant properties, CoQ_{10} has been investigated worldwide for a number of degenerative and age-related conditions that are neurological and cardiac in nature. As all supplements in the United States, it's not FDA approved to prevent, treat, or cure any disease. In Japan, it has been investigated since the 1960s and approved for congestive heart failure treatment since the 1970s.

Without getting into a lot of intricate biochemistry, CoQ_{10} is vitally important for energy production within the mitochondria, organelles found in most all cells. The mitochondria are analogous to the batteries for the cell; they provide the energy needed to run the many necessary intracellular reactions, as well as sustaining cellular life itself. CoQ_{10} is one of the most important coenzymes needed in the electron transport mechanism used for aerobic respiration, resulting in the production of adenosine triphosphate (ATP). ATP is basically the *energy currency* of the cell, as it is the breaking of this triphosphate bond that forms ADP (adenosine diphosphate). This provides the needed energy. You get 32 ATP molecules from 1 molecule of glucose from the oxidative phosphorylation process, which takes place in the inner mitochondrial membrane.

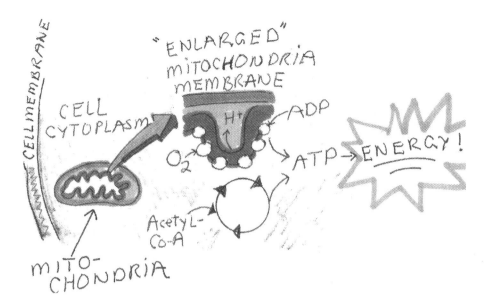

Figure 6.1. Inside the mitochondrion, CoQ10 helps convert chemical bonds to produce energy (ATP). Much like a battery, the mitochondria leak some energy (heat) during this process.

A few further points worth mentioning: One, the rate of this oxidative phosphorylation is determined by the need for ATP, or energy production. The entry of ADP into the mitochondria requires the exit of ATP, which is coordinated by ATP-ADP translocase, an enzyme carrier located in the inner mitochondrial membrane. So there are many intricate demand and supply relationships for different raw materials. Another point is that this energy production is somewhat inherently *leaky,* meaning there is an appreciable amount of free radical production. This quality increases risks for damaging all the intracellular components.

This can be compared to the surrounding heat produced by the internal combustion engine in your automobile—no matter how efficient it is. Surely, this generated energy must have a way to escape the engine compartment, namely, via the radiator, coolant, and fan. This cooling system's components must function together properly, or the whole vehicle could burn up—*rapid* oxidation. Additionally, when more fuel is forced through the engine, much as when your body takes in too much food, there is more of this oxidative damage produced. It makes sense that coenzyme Q_{10} would have some antioxidant properties to help protect the mitochondria from burning itself up.

The number of mitochondria in a cell correlates with its usual energy demands. For example, in the strong bicep muscle, there are approximately 500 per cell. You may be surprised to find that in a heart cell, there may be 5,000 or more! When you think about it, your heart is always active, using energy constantly, right? I hope so, for your sake. Either it's *relaxing* to fill up with blood, or it's *contracting* to pump blood to the rest of the body. Relaxing isn't resting though. Amazingly, it actually takes *more* energy for muscles to relax than to contract! This may not make sense at first, but think about it this way: Once we die, there's no more energy production and our muscles get stiff. Rigor mortis sets in. So muscles need energy, or ATP, in order to appropriately relax. This relaxing is very important especially when it comes to proper heart function.

The heart is basically a pump that must first expand and be filled with a certain volume of blood. If the heart is young and pliable, it can fill with a good volume. This is called the *diastolic* function. Then, the heart needs to pump this volume with a good coordinated reboundlike contraction—the *systolic* function. Conversely, in the older, stiffer heart, the stroke volume diminishes; so the heart has to contract even harder and pump faster to maintain the same cardiac output. The mathematical equation is:

$$\text{Cardiac Output} = \text{Heart Rate} \times \text{Stroke Volume}$$

Note: In order to keep output the same with less volume, the heart rate must then go up. To accomplish this, the overactive stimulation of many diverse neurohormonal systems involving adrenaline, renin, and many others take place.

Thus, the energy *demand* of the heart increases starting the self-defeating cycle of dysfunction, or congestive heart failure (CHF). As a matter of fact, early *diastolic dysfunction* can be elusive to diagnose early on, yet eventually progresses to include frank *systolic dysfunction*. Furthermore, the innermost side of the heart experiences increased pressure, as explained by Laplace's law, which further depletes the blood *supply* of oxygen, glucose, and the ability to rid lactic acid buildup.[120] This further increases the risk for myocardial infarction.

So it makes sense that optimal coenzyme Q_{10} levels help with the overall health and energy balance of the heart, matching ATP supply with the demand, all the while protecting it from oxidative damage. How much CoQ_{10} do I recommend

---

120 Basically, the greater the radius and the pressure inside the heart, the more tension there is in the heart muscle wall. This constricts vessel blood flow. See http://library. thinkquest.org under Laplace's Law for more insight.

people take? Well, it depends on the purpose. For younger, healthy individuals with a moderately active lifestyle, I would say 60 mg or more twice daily. For athletes with stronger energy requirements and reparation, I would probably almost double that. There is some suggestion that unexplained sudden death in athletes may be attributed to depleted coenzyme Q_{10} levels, be it caused by an arrhythmia or sudden heart attack.

On the other end of the spectrum is the older person suffering a variable severity of CHF. You may wonder how I diagnose *early CHF* in someone without any appreciable symptoms. Mainly I look at the risks—over forty-five years old, having hypertension, family history, alcoholism, obesity, shortness of breath, glucose intolerance, or other metabolic and hormonal disturbances. Besides an obvious stress test, there's also lab work done for cholesterol and electrolytes. A CHF marker, *beta natiuretic peptide*, may be elevated. I usually correlate this with an echocardiogram, which produces dynamic ultrasound images that can assess the pumping action, valve function, and wall thickness of the heart. Typically, early diastolic dysfunction shows minimally if there is any associated reduction in systolic function or ejection fraction, yet displays the decreased stroke volume with stiffened ventricular walls. Almost all patients I see with these early CHF findings were inappropriately told by their doctor, radiologist, or even cardiologist that the test came out "normal." It is a shame, too, because a lot can be done at this earlier point and help slow progression of severe CHF.

For those with moderate to severe CHF, I usually start out replacing with 100 mg coenzyme Q_{10} twice per day. I will then follow up with lab work in about a month specifically measuring CoQ_{10} levels, shooting for a level above 3.5 ng/dl. Of course, all the risk factors mentioned above should also be dealt with accordingly using individualized medical and nonmedical means. This includes appropriate hormonal analysis and replacement when appropriate. However, the focus of this book is on midlife, therefore, my emphasis on the prevention or detection of *early* CHF. There's some equivocal research on the benefits of coenzyme Q_{10} when it comes to CHF, but overall I believe it's a good adjunct to proper medical therapy and lifestyle improvement but, by no means, a replacement. On the upside though, there are basically no appreciable side effects or drug interactions.

A rather interesting history exists about CoQ_{10}. Supposedly, it all began when Merck first began investigating simvastatin—now the commonly prescribed cholesterol-lowering statin drug named Zocor—and noticed lower CoQ_{10} levels in muscle. Their initial drug called Zedia (not the new drug by Merck similarly named Zetia) appropriately combined coenzyme Q_{10} with simvastatin in order to help offset this abnormality. For some reason, they decided to drop CoQ_{10} and just went with the single drug. Some research suggest that the most common side effects of statin drug therapy—muscle aches, fatigue, liver inflammation, and mental changes—may be ameliorated or prevented with coenzyme Q_{10} supplementation.[121]

As a review, *all* statin drugs may cause a spectrum of muscle pathology, ranging from benign myalgia (basically only achy muscles) to myositis (muscle inflammation that can be objectively determined by CPK levels in the blood) to life-threatening rhabdomyolysis. The latter is caused by the muscle's toxic breakdown product, myoglobin, on the kidneys. The resulting cases of kidney failure and death of some patients in combination with cholesterol-lowering therapy with Baychol prompted Bayer to pull it from the market. Yet, not all statin drugs are the same. The vast majority of individuals with the proper routine follow-up and lab work are quite tolerant and do well with statin drug therapy. These do a great job lowering LDL cholesterol and in all probability save countless lives. Don't stop them unless you talk to your doctor about it. On a related issue, CoQ_{10} has also been shown to lower the cardiotoxicity of a common yet risky cancer treatment drug named Adriamycin.

Coenzyme Q_{10} is called ubiquinone because of its presence in virtually all tissues in the body. It is found not only in the heart, but especially the kidney, liver, pancreas, brain, and colon. It's ubiquitous. According to *American Family Physician*, CoQ_{10} appears promising for help with neurodegenerative disorders such as Parkinson's disease and other neuromuscular conditions. They also consider it safe with low drug-interaction potential. For us guys whose *boys* may be getting lazy, some research suggests it also helps with infertility. Since it may lower the "stickiness" of pathologically inflamed platelets, I would add some caution if taken with a blood thinner like Coumadin. Women should avoid this if pregnant, as there's no research on this matter.

I must add that some of the research indicating some benefit, as in those with Parkinson's, used uncommonly high amounts—as much as 1600 mg per day. Not cheap but, on the other hand, neither are these diseases. For further interesting reading on the history and research on this interesting supplement, I recommend *The Coenzyme Q_{10} Phenomenon* written by world-renowned cardiologist and lec-

---

121 P. Kelly did a pilot study as presented at the annual meeting of the American College of Cardiology and in the article: "Coenzyme Q_{10} relieved statin induced pain family practice news," June 1, 2005.

turer of integrative methods, Dr. Stephen T. Sinatra. No relationship to Frank, but he also believes that "fairy tales can come true … if you're young at heart." CoQ_{10} may help accomplish this.

H. Sam-E (S-adenosyl methionine) is a favorite supplement of mine that safely helps chronic arthritis and chronic pain syndromes. It's a natural antioxidant found in our bodies that's needed for adequate nervous system functioning, including the brain. Therefore, it's not really an herb or such. Relating back to the synergism of all vitamins, deficiencies in B_{12} and folate have been found to lower Sam-E levels. Numerous studies, such as DiPadova's research published in the *American Journal of Medicine* in 1987, found it to be as effective as Advil in relieving pain and inflammation.[122] In more recent research, Sam-E resulted in similar pain scoring as NSAID use, but with fewer adverse affects.[123] I like the fact it doesn't carry the serious risk of gastrointestinal bleeding associated with NSAID use. It is estimated that approximately eighteen thousand Americans die from this annually. That's about half as many that die annually from handguns. That's a pretty dire statistic and many don't have any warning. Such GI bleeding risk is increased with alcohol use and advanced age. Yet, the FDA says it's okay for Advil and Aleve to be OTC.

Now, for some needed clarification: *All* NSAIDs, from Advil and Aleve to Vioxx and Celebrex, carry the *class effect* of increased risk for worsening hypertension, asthma, liver and kidney disease, and more. For the past five years since learning about the benefits and safety of Sam-E, I have recommended it instead of NSAIDs. I may add fish oil for the inflammatory pain from osteoarthritis, rheumatoid arthritis, and other rheumatologic conditions such as psoriatic arthritis, ankylosing spondylitis, polymyalgia rheumatica, fibromyalgia, chronic fatigue syndrome, and myofascial pain syndrome. In most cases, this combination allowed the cessation or a lower dose of these riskier rheumatologic drugs. There are even some animal studies that showed Sam-E *prevented* osteoarthritis. These are good options, especially since Vioxx and Celebrex have fallen out of favor.

Studies have reported Sam-E to be up to three times *quicker* to improve mood and *just as effective* as prescription antidepressants.[124] Low levels of Sam-E are seen

---

122 DiPadova's research published in the *American Journal of Medicine* 83 (1987).

123 Soekin studied a meta-analysis of Sam-E's safety and effectiveness in osteoarthritis published in the *Journal of Family Practice* 51 (2002).

124 Brown et al. in *Clinical Practice of Alternative Medicine* (2000):1; and *Psychiatric Annals* (2002):32. The latter point was also concluded by Hardy et al. in the *Agency for Healthcare Research Quality* (2002) publication 02-E034.

with low levels of serotonin, which is a hallmark of depression. Most new prescription antidepressants work on this latter deficiency. Some studies have even found it to lower migraine headache intensity.[125] Others saw improved cognition in Alzheimer's disease patients.

Sam-E's side effect profile is similar to placebo. It doesn't have the severe side effects of prescription antidepressant drugs such as weight gain, sexual dysfunction, worsening of mood, and more. Of course, people with chronic pain or inflammatory diseases have severely increased risks for depression. Such depression, even if mild, usually lowers pain threshold in the individual, which in turn only serves to intensify pain. Thus, this cycle usually worsens if not broken. I feel very fortunate, and my patients do too, that we know of a proven, safe alternative to typical NSAIDs that treats both the depression and pain components of such debilitating diseases.

Further increasing my favor of this supplement is its additional liver support properties. Here's a substance that not only helps pain and depression, but also actually *benefits* the liver. Most pain pills do the exact opposite. It's as if it were an actor; it would exclaim, "I have come to praise the liver, not to bury it!" Studies by Mato in 1999 concluded Sam-E even decreased the hepatic injury associated with alcoholic cirrhosis.

Sam-E is reputed to be the most prescribed anti-inflammatory in Europe. Here in America, it is available without a prescription. It is OTC, which is both good and bad. Good, because you don't need a prescription. Bad, because it's not FDA regulated so you don't know if you're getting the real thing or the right amounts. Try to get the best grade you can. I recommend Nature Made, dosed usually 200 to 400 mg maximum twice per day. It's not that cheap; but considering the multiple beneficial and safe effects it has on such disabling severe and elusive diseases, it's a bargain. Use caution in bipolar illnesses, and its effects have not been studied in pregnancy or lactation. You guys don't have to worry about the latter conditions.

I. Glucosamine and Chondroitin Sulfite. Most supplement aficionados are aware of the safe, beneficial effects these have in osteoarthritis (OA), although the American College of Rheumatology doesn't. In a meta-analysis, there was less joint-space narrowing and less pain with greater mobility in as little as four

---

125 Gatto 1986. More can be found at the Agency for Healthcare Research and Quality at www.ahrq.gov, accessed 9/07.

weeks of use.[126] The dosages studied ranged from 200 to 2000 mg daily; and most importantly, adverse reactions were comparable to placebo.

Even more promising outcomes were noted for follow-up OA patients on glucosamine for three years. Their risk of receiving lower limb joint replacement within the next five years was halved. Additionally, the treated group enjoyed better overall health status and functioning with less pain and required less health-related expense and resources.[127] Glucosamine is generally thought to work by promoting anabolism (the building up) and diminishing catabolism (the breaking down) of joint tissues. This may be mediated through its inhibitory effects on metalloproteases, other related free radical generation, and pro-inflammatory mediators. I believe glucosamine and chondroitin are quite safe and worthy of a trial in patients with mild to moderate OA who still possess a good amount of cartilage. Those with sulfa allergies or on blood thinners should use caution. I would additionally recommend they first try Sam-E and fish oil as options.

J. Probiotics and Irritable Bowel Syndrome. Again, there are volumes written about various supplements. I'm only trying to give you some introduction on the pertinent ones I've found to be effective and safe. Such is the case with probiotics. Most lay persons and most doctors aren't familiar with these. First, I'll give a little background in order to appreciate what these are all about. *Probiotic* means "for life" in Latin. Outside the body, *inside* it, and especially throughout the gastro-intestinal system, there are lots of germs, both the good, the bad, and, well, not the ugly, but yeast. Optimally, this neighborhood gets along well and there are no problems. There's a proper balance.

Women are usually more knowledgeable about when this goes awry. They often get a yeast infection when put on antibiotics. In this case, the antibiotic (Latin: "against life") kills the bacteria, disturbing this delicate balance, and lets the yeast proliferate unchecked. Most gals know taking *Lactobacillus acidophilus* may help prevent this side effect. This can easily be achieved by taking a few teaspoons of acidophilus yogurt a day while they're on antibiotics. A more dangerous effect of antibiotic use by both sexes is the risk getting pseudomembranous colitis. Caused by an overgrowth of *Clostridium difficile* bacteria and the subsequent release of its

---

126 Including fifteen screened trials on hip and knee OA published in the *Archives of Internal Medicine* (2003): 163 by Richy.

127 This according to original published research by Dr Bruyere in 2001 *Lancet* and then the follow-up data being presented at the Annual Meeting of the American College of Rheumatology in 2003.

toxin, the damage to the colon can be disastrous, even fatal. Research has proven that taking probiotics helps diminish the risk of yeast infection and colitis due to antibiotic use.[128]

A pharmaceutical-grade probiotic basically contains a combination of the *good* bacteria that usually colonizes the various parts of the gastrointestinal system, not just *Lactobacillus acidophilus*. When you think about it, the GI (gastrointestinal) system is quite complex and goes through a lot of changes between the mouth and the anus. In the stomach, there is a very acidic environment. This turns more basic in the duodenum and becomes more neutral toward the colon. This makes for different populations of bacteria at each juncture, thus the need to have a properly designed pill. As you can imagine, getting this effective delivery of the bacteria is no easy task; so again, I stress the importance of getting quality supplements. This is especially so when it comes to probiotics.

Studies as far back as 2000 suggested probiotics reduce the severity and duration of acute diarrhea in children especially if caused by *Rotavirus*. Antibiotic-associated diarrhea was reduced from 26 percent to 7 percent in kids taking a probiotic. Some of the earliest research showed decrease respiratory infection rates in children with cystic fibrosis. Research presented at the 2006 Annual Meeting of the American College of Gastroenterology concluded four weeks treatment with probiotics resulted in a 23 percent improvement over placebo in irritable bowel syndrome symptoms for *both* constipation and diarrhea prominent subtypes.[129] As many sufferers have learned, IBS is a poorly understood yet very debilitating gastrointestinal disorder that is very difficult to control. Studies suggest that many IBS patients have overgrowth of hydrogen- and methane-producing bacteria. One of the studies presented suggested IBS patients have a higher proportion of pro-inflammatory mediators. Probiotic use also has been shown to help normalize such pro-inflammatory responses.[130]

---

128 G. W. Elmer et al., "Biotherapeutic agents: A neglected modality for the treatment and prevention of selected intestinal and vaginal infections," *JAMA*. 275, no. 11(1996):870–76.

129 This included abdominal pain and discomfort. It appears the *Bifidobacteria infantis* 35624 strain was the most effective. S. Faber, ACG Conference Sixty-seventh Annual Scientific Meeting, Seattle, Washington, 2002 abstract #336; M. Pimental, et al. *American Journal of Gastroenterology* 95 (2000): 3503–06.

130 This was according to research found in *Gastroenterology* (2005): 128.

The prescription drugs typically used for IBS aren't that effective and may possess very serious side effects, even death.[131] The patient usually has to sign a waiver that they understand this risk and won't hold the physician liable. I guess that's an indication of how seriously debilitating on many levels that IBS can be. On the other hand, there was generally no significant increase in side effects with the probiotic users. According to Dr. Talley, professor of medicine at the Mayo Medical School, there's general agreement probiotics are safe, overall. However, for immunocompromised patients, as those with AIDS, probiotics may warrant some increased caution.

Some physicians and researchers, including myself, believe that IBS is part of a complete spectrum of inflammatory bowel disorders, including inflammatory bowel disease (Crohn's) and ulcerative colitis. If mild symptoms and no inflammatory pathology, it's more likely IBS. If more severe, it's probably more consistent with the chronic inflammation seen in the latter two. The term used just depends on what section of the bowel is affected. This chronic inflammation can lead to progressive reactive cellular changes, even resulting in an increased risk of cancer.

I was turned on to probiotics about five years ago after investigating these diseases quite heavily and finding a lack of safe, effective prescription therapies. I also found that a high percentage of patients suffering from irritable bowel symptoms also had symptoms of *fatigue* and *myofascial pain*. These typically have undergone a negative rheumatologic workup and given the "wastebasket" diagnosis of *chronic fatigue syndrome* or *fibromyalgia*. This curiosity led me to search for possible pathological connections between these two elusive syndromes. As you know by now, I'm always trying to uncover the true root cause of a disease in order to offer a safer, effective cure. I prefer this approach as opposed to merely treating the symptoms with a myriad of pills.

It wasn't until I spoke of this with a few cutting-edge, integrative physicians that I came across the role *leaky gut syndrome* may play. First, you must appreciate that the gastrointestinal system is a lot more complex than most people, and even physicians, give it credit. It is a very important line of defense against infections, including toxic bacteria, viruses, parasites, and even more microscopic pathogens such as prions and virions. Second, it has a very complex, dynamic function of selecting what to *absorb* and what *not* to, basically acting as a complex sieve, or ionic filter. Simply put, if a particle is too large, it shouldn't be absorbed into the

---

131 Zelnorm and Lotronex (risk of ischemic colitis, liver failure, and death), are prescription treatments.

body. If these selective membranes are infected or inflamed, they'll allow abnormally large molecules to be taken into the bloodstream. Last, the GI system must specifically and dynamically *secrete* numerous molecules in order to help maintain proper electrolyte and fluid balance. As you can deduce, these integral life functions are quite complex; therefore, any disturbance in this system can have widespread, deleterious effects. Do you have to have the guts to be healthy?

Most allergenic molecules are *macroproteins*. These protein fragments may be found in peanuts, milk, soy, whey, gluten, for example. In the leaky gut syndrome, it's theorized that the irritated, inflamed gut improperly allows such macroproteins to enter the bloodstream. The immune system, trained to recognize *self* from *nonself* substances, subsequently mounts an inflammatory response against these foreign intruders. This could be in the gut wall, further worsening inflammation and creating a deleterious cycle, but can also spread into the bloodstream. When this occurs, *systemic* effects such as fatigue, achiness, depression, and the whole gambit of inflammatory symptoms coexist. This snowballing pathology can cause an avalanche if this superactivated immune system gets confused and starts attacking *normal* tissues. Similar to friendly fire in a battle, there is a lot of collateral damage from these heightened inflammatory responses. In actuality, such *cross-reactivity* is quite common, especially for an aging immune system. All of a sudden, *normal* tissues such as muscle, connective, and joint tissues become a target that must be destroyed. Unfortunately, it's not just the musculoskeletal system that is at risk, this can also involve various tissues throughout the body, even the central and peripheral nervous system. According to believers of the leaky gut syndrome, the whole host of degenerative neurological diseases such as Parkinson's, multiple sclerosis, various dementias, and just plain old depression may result.

Clinically, where does all this fit in? From my perspective, I can only partially comprehend the complexities between the gastrointestinal, immune, and neurological system. The leaky gut syndrome does make for good physiological and pathophysiological theory, but this is quite novel and not mainstream medicine. Thus, there's not much valid research; yet preliminary studies do seem promising on probiotics' efficacy in many gastrointestinal disorders, and just as important, its safety.

> Generally, I have clinically found probiotics to be quite helpful in preventing antibiotic-associated gastrointestinal symptoms and yeast infections. I've seen them help out the majority with mild to moderate cases of IBS and those nonresponders to medical therapy. Also they are helpful as an option for those who refuse prescription medication because of side effects or risks.

If a patient possesses the elusive, vague symptoms of chronic aches and fatigue similar to fibromyalgia yet has IBS-like symptoms, then I'm more apt to suggest a probiotic as part of a therapeutic trial of treatment. (This is, of course, only after the appropriate medical workup has been done to rule out the other potentially serious causes for such symptoms. In these individuals with leaky-gut-syndrome-like symptoms, there should be a full gastrointestinal and possibly additional neurological and rheumatological workup done to first rule out more pathological causes.) I have also found food allergy testing and its corresponding recommendations to be a helpful and a safe, effective modality either singly or in addition to probiotic supplementation in such individuals. More help may be found from International Foundation for Functional Gastrointestinal Disorders at http://www.iffgd.org.

K. Sports-Related and Miscellaneous Supplements that may help improve *body composition* follow:

Chromium may help some with mildly impaired glucose metabolism. Low chromium levels have been found in diabetics, although such supplementation has had equivocal outcomes. Regardless of this, I do recommend chromium, as well as L-carnitine for those wishing to lose weight and improve body composition, as both are safe and without appreciable side effects. L-carnitine has been shown to help improve *fat metabolism* in the mitochondria, basically the battery or energy producer, of the cell. It also acts as an antioxidant, decreasing apoptosis, or cell death.

Better yet, according the recent research, L-carnitine was more effective than testosterone for improving typical male aging symptoms such as ED, depression, and fatigue. Testosterone is thought to partially modulate its effects through increasing tissue carnitine concentration.[132] I find it quite interesting that 2 grams daily of L-carnitine didn't significantly raise prostate volume, testosterone levels, or lower

---

132 According to Italian reproductive researchers who studied 120 symptomatic healthy men with a mean at age of sixty-six for six months. *Urology* (April 2005).

LH (luteinizing hormone). There was no rise in PSA in either group. This may make it a good option for those men with prostate cancer that shouldn't have TRT yet desiring improvement in body composition. More interesting was that the carnitine-treated group had better scores for orgasm and sexual well-being. Figure that one out! I generally recommend 1 gram of L-carnitine supplementation per day.

Although **creatine** is mostly known by most athletes for its muscle-building capability, there is some research to suggest it may also improve the mind. According to findings by Dr. C. Rae published in the *Proceedings of the Royal Society*, university students taking five grams daily of creatine for six weeks had improved memory and intelligence scoring. Adding some sense to this mind-body connection is the fact that both the muscle and brain-stored creatine. Although this supplement is banned in France, it is readily available OTC in the United States, Canada, and allowed by the International Olympic Committee. The long-term safety of creatine supplementation is unknown; the most frequent complaint is flatulence and related gastrointestinal symptoms—lots of it apparently—which makes me jokingly wonder if those who took this supplement could better concentrate since they had then no nearby friends to distract them. At any rate, this may help to explain some of the random grimaces expressed by some athletes. Because of the resulting stink that may be raised, they may not be the best team players to have around.

I personally—yes, I admit it—suffer from bloating and flatulence when taking only one gram of creatine. Because of strong requests made by my wife and family, I had stopped it.. One point worth mentioning though, it seemed I had less trouble with the encapsulated time-release preparation than the loose powder. Yet, if you tolerate creatine and, like most healthy young men, you don't suffer from kidney disease, one gram daily, cycling six weeks on and two weeks off, is probably quite safe. Remember to also take in a lot of fluids.

As expected, supplementation mostly helps those who are found clinically low in creatine. Unfortunately, this is quite hard to objectively measure. Most wouldn't want to undergo the needed muscle biopsy. However, if you find you gain some muscle strength, endurance, and some healthy weight while using it, you're probably getting some benefit. Again, there is no one magic supplement out there; and it's much more important to concentrate on a properly balanced diet and exercise regimen.

In closing, there are some tidbits about a few other supplements I feel worth mentioning. Feel free to investigate these further.

- **Green Tea.** A great natural antioxidant that also helps lower cholesterol, prevents diabetes, boosts the immune system, helps rheumatism, and may even help prevent carcinogenesis. In July 2003, researchers at the University of Rochester in New York found the catechins and similar compounds found in green tea inhibit the aryl hydrocarbon receptor and thereby inactivate some cancer-causing genes. This would be the exact opposite effect smoking tobacco has on this receptor. Most beneficial research used amounts of extracts you realistically can't get from merely drinking tea. If this goal is desired, probably taking a supplement would do the most good.

  I recommend drinking a few cups daily anyway. One tip to avoid the bitter taste found in green tea is to steep it properly. Only heat the water until it is about to boil and then steep it for a longer time than black tea. While on that subject, I also believe *all* teas have about the same health benefit, be they black, green, or white. Black has the most caffeine and white, the least. Nonetheless, I would avoid any caffeinated beverages before bedtime. Lastly, avoid *bottled* teas, which typically contain a lot of sugar. So what does all this boil down to? Probably, tea does contain a lot of antioxidants and mixes quite well with an overall healthy lifestyle. Add some honey and lemon for some additional taste and antioxidants, what the heck!

- **Iron.** There's been a lot of focus on iron the past few years. Most people are familiar with the deficiency-causing microcytic anemia, or iron-poor blood. However, there is an increased interest that *minimally high* iron levels may increase risks for some other common diseases, though most of what I've researched shows an *association*, not necessarily cause and effect. I'm not aware of any research concluding that when such minimally high iron levels are lowered, any of these diseases improve. For example, in metabolic syndrome, there is usually an increase in inflammation, which is marked by a jump in what's called acute phase reactants. Since these also carry iron in blood, this would *artificially* raise iron measurements.[133] Far better indicators for metabolic syndrome would be family history, being overweight, and increased abdominal girth. My take on iron levels

---

[133] There is an inherited iron-storage disease called hemosiderosis that causes *very abnormally high* iron levels and results in frank diabetes; that's not what I'm talking about here.

for right now is that they should be in the midrange, not in the low-normal or high-normal range.

Again, it's very hard to cherry-pick a few magic supplements and expect these to be the magic pill. They offer no substitution for the proper lifestyle; and unfortunately, there are still no shortcuts. On the other hand, if you're careful and you choose quality supplements, you may find there are some that may safely offer some synergism in improving longevity and decreasing risks for many diseases, multiple medications, and operations. According to the November 22, 2004, issue of the *Archives of Internal Medicine*, a low-dose antioxidant vitamin and mineral supplementation lowered all-cause mortality in men. I usually recommend the lowest individualized supplementation combined with the proper diet, exercise, and hormonal optimization. If you take a megadose of one vitamin, you may be doing more harm than good because the relative ratios of vitamins are either beneficial or antagonistic to each other. This reflects the importance of a balanced diet—eating all kinds of healthy foods, such as fruits and vegetables, for example. Additionally, the same way that one man's meat is another man's poison, a supplement's beneficence may depend on your specific genetic makeup. The study of such interactions between nutrition and genetics is nutrigenomics. What's good for the goose may not be good for the gander, after all.

Besides looking for the *official* GMP label, you can go to the FDA and USDA Web sites mentioned above. I personally take the Men's Optimizer and the Men's Nutrients from Cenegenics listed in the appendix. You can also subscribe to http://www.ConsumerLab.com for an annual fee, or go to http://www.usp.org, a freebie. As presented in the introduction of this chapter, supplements aren't FDA regulated, so you have to trust the manufacturer to honestly present what's in and *what's not*, in the bottle. Nowadays, over 60 percent of Internet users search for health information with over half of these looking into so-called natural, holistic, or complementary therapies. Although illegal, over 80 percent of sites expressed health claims *to treat, prevent, diagnose, or cure specific diseases.* Additionally, many lacked warnings about potential adverse effects. Be careful, there's a lot of quackery out there, especially on the Web. In August 2006, the FDA found fake versions of Lipitor and other widely used prescription drugs ordered through ten Web sites linked to a Canadian pharmacy. These included http://rxnorth.com/, http://canadiandrugstore.com/, and http://rxbyfax.com/. It's your health—your best asset. As such, do your research and invest in it wisely.

Chapter 6. MAG adds a GMP-certified multivitamin and 100 mg coenzyme Q_{10}, twice daily. Niacin, 1000 mg, is taken before nighttime to help lower his triglycerides and raise his HDL. His B_{12} and folate level wasn't optimal, so he adds a B complex on top of these. He now drinks tea as opposed to coffee. Feeling as he did in his thirties, he's lost two inches off his waste and ten pounds overall. His coworkers notice his improved performance and he gets a promotion!

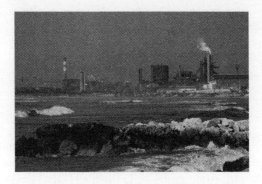

VII.

Fluids and Toxins: Detoxing Your Way Back to Health.

Basically, we're all bags of water; just some are bigger bags than others!

In this chapter, we'll review the importance of hydration under normal situations and when undertaking a more aggressive exercise regimen. Additionally, methods for avoiding toxin exposure as well as detoxification methods will be introduced.

A. First of All, Water. Life probably evolved in water and ever since can't exist without it. Water is indeed ubiquitous, existing in three phases; gas, liquid, or solid. Most of you know that the body is about 70 percent water. So we're all bags of water, just some are bigger bags than others! H_2O is used in almost all reactions occurring in the body, including keeping us cool and ridding of toxins. We could live for a week without food; yet serious health problems start to occur if we don't drink water for just *one day*. In undeveloped nations, clean water is a most expensive commodity. In industrialized nations, clean water is available; yet because of the resulting pollution, there are many other inherent dangers. So water is integral to our very existence as well as to our optimal health.

It would be difficult for a normal, healthy individual to drink *too* much water. The body has an excellent system in place to balance electrolytes and fluids. Only in extremely rare circumstances or if you suffer with kidney or heart problems can this become a problem. My basic advice, under normal circumstances, is to drink about a gallon of fluids throughout the day. What fluids? Well, basically, just plain filtered water is best. Some iced or hot tea is fine. I prefer you get your fruit juice *from the actual fruit itself* because juices typically have a lot of natural sugar—which results in a high glycemic index—and less of that important disease-fighting fiber we mentioned. Vegetable juices are minimally better; however, check for the usually higher salt content. Because of such, we basically don't advise drinking any processed juices at all! (Please review the diet chapter for the implications of foods with a higher glycemic index. They basically raise your insulin and cortisol levels, creating metabolic disturbances and lowering HGH release.)

If you must, a daily glass of wine or beer is okay, provided you don't have problems with alcohol addiction. Of course, I prefer you partake a dry red wine or a low-carb beer because of the relatively lower glycemic index. Even one cup of coffee is okay in the morning. But I would hold off on such stimulating drinks containing any caffeine before bedtime, including any teas. Surprising to some, alcohol may help you *get* to sleep but causes many to wake up in the middle of the night. Avoid all bottled drinks with high sugar; read the labels.

What about if you plan to exercise a lot? First of all, you should use some common sense to *prevent* heat stroke and dehydration. Don't work out in the heat or direct sun for extended amounts of time. Plan your workout indoors or under the shade; it may be early in the morning or in late afternoon. As a general rule, you should drink some fluids before exercising, but not too much as you may get nauseated with those fluids sloshing around in your stomach. A good protein drink or bar, or simply having a balanced meal, about an hour or so before may help. During the workout, depending on how long it is, *sipping* on a low-carb protein drink may help you from "hitting the wall" toward the end. (Some marathon runners drink too much plain water and actually suffer from hyponatremia [low sodium] that can lead to serious neurological problems.) Afterward, just finish that protein drink. I may fix a concoction of a little orange juice with whey protein and some creatine. If it's about time to eat a meal, I'll naturally just eat that to replenish things. I may also fix some chocolate skim milk as an option. The protein is good for muscle repair and the little bit of sugar replaces the used-up glycogen stores. This agrees with recent advice from most exercise and nutrition gurus.

Because of the expansive nature of water, there is correspondingly about as much written about it. I often get asked or come across ads about the importance of attempting to make your body more *basic* in pH. These claim to help your body maintain a better pH and help avoid it becoming too *acidic*. I've never found any good scientific evidence supporting this, yet there are a lot of products and paraphernalia claiming benefit. With the exception of those suffering from severely acute lung, heart, or kidney failure, healthy individuals shouldn't have any problems with acid-base balance.[134] I find that most of the statements used by manufacturers of such deacidifying supplements have inappropriately extrapolated what may be appropriate for only severely end-stage sick individuals. They have then marketed this to gullible, uninformed individuals that may be neurotic about their health or perceived conditions. The Church Lady would say, "How convenient!" Your kidneys and lungs are quite adept at maintaining the proper pH. At the very least, since there is no established *benefit*, you may be exposing yourself to unnecessary *harm*. Remember, supplements aren't FDA approved to treat, cure, or prevent any disease or condition. Don't waste your money.

B. What about Toxins? Whew, there is just *so* much about this topic.

Currently, over 4 billion pounds of toxic waste are produced and more than 1.2 billion pounds of pesticides used annually in the United States. Indeed, because of the Industrial Age going on in the United States for well over a hundred years now, it's understandable there's been an enormous amount of pollution and toxins dispersed into our atmosphere, ground, and water. There is even *e-pollution*, the deposition of all the lead, mercury, PCBs (polychlorinated biphenyls), battery material, and cadmium from old discarded computers! Aaaahhhhhh! Because of us humans being at the top of the food chain and having a relatively long life span, we unfortunately have a resulting great potential of lifetime toxin accumulation. I imagine this is part of the price we pay for all these modern conveniences. A growing problem today is the *rest* of the world now becoming developed and industrialized. They're contributing to the demise of the world as we know it too. Their polluted air is now blowin' and a flowin' over us! How dare them! I will now try to give you a few important tidbits to *live* by.

The best way to avoid getting toxic is, of course, to avoid toxins in the first place. Drink only filtered water, preferably out of a glass. Just because water comes in a bottle or a jug doesn't mean it's safe. Remember Perrier bottled water and benzenes a while back? Installing a large filter for your *entire* home's water source is a good idea. Then, get a multistage or reverse osmosis for your *drinking* faucet, usually in the kitchen. Remember to replace the filters regularly. Run the water first for a few seconds before collecting it. As far as the container is concerned, try

---

134 Only severely sick individuals, such as those in the ICU, may have severe acid-base disturbances because of organ failure, medications, or fluid imbalances resulting in a build up of lactic acid, and in only a few instances, may require some bicarbonate given directly into the veins. Even this modality hasn't shown much benefit and may even worsen acid-base balance within the cell.

to find ones made in the United States or Canada having higher manufacturing standards that meet established lead safety standards for glazes. Good luck! Most are from Asia or such, where it's much more lax. If it's from outside the United States, it probably contains some lead or other heavy metals.

C. Get the Lead Out! I recall a patient that was suffering from vague symptoms of lead poisoning, the source of which was quite puzzling. We eventually traced it down to his coffee mug made in Malaysia that he sipped from every morning! If you find a white powder forming on any glazed ceramic ware, you should immediately throw it away, or utilize lead testing kits from the local hardware store to ensure safety. You can find more information and order kits from http://www.leadtestkits. com or get water-testing kits from the nonprofit group, Clean Water Lead Testing Inc. Try to avoid styrofoam, plastic, or aluminum containers, especially if it's going to hold a hot or acidic beverage. This may promote the dissolution of these materials. Oh, and just because the water tastes great, doesn't mean it's safe either. Arsenic and many poisons can have a sweet taste, too Test it.

Sometime around 1971, it became illegal in the United States to manufacture paints with lead. Regardless, lead poisoning should continue to be significant concerns as one-quarter of homes with kids under six still contain lead-based paint. The lead paint can be found under the newer paint and then released with any repair or reconstruction. Traditionally, doctors were just concerned of lead levels above 60 micrograms (µg) being dangerous; however newer research lowers this to 10 µg or less—the previously *normal,* acceptable range. Research from the Boston's Children's Hospital and the Harvard Medical School studied about 250 middle-class children's lead levels from birth to ten years. They found proportionately *greater* harm with lower levels of lead previously considered safe. This was reinforced by findings in the April 2003 *New England Journal of Medicine* that suggested *any* amount of lead is harmful to a child's brain. Unexpectedly, *greater* damage seems to occur at levels *below* 10 µg than above it. Similarly, psychologists at Cornell University that followed kids from six months to five years found that for every lifetime average lead level below 10, there was a decline of seven IQ points.[135]

Related studies also found a bad link between increased lead levels and teenage boys' behavior. They were more likely to have committed antisocial acts such as bullying, vandalizing, committing arson, shoplifting, and more.[136] Lastly, early lead exposure

135 Dr. R. Canfield, developmental psychologist at Cornell.
136 Dr. Kim Dietrich, from the University of Cincinnati, has been following three hundred children since 1981.

has been shown to slow the brain's recovery after injury as well as to impair the immune system as a whole.[137] Research has shown that lead can increase a man's risk for getting cataracts threefold. Cataracts are a leading cause of vision loss in the United States.[138] Large studies have shown that even *moderate* elevations in lead are associated with a 39 percent increase in mortality from all causes. There was a 46 percent increase in mortality from cardiovascular diseases and an appreciable 68 percent increase in mortality due to cancer. Even *lower* levels were associated with significant increase in these conditions.[139] Dementia in men is also increased with higher lead levels, prompting the new term *accelerated aging*.[140]

The above points are quite important. As I stress in my practice, there is no *safe* lead level at *any* age. Even in the rare case where you were tested for lead as a kid and your mother *may* recall being told it was normal, it doesn't mean it really *was* then, or *is* now. Lead-toxic boys become lead-toxic middle-aged men later on and may suffer from the many vague neurological, cognitive, pathophysiological, and even sociopathic conditions mentioned. We midlife men also have kids, siblings, or parents who may be suffering from these symptoms of heavy metal poisoning. The only way to know for sure is to get tested. It's important to note blood tests for lead only reflect your exposure the past three to four months. Bone levels, though more expensive and inconvenient, indicate your exposure and storage of lead for preceding decades.

Unfortunately, but according to research, chelating kids with heavy metal poisoning doesn't help restore the *lost* intelligence; although I would find this hard to define and subsequently measure. At any rate, I would say the earlier a person is checked and treated for any amount of heavy metal toxicity, the better the out-

---

137 Presented by researchers from the Jefferson Medical College of Philadelphia to the Society of Neuroscience's annual meeting, October 25, 2004.

138 D. Schaumberg, assistant professor Harvard Medical School.

139 Data taken from Dr. Mark Lustberg of the University of Maryland School of Medicine and Ellen Silbergeld of Johns Hopkins University. 2002. (They compared data from the 2000 census in the massive Third National Health Nutritional Examination Survey, NHANES-III.) "Blood lead levels and mortality," *Archives of Internal Medicine* 162: 2443–49. P. Muntner, *Circulation* (2006): 114. Analyzed data revealed subjects with levels above 3.62 µg per deciliter at higher were 55 percent more likely to die from all causes and cardiovascular etiologies than subjects below 1.94. Even low levels increased risk substantially.

140 *Epidemology* 14 (2003): 713. Also taken from the Normative Aging Study and from the Baltimore Memory Study, Brian Schwartz.

come. In the end, it may be that your exposure as a teenager to that heavy metal your parents warned about was indeed correct—only it wasn't the musical form!

> Even what's considered mild lead poisoning can cause irreversible neurological harm and many other serious health risks.

D. Miscellaneous Toxins.
As far as food goes, I must reemphasize you should eat the most natural products you can get your cleaned hands on. Shop the perimeter of the store—all the veggies, fruits, lean meat, diary, and such. Reread the diet chapter if you need a refreshing. Avoid processed, packaged foods in a box, can, or jar. These invariably have preservatives, saturated and trans fats, lots of sugar and salt, MSG (monosodium glutamate), and whole host of junk for your mind and body. Acrylamide, for example, is a known animal carcinogen commonly found in potato chips, french fries, cereals, breads, and even baby food. It's well known to damage DNA.[141] Even with natural foods, you need to observe some precautions. Wash all fruit and vegetables with a soap solution, even banana peels! Pesticides are *fat soluble,* so just rinsing with water doesn't do much. Suffice to say, pesticides are really bad for you. They accumulate in your body and can cause cancer. Most act as a form of *xenohormone.* These *unnatural* hormones act in an improper and unpredictable nature to the many hormonal receptors found throughout your body. They may over- or understimulate them, possibly causing a cascade of metabolic and cancer-causing derangements. I opine—and there's good research to back this up—these contribute to the increased risks for hormonally sensitive cancers such as *prostate* and breast we are seeing in the United States. Some researchers even blame this for the much earlier onset of puberty seen in today's young girls. Since 2003, the majority of Canada has banned the outdoor use of pesticides, including all herbicides, fungicides, and insecticides.[142] Why haven't we?

> Pesticides can real havoc on your hormonal system and increase risks for cancer. Since they're fat soluble, wash your fruits and vegetables with soap and water.

What about meat? Fish is better for you, yet there is a valid concern about *mercury.* According to the CDC (Centers for Disease Control), fish is to be avoided by kids

---

141 FDA sources.

142 *Toronto Star,* November 18, 2005. Canada's top court backs precedent—setting pesticide ban in Toronto despite industry opposition.

and childbearing-aged women. According to recent report from a University of North Carolina lab, swordfish samples taken from supermarket chains including Safeway, Shaw's, Albertson's, and Whole Foods contained mercury levels above the legal limit. Quite a shame, isn't it? If you then switch to eating more chicken, especially if you like crunching on that crispy outer skin, you may be exposing yourself to arsenic—as in the old play, *Arsenic and Old Lace*. It's commonly and universally used as a form of infection prophylaxis in most poultry farms and builds up in the chicken's subcutaneous fat. So *avoid* the skin. All this bad news makes us think that eating lean beef may not be that bad after all.

Well, besides the obvious saturated fat issue, I have concerns about the anabolic injections livestock receive to fatten them up about six weeks before going to the slaughterhouse. Many believe that once ingested, these nonhuman anabolic hormones also act as xenohormones and further contribute to the increased incidence of the metabolic, hormonal, and cancerous conditions we Americans have. What then is a health-conscious big-meat eater to do? Well, at least avoid processed and fast food meats with all their nitrates and other preservatives. At the least, if you can pull it off in a nonconspicuous, socially acceptable way, try to pat the meat with a paper napkin to absorb some of the excess grease.

We must not forget to promote the healthy, normal detoxifying and cleansing your body is quite adept at performing. When you think about it, animals and humans ingesting and being exposed to potentially toxic substances is nothing new; we've been doing it for eons. On the other side, our bodies have probably not had anywhere near the needed time to adapt in order to effectively deal with these newer man-made toxins. For now, simply drinking a lot of water to perfuse the kidneys and sweat glands will do a world of good. After working out, rinse off that *toxic* sweat using soap in a shower. Have a good BM (bowel movement) at least once per day. (Some naturopaths suggest three BMs per day. I find that hard to do logistically, thus the modifier *good* before BM.)

The diet we recommend has many of the antioxidants and fiber to help naturally prevent free radical damage and routinely help eliminate toxins. The liver is another very important organ for detoxifying our bodies, so don't overstress it by using too many drugs and booze. Artichokes contain Silymarin that may help support the liver. Apples contain quercitin, another very important antioxidant that helps the liver and immune system. This probably accounts for the saying, "An apple a day keeps the doctor away." Similarly, all vegetables and fruits with their fiber, by their very nature, help detoxify the body. Just the same way you clean your skin daily, these fibers should be scrubbing out the waste inside your GI tract.

> Consuming any type of meat has its risks. To avoid toxins, shop wisely and cook healthily. Keep your diet balanced with fiber and complex carbs. In order to help your body's natural detoxing, drink plenty of water, have a daily bowel movement, and don't abuse your liver.

I was even surprised to find out air pollution in U.S. cities causes twice as many deaths from heart disease as it does from lung cancer and other respiratory ailments.[143] The pollution risk is from what scientists call combustion-related fine particulate matter, which is basically soot, emitted by vehicles, coal-fired power plants, and factories. Maybe Mr. and Mrs. Oliver Windle Douglas were right after all when they moved from Park Avenue to a small farm in Hootersville. "Fresh air!"

Besides the pesticides which all animals absorb from the environment, only mercury, lead, and polychlorinated biphenyls (PCBs) are currently proven to cause health problems in levels that accumulate in the body. A fourth, PBDEs (polybrominated diphenyl ether), basically the flame retardants found in plastics and foams used in furniture and electronic equipment, will be banned in California starting 2008. Canada and the United States account for half of the worldwide use of this neurotoxin.[144] Apparently, the European Union—acting quickly on a Swedish study that reported PBDE level increased in breast milk in Sweden fortyfold from 1972 to 1997—banned these compounds years ago. Even China and South Korea are considering bans. Only a handful of the estimated seventy-five thousand chemicals found in the United States have been tested for their health effects. Although PCBs and DDT (dichloro-diphenyl-trichloroethane) were banned decades ago, *biomonitoring*, which checks human samples of urine, blood, and breast milk for the accumulation of pollutants, reveals these toxins still substantially exist in our environment. This results in what's now called the *body burden*. This is essentially the buildup of such toxins in the body during the entire lifetime.

The results are quite scary. San Francisco area women have three to ten times as much PBDEs in their breast tissue as their European or Japanese cohorts.

---

143 According to C. A. Pope in December 16, 2003, *Circulation*, the journal for the American Heart Association.

144 "Body burden: The pollution in newborns," *Environmental Working Group*, July 14, 2005, summary. Go to http://www.ewg.org for more information.

Adding fuel to the fire—no pun intended—Indiana's and California's women and infants' PBDE levels were twenty times higher than those in Sweden and Norway! Recently, the CDC released data from twenty-five hundred volunteers and found many chemicals—among them were mercury, uranium, and cotinine, a metabolite of nicotine. Additionally, it appeared our black children are probably exposed to twice as much secondhand smoke and that Mexican American children possess three times the amount of DDT derivatives than other children. Thank god, we finally banned wood decking sealants, huh? With the exception of Al Gore, it seems like America is always lagging behind the rest of the developed countries when it comes to addressing pollution and preserving the environment. Not that we've had some subtle warnings. Remember the 1960s commercial featuring a Native American Indian crying when he looked at the extensive litter scattered on the mountainside? Rachel Carson helped raise the awareness of environmental protection way back in 1962 with her book *Silent Spring*. Where's a good hippie today when you really need one?

E. Mercury is Rising. I covered how to buy fish that's lower in mercury in the diet chapter. Avoid farmed or bigger-sized predator fish. Basically, mercury is emitted into the atmosphere from various factories and power plants. Rain and gravity eventually gets the mercury into the soil and water supplies. Smaller fish and land animals assimilate this heavy metal into their bodies. Larger animals, including us, then eat these smaller, toxic animals. Simply put, the EPA (Environmental Protection Agency) and large corporations have made deals to get around the recent Clean Air Act. If implemented as planned, 90 percent of mercury emissions would be eliminated by 2008. The AMA (American Medical Association) is pushing hard to lower the global mercury burden by raising U.S. emission standards. It may be better to enact the laws we currently have.

Additionally, silver-colored teeth fillings contain mercury. My opinion is that some people may do quite well with such fillings. However, many individuals may not, depending on many factors. How the amalgam was made? How old is it? What's the environment inside the individual's mouth? Is it acidic, or highly enzymatic? The amount of mercury in an average filling would be enough to label most lakes unsafe to swim in. Recently, the FDA advisors voted to keep studying the role that mercury-laden "silver dental fillings" may play in heavy metal poisoning. Personally, I had all my silver fillings taken out and replaced with composite ones. It was relatively cheap. You would need to find a dentist experienced in removing these fillings without spilling the mercury shavings and particles that fly about. (In my opinion, having a positive hair analysis would be enough to warrant this dental procedure.) There's also the concern of mercury, in the form of thimerosal, in many childhood vaccines.

The symptoms of mercury poisoning are very similar to lead poisoning mentioned above. Again, these are usually very vague yet very common complaints. Complicating matters is the fact that physicians aren't trained to diagnose or treat these disorders. Mercury is a neurotoxin, so any nerve related complaint or disorder could be, at the very least, complicated by heavy metal toxicities. Vague concerns would include fatigue, nervousness, depression, insomnia, forgetfulness, and such. More severe disabilities would include neuropathy, dementia, mental retardation, ADHD, learning disabilities, tremor, anemia, physical deformities, and much more. Do you think society is seeing any increase in these maladies lately? For more horrific insight into the political and historical aspects of heavy metal—including mercury—poisoning, you may want to read W. Eugene Smith's classic book, *Minamata: Words and Photographs.* It describes the challenge faced by townspeople against the corporate giants responsible for the massive mercury poisoning of residents. More information may be found at the American Board of Clinical Metal Toxicology Web site at http://www.abcmt.org.

Get routinely checked for heavy metal poisoning—especially mercury and lead. You can check lead by a simple blood test; however, mercury is best checked by hair analysis. Such kits are relatively inexpensive. Unfortunately, most medical doctors' offices don't have these, nor would the average doctor even know what to do when it comes back abnormal. Recall the saying, "Mad as a hatter"? This probably came from the old days when hatmakers would rub mercury into black hats to make them shiny. I imagine some absorbed too much mercury through their skin and began to exhibit the neurological and mental symptoms. When forensic analysis on Andrew Jackson's remains was done recently, they found he probably suffered from such poisoning when he wigged out in his old age. I wonder what they would find if they dug up other mad presidents? Well, if you grow up to be president one day and then become curiously sick, let's not wait until you're exhumed hundred of years later to find out why—it'll be much too late to do anything about it.

I have found many patients, from the very young to the very old, who suffered with vague, elusive complaints such as fatigue, neuropathy, depression, anxiety, and even ones misdiagnosed with ADHD, Parkinson's, multiple sclerosis; and I could go on and on … Once appropriately tested, they exhibited abnormally high heavy metal levels. (Some also had additional ill effects of medications, allergies, and vitamin deficiencies.) They had previously seen many respected, traditionally trained specialists and had all negative tests. "If you don't know how to look for something, you won't find it," advised many of my wise medical mentors. Disheartening in many cases, these patients were then relegated to taking prescription drugs that provided only symptomatic relief, at best. Each drug added its own host of adverse symptoms. Once we forged ahead with a more integrative approach, which included heavy metal detoxification, the person appreciably improved and was able to wean off most medication.

The symptoms of heavy metal poisoning are quite varied yet quite common. Some resources estimating over 25 percent of the U.S. population suffers from such poisoning. Fill out the detoxification questionnaire in the appendix to see if you may have the symptoms of heavy metal toxicity. Whether these complaints are solely caused by heavy metal toxicity or merely coexisted with those many other diseases is hard to say. Regardless, by treating these comorbidities, the patients got a new lease on life.

You may now ask, "Just how do we rid of this heavy metal? Well again, it depends on the clinical picture. Mostly, I try to steer away from IV chelation because of the questioned benefits and the unnecessary risks of allergic reaction, and kidney and liver failure expressed in much of the scientific literature. Besides, the oral chelation I generally use is proven effective, yet with fewer risks. I haven't had any problems in the past five years of chelating patients this way. Some may have mild gastrointestinal symptoms, as expected. I may use DMSA (dimercaptosuccinic acid) or a milder concoction of detoxifying substances, the dosing of which depend on the particular situation.[145] Personally, because of eating so much fish and repairing so many old houses when younger, I undergo oral chelation for about six weeks twice per year. If it's good enough for you, it's good enough for me!

Like lead poisoning, the many common symptoms of mercury toxicity can be quite elusive. Blood tests are of minimal value, yet hair analysis may help in making the diagnosis. Chelation can be performed to help eliminate this heavy metal.

145 DMSA, Dimercaptosuccinic acid, is an oral heavy metal chelation drug.

In summary, there are unfortunately a lot of reasons why we *should* be appropriately neurotic about today's toxic environment. Given the hundred years or so of the Industrial Revolution, combined with the panoramic presence of pollution, today's population is constantly being bombarded. The symptoms caused by these toxins are vague, and the proper diagnosis can be quite elusive. This makes targeted therapy uncommon. I wonder how much of the increased psychiatric, behavioral, neurological, and cancer problems we see in today's society, especially in our children, are due to the toxic environment we live in. Each toxin, by itself, may not be the sole cause, but all these exposures serve as yet another "hit." These eventually add up to increase the risks of genetic mutations and getting many cancers and diseases. One of the best ways to stay healthy and avoid getting toxic is to avoid them as much as reasonably possible in the first place. As usual, this involves a proactive, synergistic lifestyle along with the integrative modalities we introduce in this book. I truly hope my advice helps you. There are volumes more I could cover; it would just be beyond the scope of this one book.

Chapter 7. MAG gets a water filtering system for his home and only drinks out of glass. He washes all vegetables and fruit with soap. He had his lead level checked and he had a positive level of 6. Oral chelation with DMSA was initiated, and MAG then scheduled to get his mercury amalgams removed. Lastly, he uses only organic pesticides in the home and yard. He and his wife notice improved energy, mood, and creativity.

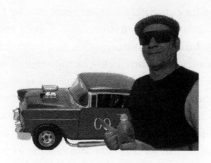

VIII.

Andropause and the Aging Man: Fact, Phallic Symbol, or Fallacy?

I always put "Hi-Test" in my rod ... makes my engine run hard and last longer!"

—"anonymous" race car driver

A. Introduction. In these next few chapters, we'll cover the hormonal changes, which occur in aging men with more detail and references. Let's expound on that paradigm shift in thinking, which promotes *health span* versus merely *life span*. This is a measurement of your potential health that can result from maintaining optimal hormonal balance and the proper lifestyle. It's more about *how well* you live, than just *how long* you live. It's about having less disability and sickness in the end, or *morbidity compression*.

Please refer to the graph below: Quality of Life vs. Time (age). Let's say a male starts life out as a healthy child with rather okay genes, parenting, environment, and so on. This would be represented by curve A. He would reasonably be expected to reach peak *physical* performance and health anywhere from about eighteen to twenty-eight years old. Recall the saying, "Life begins at forty." Well, it's really more like life begins *to fall apart* at forty. Of course, the spiritual, emotional, artistic, and many other facets of his whole being, can hopefully improve with maturity. Yet, because of decaying overall health and the ill effects this will have on his brain, chances are these cognitive and mental qualities will probably decline, too. Regardless, the important point is that the *pattern* of this bell-shaped curve, with its normally increasing health status associated with youth and its decreasing nature seen with older age, can be manipulated in either a good or a bad way. Additionally, the apex, or the maximum vitality, he obtains in life can be improved … or diminished. The earlier he starts focusing on proactive age-management therapies, the better off he is throughout his lifespan. Yet if he's a late bloomer when it comes to being more proactive about health, it's never *too* early or absolutely *too* late to start improving things. Let me show you what I mean.

Two more scenarios—one better and one worse: The first is curve B in which the same boy improperly ate a pro-inflammatory diet, had a more sedentary lifestyle, and was exposed to toxins and then smoked. This guy would probably begin midlife obese with increased visceral fat. With these come risks for metabolic syndrome, peripheral and coronary artery disease, erectile dysfunction, fatigue, depression, shortness of breath, and a whole lot more. As you can see, he never reached the optimal health (apex) he could've experienced in middle age. His older years weren't as healthy or as long. Life was instead blunted, shortened; and the end of his life was spent with more sickness and disability. He ignored my often-repeated advice, "You only have one life, be there!"

The second is curve C. Here, a more proactive approach yields even better results than curve A. In this case, the boy had been taught better coping mechanisms and developed more effective ways of dealing with stress. He rested better and had less exposure to toxins, pesticides, and heavy metals. He lettered in sports, which resulted in improved body composition—more muscle and bone mass, and less visceral fat. His parents pushed a cancer-fighting diet that focused on natural vegetables and fruits, less preserved meats, and more fish. Lastly, neurohormonal replacement was instituted and maintained at optimal physiological levels starting in midlife. The expected result is a healthier start in childhood, better optimization of midlife with the prevention of early disease risks, and increased *health span* and *life span* in old age. This resulted in *morbidity compression*, living life until the very end. Clearly the best way to go of the three scenarios, wouldn't you say?

It's like being a contestant in the old TV game show, *You Bet Your Life!* Are you going to choose, curtain A, B, or C? Where do you see yourself on the curve *now*? Going on that path, how do you expect to feel in ten years? Instead, where would you *want* to go from here? These next few chapters will show the facts and the methods to achieve optimal health and longevity. When Father Time's whip comes down, you got to be prepared or else it may be curtains!

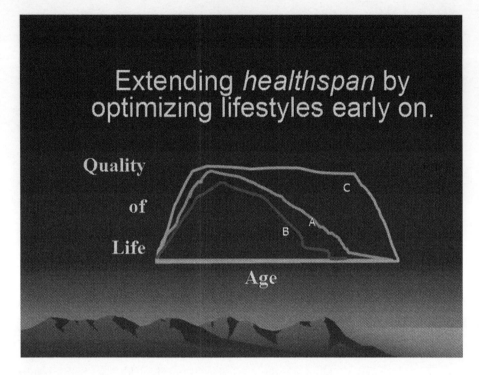

Figure 8.1. Depending on how proactive you are, you can extend your life span and health span.

I'm often asked the following: When is the best age to start these age-management modalities? Am I too old to start anything to do with improving my age? My short answer is, "It's never too early or too late to get healthier." It has been shown many times over that being more proactive with diet and exercise has tremendous health benefits for children as well as adolescents. In today's world of early-onset adult diabetes in our teenagers, now more than ever, we need to get aggressive in order to help prevent future health complications. Research has shown that effective intervention in children and adolescents has a beneficial effect in improving such metabolic disorders, obesity, self-esteem, mood, and much more. As suggested before, we parents should lead by example.

In my practice, I have patients starting in their midthirties desiring age-management modalities. I also have ones in their nineties that pole-vault a few times a week! Basically, the *first* type is a health-conscious individual who's currently looking and feeling great. He has read a lot on his own and wants to keep feeling this way. The *second* type may be an executive in his early forties like our MAG, who now finds it a little more difficult to keep up his previously excellent edge, performance, and endurance. This is despite the fact that he may be relatively okay with the proper diet and exercise. (However, I usually find the diet and exercise regimen needs some work still.) They may be used to feeling great when younger, but now feel, well, okay. Sort of like used to getting an A in life, but now they're getting a C. Men will typically complain of that middle-age spread, sexual concerns, and/or weight gain. Upon further history, there may also be mood and cognitive complaints. These may range from irritability, poor concentration to insomnia and such. (His similarly aged spouse is feeling a lot of this too. She's not the purring sex kitten or the tigress-on-the-prowl she used to be. Thunder thighs and cellulite-textured buttocks may be her concerns, as well as mind or mood issues.) A healthy lifestyle is, of course, most beneficial when started younger—the earlier the better. If you've slacked off since, as many obviously have, early midlife, it is best to get down to the nitty-gritty and become proactive again. It's time to get your life happening.

The third type may be a man in frank middle age, or his wife that's now peri-menopausal. Again, this is a time when neurohormonal changes tailspin further out of control, making it even more difficult to retain that younger vim and vigor. These subtle and not-so-subtle changes may have worsened a few or more times, but a routine lab work from the OB-GYN turned out to be normal. "There's nothing wrong, you're just getting older and have to *get used to it*. Welcome to the club!" And as the eyeglass-wearing doctor patted his large belly, the visit may have ended with, "You just need to do more exercise and better dieting." He's obviously at a loss for the expertise and time needed to properly counsel and help you. Why else would *he* feel so old, cranky, burnt-out, and fat?

So the average Middle-Aged Guy, MAG, will try some good old-fashioned diet and exercise. Usually, he gets minimal results though. Why is that? I've most often found this to be due to the following:

- Usually, MAG doesn't know *beans* about the proper diet. It's paramount that he reads our diet chapter to find out how to start lowering insulin and cortisol, the so-called *aging hormones*. This lack of knowledge isn't too surprising; even well-educated physicians receive minimal nutritional training. Remember, we doctors are mostly trained to *treat* diseases, not *prevent* them!

- The exercise is inappropriate too. MAG will invariably try to resume suddenly the physical activities he did as a teenager. But this is twenty years later, and his body isn't anywhere close to the condition it used to be in.

He and his younger weekend-warrior cohorts will quickly injure themselves, which only undermines any further proper physical conditioning. "Too much, too soon, and too often" is the usual catchphrase for this overuse injury. See the exercise chapter for tips.

- Lastly, MAG and his spouse may have even been proactive enough to join a gym or attend a weight-loss course. They soon found out these tricks didn't work long-term or was simply impossible to maintain with their social life. After that failure, they may have tried some magical OTC herbs that guaranteed to burn off the fat, or may have tried more fad diets. In the end, MAG feels it's just no use and gives up. Yet, lifestyle *must* be improved to effect any real change; that's a given. Basically, there are far too many *lose-weight-quickly* gimmicks out there. MAG needs to be duly and truly committed to the real deal. Yo-yo (dieting) is a no-no! There are no short cuts or magic pills. Don't give up though. Here's the other piece of the puzzle you're probably missing.

So what else is happening? Well, Mother Nature has begun her sneaky duty. As a male of the species, you have now lived past *reproductive* age. You passed on your genes and lived long enough to raise your young. Your job's done as far as Mother Nature is concerned. But exactly how does she do us in? As I've said before, it just happens as we age; the hormones you wish would go up, go down. The chemical messengers associated with youth by keeping muscle mass up and fat mass down, decrease. These would include the *natural sex hormones* (for example, see below). The ones involved with *catabolism*, mainly insulin and cortisol, go up. This *breaking down* of the body eventually wears it down to become a frail fraction of what it once was; it magnifies inflammation and blunts the immune system. Sarcopenia, osteopenia, obesity, infections, and more ensue.

Specifically in men, testosterone (T), DHEA, pregnenolone, HGH (human growth hormone), and thyroid hormones variably go down (see below). Melatonin has also dwindled, reflecting more sleep complaints expressed by the aged. Estrogen is the only sex steroid, which has relatively gone up. (This fact may help explain why older men's breasts enlarge and sag.) Old guys do become more androgynous and, well, less competitive or has less machismo. Less studlike, they begin to don aprons, do gardening, gossip, cry watching the soaps, and cook more—maybe even buy a DVD copy of *Brokeback Mountain*. (Interestingly enough, some newer research points it may be this decrease in T and increased estrogen levels, basically a reversal of their earlier fortune, that increase the risk for prostate cancer in older men.)

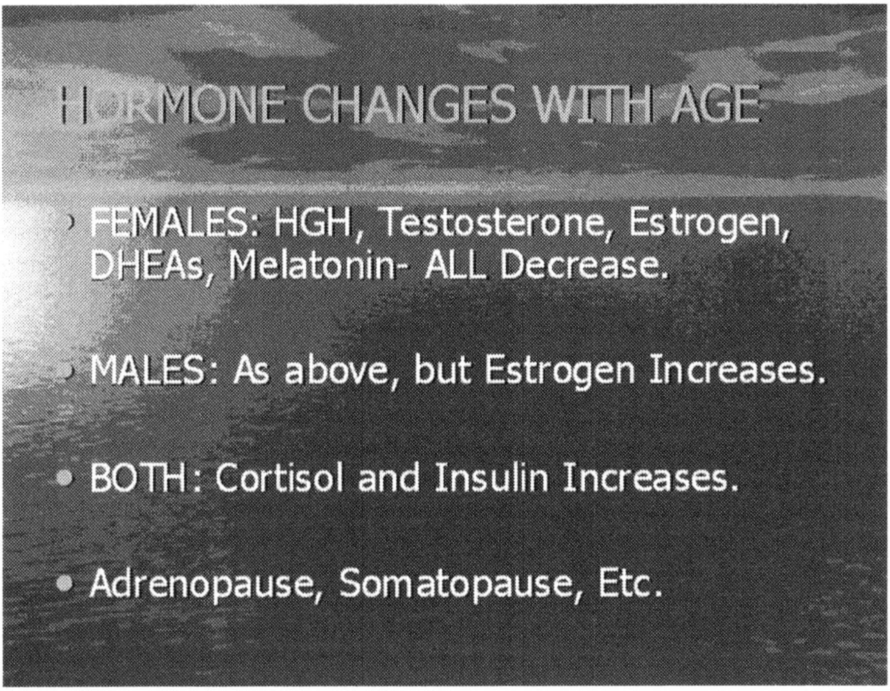

Figure 8.2. Hormonal changes seen as we age.

It's again important to understand that different people physiologically age at different rates, some faster than others. As the Subliminal Man on *Saturday Night Live* may put it, "We have all been to reunions where some colleagues looked older—Cool! That's hip—than we did. Yet, some looked younger—Oh no! Bummer!—than their *chronological* age." Early in life, good genes can help. The many proactive modalities we promote will only have beneficial effects on all these parameters. Conversely, if someone hasn't lived healthily, the effects are exponentially detrimental—much as one plus one equals three, in either a good or a bad way.

Getting your hormones optimally balanced will help solve Mother Nature's riddle of premature aging. Along with a healthy lifestyle, this will help increase your *health span*.

B. The Hormonal Cascade. Hormones can simply be considered nature's conductors in the body. They help maintain your optimal health. We need to understand their normal functions and then what happens when these *good* hormones go *bad*. I will review some basic biochemistry and the synthesis of the sex hormones. Although this may seem daunting at first, you need some basic knowledge to help determine fact from fiction when trying to weigh the pros and cons of starting various hormonal replacements.

All hormones work in concert with each other. Like the players in an orchestra, they must first know the right piece of music. In addition, they must play the right key, tempo, and volume. Lastly, they must intuitively respond to each other's groove and nuances. Only in this way can all the multiple individual players, all with their own personalities, create a masterpiece. Indeed, the whole is more than merely the sum of its parts. *Optimal* hormonal balance achieves this goal.

Looking at the diagram below, let's start in the brain. Inputs from the conscious, subconscious, and unconscious mind affect the *thalamus*. Hormonal levels, metabolic state, genetics, toxins, and more also have roles here. Eventually, the *hypothalamus* deciphers all this and sends out the first wave of hormones, its *releasing factors*, to the pituitary gland. An example would be gonadotropin-releasing factor. From here, many *stimulating hormones*, such as thyroid-stimulating hormone or follicular-stimulating hormone, represent the second wave. These then have diverse effects on many target glands and tissues throughout the body. Eight major endocrine glands comprise this system, communicating from various points throughout the body. Although all glands have secondary and tertiary functions, the following list focuses on their primary ones.

- pituitary gland—regulating other endocrine glands
- pineal glands—regulating biological rhythms and moods, and stimulating puberty
- thyroid gland—regulating metabolic rate
- parathyroid glands—regulating blood calcium
- adrenal glands—regulating fluid and sodium balance, as well as warning of stress
- pancreas—producing hormones, such as insulin
- gonads—testes or ovaries involved in sex organ functions and secondary sex characteristic development

The end effects of these hormones and the diverse metabolic parameters resulting from these glands then feedback to the brain in order to maintain proper balance. If a particular player is playing his instrument too loudly, the conductor will lower his hand to instruct him to play softer. This is called *negative* feedback. Conversely, if a crescendo is needed, the conductor raises his hand to encourage the needed higher volume. This is called *positive* feedback. This analogy is quite simple compared to what actually happens in the body. Nonetheless, you can still appreciate how all the hormones have their individual parts to play that must then come together to make one beautiful symphony. There are slow and fast parts, quiet and loud parts, key changes, solos, and more. They must play off each other and know when to sit out a spell. No two concerts are exactly the same, yet they all sound great in the end.

What do you think would happen if only a few fake players showed up to perform and an inexperienced director asked them to just play louder in a vain attempt to compensate for the missing ones? It would become nothing less than a train wreck. The audience's ears, used to hearing a beautiful symphony, would now hurt. The players would get lost in the music and make many errors. The crowd would shriek and would want to leave early. If they couldn't escape from this torture, they may then become psychotic and start to tear up the place. Some spectators may want to curl up and die. This is similar to what happens in your aging body when inexperienced doctors attempt to nonsensically replace only a few hormones with artificial ones. "Heck, any dose will do. Let's roll the dice and see how you do." Thinking cavalierly, he can cause total anarchy in your body! Thus is the logic behind using only *balanced*, bioidentical hormonal replacement therapies instead. Anything less will give your body one hellacious case of stage fright!

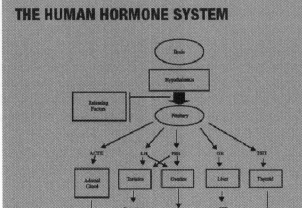

THE HUMAN HORMONE SYSTEM

A Cascade of Events

- At the top of this cascade is your brain, followed by the
  pituitary gland and target organs (i.e., ovaries, thyroid,
  testicles). Physical and mental functions follow (e.g.,
  skin thickness, menstrual periods, sex characteristics,
  aggression, hair distribution, etc.)
- Hormone release originates in the hypothalamus, part of the
  brain. It starts a cascade, secreting "releasing hormones,"
  which activate the pituitary "master gland." The pituitary,
  at the brain's base, communicates directly with the
  hypothalamus via special nerves and blood vessels.
- Releasing hormones stimulate formation and release of
  pituitary hormones into the circulatory system. Pituitary
  hormones exert their effects on many parts of the body, such
  as the thyroid gland, adrenal glands, testicles, ovaries
  and breasts.
- Pituitary hormones have effects on specific targets, which
  release hormones of their own. Thus, pituitary hormones act
  as traffic controllers, determining what is needed and telling
  the organs in the body when to release other hormones.

Figure 8.3. The hormones are a cascading, complex, well-concerted, dynamic system! (Adapted from Cenegenics©)

C. Testosterone Synthesis. First of all, it's interesting and pertinent to learn that virtually all cells (and subsequent tissues) have receptors and thereby respond to the sex hormones. Because of such, sex hormones have many varied and widespread effects in the body. Since testosterone (T) is considered the *man's* sex hormone, let's go for it first. As the below diagram shows, sex hormones such as T have a steroid structure and, as such, are derived from cholesterol. In men, the majority of T is produced by the Leydig cells in the testes; however, small amounts are produced by the adrenal glands.

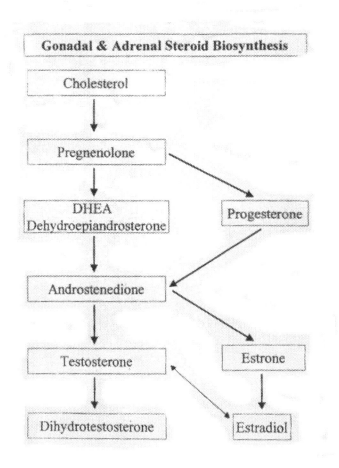

Figure 8.4. Derived from cholesterol, all these prohormones have their own multiple functions and feedback mechanisms. These are then converted into the sex hormones such as testosterone, estrogen, and progesterone.

Secondly, the majority of the sex hormones are bound to a "carrier" in the blood, which makes them an inactive form. Therefore, the "free" or active component is what's more metabolically active and important. For example, nearly 98 percent of T is bound. Therefore, only about 2 percent is active. This level of free testosterone (FT) is what's clinically useful yet commonly overlooked.

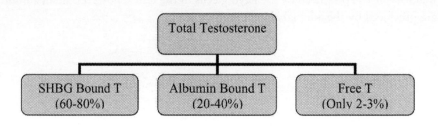

Figure 8.5 Total vs. free testosterone. Bioavailable T is a combination of "loosely" albumin bound and free T.

Measuring merely total testosterone, TT doesn't provide us a full picture of gondal function. The active fraction, free testosterone, FT needs to assessed as well.

In the below diagram, we see how T is produced by the Leydig cells found in the testes. Basically, there is a *feedback loop* between the pituitary gland and these cells. In cases of *secondary failure,* the pituitary in the brain has failed. In this case, we see very minimal, if any, luteinizing hormone (LH) produced. Therefore, there is no stimulation to the testes to produce T. LH and T levels are both low. Typically, we see this in a *minority* of patients. Usually, there may be a history of head trauma; and because of the other accompanying hormonal deprivations resulting from such pituitary failure, there tends to be more severe and widespread symptoms.

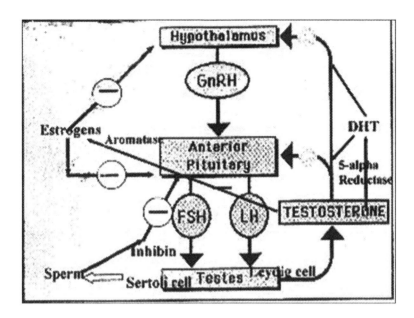

Figure 8.6. Primary versus secondary testicular failure. In primary failure, the testes don't produce enough T; therefore, LH increases to try to stimulate the testes to make more. In secondary failure, there is no LH production, therefore, any stimulation to the testes to make any T.

The commonest scenario we see follows. As T production decreases in the *early* middle-aged guy, LH will appropriately increase in order to stimulate the testes to make more. As men age further, this feedback loop becomes somewhat lazy, or insensitive. Therefore, we may then see an inappropriately "normal" LH level, although the T is actually low. Remember, there is great variability between men as to exactly *how much* and *how soon* testosterone will drop. This is called *primary failure*—the testes simply don't make the T they should. As you will find out, T in the upper one fourth of "normal" levels helps reduce risks for most age-related diseases and frailties, even death. The only real way to find out if you're low in T or is at such risk is to get checked by a doctor knowledgeable in testosterone replacement therapy (TRT).

> As men age, testosterone levels generally but variably decline due to the slug-gishness of the hormonal feedback loop.

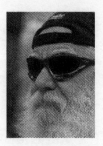

D. Why is Testosterone Important? Many reasons, and there are just as many books and references that go into greater detail than I can in this one book. For one *killer* reason, men with low testosterone have a 75 percent increased mortality rate. The *Archives of Internal Medicine* published an eight-year study of men with low testosterone aged older than forty, and found a mortality rate of 35 percent versus 20 percent in those with normal levels.[146] "Low testosterone is a common condition in aging, associated with decreased muscle mass and insulin resistance."

As I preach, older adults succumb more to the *frailty syndrome* than the many actual age-related diseases themselves, i.e., cancer, infection, dementia, emphysema, and unfortunately a whole lot more. Falls are the number 1 accident killer of older adults.[147] Also, the increased insulin resistance seen with low T is a risk for diabetes, hypertension, hypercholesterolemia, heart disease, erectile dysfunction, and more complications.[148] This adds credence to what I'm promoting—a paradigm shift that identifies and treats the root causes of such age-related diseases. It's proactive and not reactive, a much better course in life! I will present a few of the best-known important benefits below.

---

146 M. Shores, "The Geriatric Research, Education, and Clinical Center; VA Puget Sound Health Care System," *Arch Intern Med.* 166 (2006):1660–65. This was concluded even after adjusting for all other risks for mortality including age, medical comorbidities, and other covariates. Also, first year results were excluded to rule out acute disease as a cause for an early death.

147 November 20, 2006—The U.S. Centers for Disease Control and Prevention (CDC) reported in the November 17, 2006, issue of the *Morbidity and Mortality Weekly Report* on the increased rate of fatal falls among elderly men.

148 Men with diabetes aged forty-five and older may be more than twice as likely as nondiabetic men to have low testosterone levels, according to new data announced at the American Diabetes Association Annual Meeting and Scientific Session in San Diego, 2005. Results of this multicenter study, which screened more than two thousand men, also found sexual dysfunction to be the most common symptom experienced by men with diabetes and low testosterone (known also as hypogonadism, or low T). These data are a subset analysis of the Hypogonadism in Males (HIM) study.

Ask any young person to imitate an "old geezer." He will bend over, shuffle his feet, move unsteadily slow, and usually have a Parkinsonian-like tremor. He would annoyingly ask the same questions many times and would be sporting a hearing aid and thick glasses. This constellation would be identical to the many aging outcomes presented previously, i.e., osteoporosis, the neuro-degenerative disorders, sarcopenic obesity, and such. The young thespian has just acted out the physical characteristics of the frailty syndrome.

Osteoporosis and the Frailty Syndrome; I've fallen and can't get up. Laurence Katznelson, MD, reviewed a lot of what is presented above in *Testosterone Therapy in Men: An Update.*[149] He focused on T deficiency being a most important risk factor for osteoporosis, and the resulting fractures and morbidity seen in men. Men over sixty-five years old have a hip fracture rate of about five in one thousand, and it may surprise you to find that approximately one-third of all hip fractures do occur in men. Such T-deficient men have significantly decreased trabecular, or *middle bone*, density, making up over half of those presenting with a hip fracture. TRT leads to a significant increase in skeletal mass and strength. Many others have since reinforced these positions.[150]

Other underappreciated ramifications of osteoporosis include the following: The chronic debilitating pains alluded to above and the subsequent risk for depression. There's also restrictive lung disease. Some patients initially present just complaining of shortness of breath. This is because of the stooped over, or kyphotic, posture that restricts good lung expansion during inhalation. The lungs are literally squashed. This, in turn, increases risks of getting pneumonia—the biggest infectious killer in America. These limitations, along with the other age-related losses in strength and coordination seen with low T, add further to the debility of so-called *normal* aging. Overall, men do a lot worse than women after having a hip fracture. Think back to the example I gave of the younger person imitating Mr. McGoo. Is this really what you want to become?

---

149 L. Katznelson, 2000. Testosterone therapy in men: an update. *MGH Neuroendocrine Clinical Center Bulletin* (6)2 (2000) retrieved from Harvard University Medical School, June 12, 2003. L. Katznelson, *JCEM* 81 (1996):4358–65.

150 P. J. Snyder et al., "Effect of testosterone treatment on body composition and muscle strength in men over 65 years of age," *Journal of Clinical Endocrinology and Metabolism* 84 (1999): 2647–53, presented these such benefits, too. He also suggested proper replacement including the monitoring of levels and side effects are very important. Christian Meier, MD, from the University of Basel in Switzerland. ASBMR 28th Annual Meeting: Abstract 1020. Presented September 16, 2006.

Most patients are surprised to learn that men, in fact, do get osteoporosis. Risk factors include smoking, steroid therapy, lack of the proper diet and exercise, along with any disabling disease, as well as just old age. Men generally lose bone mass at about the same rate as women; however, we have more bone mass to begin with. Basically, I state that men get osteoporosis; they're just about ten years behind women. When you look at it, even without risk factors, any man over sixty-five is at risk. Get a bone density test and find out now. As in heart disease, you wouldn't want to wait until you have a heart attack to find out you're at risk; don't wait until you have osteoporosis or, worse yet, a fracture to seek treatment. And you should check calcium, magnesium, TSH (thyroid stimulating hormone), and 25-hydroxyl vitamin D levels. Lastly, if you don't use it, you lose it; so remember to do those resistance exercises. If you don't get sarcopenia, then you probably won't get osteopenia!

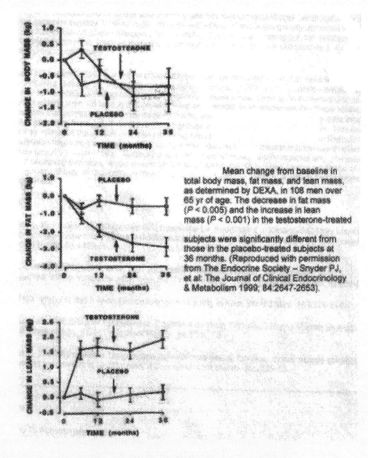

Mean change from baseline in total body mass, fat mass, and lean mass, as determined by DEXA, in 108 men over 65 yr of age. The decrease in fat mass ($P < 0.005$) and the increase in lean mass ($P < 0.001$) in the testosterone-treated subjects were significantly different from those in the placebo-treated subjects at 36 months. (Reproduced with permission from The Endocrine Society – Snyder PJ, et al: The Journal of Clinical Endocrinology & Metabolism 1999; 84:2647-2653).

Figure 8.7. Effects of T on body composition by Snyder et al., *JCEM* 1999.

Most elderly suffer from the *frailty* of getting older. The immobility and dependence are worsened with illness. In the end, the resulting frailty is worse than the diseases themselves. TRT, if appropriate, along with a healthy life-style can help fight this and keep you active in today's mobile society.

Depression and Dementia: Are mind games being played? The mind is probably less likely to proceed to dementia or depression if there are upper range T levels.[151] Most basically know women outlive men, and nowadays both can expect to live longer than their parents. The average life span of men is 11 percent less than that of women. At age sixty-five, life expectancy for women is 25 percent greater than men. But what good is it for any of us to be around if our minds are gone? Remember, we also want *quality* with this quantity of life. Let's look at this in further detail.

This increased death rate is not just from vascular and the other diseases we often think about, but virtually an epidemic of suicide as well in men older than sixty. Thus as men pass fifty, they face the increasing prevalence of life-threatening diseases that greatly impair their quality of life. Mostly, these are cardiovascular or stroke related; but sexual dysfunction, hypogonadism, and suicide are all strongly associated with depression. After sixty, women no longer outnumber men diagnosed with depression. This reflects the profound increase in comorbid health problems men get with age.[152]

Suicide *is* the eighth leading cause of death in the United States, increasing in men aged over sixty. This incidence is expected to be underestimated, and men are more likely to die from suicide attempts than women. The highest rate of suicides in America is among white men older than eighty-five. Worldwide, the aging male is at increased risk as well. This probably reflects his overall poorer health status. Regrettably, despite more effective modern therapies available, there's been no dramatic reduction in the rate of suicide in men over sixty. Probably, better screening by physicians may help identify aging men at risk, as 70 percent see a physician in the prior month. It's a shame that a lot of these men are middle-aged,

---

151 According to a research article published in the *Archives of General Psychiatry* 61 (2) in 2004, hypogonadal men appear to have a *fourfold* increase risk of depression. The mean life expectancy at age seventy-five is 9.4 years for men and about 12 years for women.

152 Facts taken from *Men Over 50: An Endangered Species.* http://www.medscape.com, accessed 5/2007.

in the peak of their workplace and earnings performance. Addictions to alcohol and drugs may contribute as well. I've known two midlife male patients die within the past six months from suicide, none from heart disease. One by a self-inflicted gunshot wound, the other by drug overdose.

The *convergence of evidence* points toward TRT benefiting dysthymic (overall feeling blue or depressed personality) or depressed hypogonadal men. There is understandably some conflicting research concerning TRT's effect in depressed men. Without going through all the trials, I will give a summation. Probably, if the depression began in his early twenties, he wouldn't be hypogonadal. This would be considered early-onset depression. TRT also shouldn't be expected to help if T levels aren't abnormally low. (No hormone should be replaced if it's not deemed deficient.) Part of the workup for mood disorders may include other hormonal testing as thyroid and cortisol. Testing for heavy metal toxicity, sexually transmitted diseases, and psychological aspects may also be necessary. However, in mid- or late lifers with depression, T levels should be checked, and properly replaced if clinically indicated. In older men, when there are many other comorbid factors along with multiple medications having depressing side effects, hypogonadism should be strongly considered. TRT should be initiated for them if the benefit outweighs their personal risks.

Heart disease and depression link. Way back in 1993, Frasure-Smith and colleagues out of Québec brought attention to the comorbid association of ischemic heart disease and depression. They reported that depressed post-MI patients have a higher risk of cardiac mortality at six months. The mortality rate was 17 percent for depressed patients compared to 3 percent for those not depressed. More important was that this increase in mortality affected not only those with *major* depression, but also those with only *moderate* depressive symptoms. Even at eighteen months, those scoring high on the Beck's Depression Scale (a common depression questionnaire) yet with no overt depression symptoms, died at the same rate as those diagnosed with major depression. Other studies also indicated even mild depression's ill effect on increasing ischemic heart disease. Lastly, I find it interesting to ponder the probability of reciprocal predisposition. Did the comorbid factors and ischemic heart disease bring on the depression, or was it vice versa?

---

153 N. Frasure-Smith, "Depression following myocardial infarction: Impact on six month survival," *JAMA* 270 (1993), 1819–25.

At any rate, depression should *not* be considered a normal aging process in men with or without heart disease. The neurohormonal changes seen with depression are associated with hypothalamic-pituitary axis hyperactivity, as indicated by elevated cortisol levels and a disturbance in its diurnal pattern. (Physicians are well aware of how corticosteroid treatment worsens cholesterol, hypertension, osteoporosis, diabetes, and other maladies.) Additionally, the increase in sympathomimetic activity seen with depression, i.e., increased adrenaline, may contribute to the pathology of arterial disease. These include vasospasm, increased platelet aggregation, and resulting clot formation. The accompanying increased risk of arrhythmia with such hormonal dysregulation may also contribute to sudden death. That really bites. So there's some evidence for depression actually *inducing* vessel disease.

In November 2002, Raymond Niaura in *Health Psychology* commented on the connection between hostility, the metabolic syndrome, and incident coronary heart disease. It's well known that irritability, anxiety, and similarly grouped psychiatric conditions generally increase during middle age. Based on data from the Normative Aging Study that looked at 774 healthy men, high hostility scores and low HDL predicted incident coronary heart disease better than most commonly known risk factors such as lipids, hypertension, smoking, and such. We all have heard the saying, "Stress can kill you." This research suggests risks for sudden coronary disease include more diverse risk factors than what's currently commercialized.

Many studies have proven the connection between *low T* and *dementia*. And again, this is probably a cyclical relationship, i.e., brain damage causing pituitary disturbances, giving a secondary cause for hypogonadism. But if indeed primary hypogonadism precedes Alzheimer's disease (AD), TRT may be considered more useful for the *prevention* and *treatment* of AD in hypogonadal men.[154] Eventually, people suffering with AD, or any other neurodegenerative disorders for that matter, usually succumb to the frailty syndrome. With this gradual yet steady decline, the person's dependency and disability become overwhelming. This becomes a tremendous burden on the spouse and entire family. This twenty-four-week study concluded that applying T gel improved overall quality of life for AD patients in as early as three months. Yet, only about 20 percent of these patients were truly T

154 This suggestion was presented by the *Neuro Endocrinology Letter* in June–August 2003. Further researching the complexities of these relationships was research posted in the *Archives of Neurology,* December 2005, by Po Lu et al.

deficient in the first place. Regardless, even this form of T *augmentation* resulted in better visual-spatial scores than placebo.[155] That's nice to know, but I would predict only AD patients low in T would benefit the most from TRT. It makes me wonder how they defined low levels of T. I would imagine almost the subjects studied had *suboptimal* T levels. As mentioned, low T could help cause, or be a result of, these chronic, complex maladies. Low T and frailty probably represent a viscous cycle. This makes for common sense. One of the best ways to prevent becoming disabled is to start peddling on the other form of a cycle now.

Also, dementia is hard to diagnose, especially in the early stages. There are many subtypes. Accordingly, there is no one specific lab test or imaging study that clinches the diagnosis 100 percent. The lack of an early diagnosis or an accurate one usually impedes proper, early treatment. Since there's currently no real cure for dementia, we should focus on delaying the inevitable decline. Hopefully, this would improve the quality of life in the interim. Other easily treatable causes for dementia, such as medications or heavy metal toxicity, should be fully investigated. It's very difficult for the physician to differentiate true dementia from depression, often called *pseudodementia*. For example, if somebody's depressed, he may not even care enough to receive or recall the information being presented to him. This results in a perceived forgetfulness. In pseudodementia, a cure is readily available. Unfortunately, I often find that both conditions coexist. Further complicating matters is the usual age-related decline in function of all the senses—hearing, vision, smell, touch, and taste.

Lower T occurs variably in all older men. Some of these have AD alone, or with Parkinson's disease, PD. Research published in *Neurology* in 2004 suggested men with the lowest levels usually suffer more dysfunction. Testosterone deficiency may act as a "second hit" to further cognitive impairment. Another common aspect of PD—apathy, is inversely correlated with T levels; proper replacement also helps. As presented above, TRT has been shown to improve both the motor and nonmotor functions of PD. These commonly overlap—the decreased enjoyment of life, lack of energy, increased sexual dysfunction, and depression. Thus, I believe T testing and, if appropriate, TRT should be instituted for all PD patients. Low T could be considered a coexisting disease with PD or even play a role in the pathophysiology. This was expressed in the *Archives of Neurology* back in 2002. Whether

---

155 Naturally, guys tend to do better at directions than women, helping to define our sex role. Women are better at expressing emotion and language skills. We don't ask for traffic directions; they like to watch soap operas and gossip. It's a fact of life.

T is the chicken or the egg, it's almost a moot point, as TRT can help delay a lot of the disabilities experienced by men with AD or PD.

> Low testosterone can help mitigate and aggravate many diseases of the mind—namely depression and dementia. The ramifications of these can be quite serious. TRT has been shown to help even hypogonadal midlifers improve these conditions.

Neurological conditions related to low T—No stroke of bad luck! A stroke, or *brain attack*, basically has the same cause as a heart attack—basically, a blockage of blood flow to the specific end organ. Similarly complicating matters, most research shows up to 50 percent of stroke patients become acutely depressed. Unlike the heart though, it depends more on which part of the brain suffered the structural damage. This may be akin to the increased risk of depression in *Parkinson's* patients. There is also increased depression seen in patients with *vascular dementia*. This common from of dementia is caused by silent, but multiple, "mini" strokes in the brain. Unfortunately, this depression is usually recalcitrant to medical therapy and is more insidious in nature because of its underlying irreversible structural damage. *Seizure,* or epilepsy, is also common result of having a stroke. All this is in addition to the obvious neuromuscular loss or paralysis resulting from a stroke. Of course, there is also the substantial loss and burden to the family, as well as to society as a whole, to consider. Most patients would rather die or have a heart attack than to suffer a stroke because of the likelihood of becoming a fraction of the former self and the loss of independence.

In 2003, interesting research done by Fukui, MD, further proved free testosterone (FT) is inversely related to carotid atherosclerosis.[156] This means the lower the FT, the higher amount of vessel disease. Such blockages would increase one's risk for stroke. Carotid intima-media thickness (IMT) has long been used to assess the plaque burden in the carotids and is also one of the best predictors of coronary vessel disease. The thicker the vessel, the higher are the risks. Research published in the *Journal of American College of Cardiology* specifically reiterated these points. Again, measuring IMT brought conclusions to a new, higher level of understanding. I say this because it parallels what we mostly see with HRT in healthier, younger menopausal women. They concluded that *middle-aged* men with symptoms of andropause, together with absolute or *compensated* (as reflected by high

---

156 M. Fukui, "Association between serum testosterone concentration and carotid atherosclerosis in men with type 2 diabetes," *Diabetes Care* 26 (2003):1869–73

normal to elevated LH) T deficiency, show increased carotid IMT. This suggests that *optimal* T levels offer protection against the development of atherosclerosis in middle-aged men. This was based on the Turku Aging Male Study, which looked at ninety-nine hypogonadal men, aged forty to seventy years.[157]

We must remember, cholesterol is just one risk factor for age-related vessel disease. We must not "miss the forest for the trees." Visceral fat, diabetes, hypertension, inflammation, and other markers or mediators put the so-called *nail in the coffin*. So in midlife, the *convergence of evidence* shows androgen *deficiency* increases your risks for many serious illnesses. Research shows proper TRT prevents and treats all these in a more encompassing yet more natural, safer approach. Given the above, it would be reasonable to expect TRT would also help prevent strokes in men with androgen deficiency.

Testosterone has a direct favorable effect on keeping vessels disease-free. Men with low levels have been shown to have an increased risk for stroke and cardiac disease.

Diabetes and low Free Testosterone: A bittersweet connection. As far back as 1992, the December issue of the *International Journal of Obesity* reported TRT in *middle-aged* hygonadal men results in less visceral fat, improved diabetic indices including insulin, and improved blood pressure. They reiterated T levels in the *mid-normal* range for healthy young men are consistent with *optimal* cardiovascular risk profile at any age, and having *low* levels may *increase* risk for disease. Many of these earlier studies may have exhibited some conflicting results because only *total testosterone* (TT) levels were measured. As mentioned above, only about 2 percent of the TT is free testosterone (FT), the *active* component. The other 98 percent or so is bound, therefore inactive.

Low FT levels correlate best with risk for diabetes, for example. The percentage of FT can vary and be quite under 2 percent, which would make this active portion even lower.[158] For example, I've seen many older men that had prior TT levels

---

157 J. Mäkinen, "Increased carotid atherosclerosis in andropausal middle-aged men," *Journal of the American College of Cardiology*. 45, no. 10 (2005):1603–8.

158 This was reflected in research by Dhiendsa, MD, of State University of New York at Buffalo and Glenn Cunningham, MD, professor and vice chairman of research at Baylor College of Medicine in December 2004. One in three diabetic men had low sex hormone levels. N. Makhsida, "Hypogonadism and the metabolic syn-

around 500—not that bad. They were suffering from all the symptoms of low T, but were told by their previous inexperienced doctor their T was great! These concerns had to be simply due to something else. Yet, *something else* was never found. In actuality, their doctors didn't really know because FT wasn't ever appropriately measured. Once checked, the FT was, in fact, pathologically low. Once TRT was properly initiated as part of a total integrative approach, the men dramatically improved. So it's important to compare apples to apples to know what's, or what's not, going on. You should get FT and TT levels checked as part of the work up for andropause. It's the only way to know what you're truly missing.

I see this more often in midlife or older obese men with glucose intolerance or other morbidities, who's sex hormone binding globulin (SHBG) is typically higher. (SHBG is what mostly binds up testosterone, making less FT available [see figure 8.5].) Low FT can either mitigate or worsen their problems. As mentioned above, the resulting loss in muscle mass and gain in fat mass only makes diabetes and all its complications worse. The above authors reiterate, "I advise all diabetic men to check (their) FT, not total testosterone … we are screening all diabetic men for low testosterone because the symptoms are very nonspecific. Anyone can have erectile dysfunction or a mood problem. And most diabetics with low testosterone do not have any symptoms. They are surprised to find they have low testosterone."

Tying a lot of the above together was an excellent article in the *Journal of Clinical Endocrinology and Metabolism* describing the relationship of androgens, insulin resistance, and vascular disease in men.[159] It deeply explains what goes awry in this terrible triad of diseases and how these are set in motion with low testosterone. This is quite cutting-edge research, so it's mostly underappreciated by the current medical community. Type 2 diabetes is now in epidemic proportions worldwide and is a big risk factor for both peripheral and coronary heart disease. In diabetics, the insulin resistance and glucose intolerance add up to increased glycosylation and the production of those AGEs presented earlier. This only serves to increase inflammation and the accompanying disorder—sort of like adding fat to the fire. The relationship between low T and the increase in visceral fat, the *apple* shape, was also explained. Besides making the older man a *manly* man, visceral fat is one of the biggest risk factors for all vascular disease.

drome: Implications for testosterone therapy," *Journal of Urology* 174, no. 3 (2005): 827–34.

159 D. Kapoor, "Androgens, insulin resistance and vascular disease in men," *Clinical Endocrinology* 63, no. 3 (2005): 239–50.

The typical woman is *pear*-shaped. This reflects the general increase in *peripheral* fat as she ages—generally, in the butt and thighs. Peripheral fat is different than the centralized, visceral fat found in men. We're talking about that hard keg where that six pack use to be. This distinction is very important when it comes to disease risks. Here's why. *Peripheral fat* drains into the usual peripheral and then into the deep venous system. Not a big deal. But *visceral* fat drains from the intestines *through the hepatic portal venous system and then directly into the liver.* The liver is then exposed to these increased free fatty acid levels. This causes some very unhealthy metabolic changes to occur. Because of the higher fat concentration, the liver mistakenly believes the body is in a starvation state and, as a result, releases glucose. This process is called *gluconeogenesis.* Please refer to the below diagram.

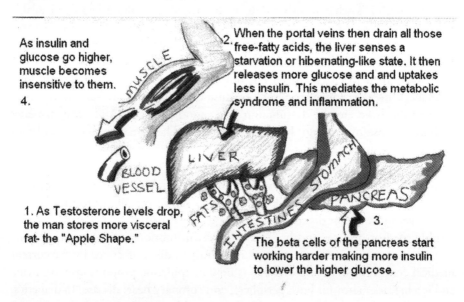

Figure 8.8. The low T–apple-shape diabetes connection. With low T, visceral fat increases and sets the self-defeating cycle of increased insulin, glucose, and fat. Insulin worsens vessel disease.

This leads to decreased insulin uptake by the liver, resulting ultimately in higher insulin levels and muscle insulin resistance. This causes further release of insulin with even higher glucose levels. The cycle continues until the person eventually has diabetes. Recall what I've said about insulin being one of the biggest inflammatory mediators in the body. The resulting *apple shape* from visceral fat correlates best with man's increased risk of earlier mortality and cardiac disease.

There are other abnormalities such as increased inflammation and decreased levels of leptin, a hormone that induces satiety. If leptin is high, the person has less appetite. Other mediators such as *fibrinogen* and *adiponectin* are also increased. Together, all these are termed *adipokines*. I believe this *modus operandi* is how Mother Nature arranged for men to generally have a shorter life span than our rib-derived descendants of Eve. (As any consolation, Mother Nature allows us men to be able to reproduce our whole lives.)

If you look around, you'll invariably see that men risk gaining this middle-age spread, i.e., visceral fat, as they age. Accordingly, FT levels decline as men age, causing that loss in muscle mass and increase in fat mass. Older men have to put the belt loop of their pants above or below this mound. They may have to wear suspenders because there are no more butt cheeks to help hold their pants up. Obese men are at increased risk of diabetes and of having low T. (Conversely, weight loss, which can be achieved with the proper diet and exercise, naturally results in higher T levels.) As usual, these relationships are cyclical in nature, so it's another case of "which came first, the chicken or the egg." This age-related fat increase also raises aromatase activity, which causes an increased conversion of testosterone to the estrogens, the female sex hormones. This may play a role in the increased fat, as well as breast size in older men. With this, LH pulses from the pituitary, which tells the testes to make more testosterone, are usually diminished. This further lowers testosterone levels, thereby increasing fat. And so the cycle continues. These relationships further illustrate the complex associations between obesity, low testosterone levels, depression, dementia, and diabetic complications.

Recently, the 2005 Annual Meeting of the Endocrine Society promoted the above points, adding that muscle strength and overall sexual functioning are improved in healthy older men with TRT. A related presentation reported subjects on TRT had *decreased* their visceral fat by 7 percent versus a 17 percent *increase* in the placebo group. Importantly, all were *nonobese* men. This suggests that even non-obese men may receive the cardiovascular benefits and lower visceral fat from TRT. That's good news for all us "not-so-phat" MAGs!

> Men with low testosterone are more apt to have increased visceral fat—the apple shape. A waste circumference over 35 inches or having one larger than his hip's puts him at risk of the metabolic syndrome. TRT will help reduce his waist size as part of a comprehensive lifestyle approach.

Ya' gotta' have heart! Decades of research shows that proper TRT in the hypo-gonadal male improves heart function—even on those with severe disease. We cover this aspect more in the Special Topics chapter. Concerning congestive heart failure (CHF) research presented at ENDO 2005, the Eighty-seventh Annual Meeting of the Endocrine Society, it was concluded that TRT significantly improved exercise capacity and quality of life in men with moderate to severe CHF.[160] The author brings up a very important point about previous research and policies that questioned the safety, or even contraindicated the use of, TRT in patients with CHF. I agree with Dr. Jones when he points out that the only research that contraindicated TRT with CHF were ones that used *supraphysiologi-cal* dosing, which would result in some previously reported undesired side effects such as increased edema. This twelve-month study with proper *physiological* dos-ing of T resulted in 35 percent of patients improving by at least one NYHA (New York Heart Association) class and about an 18 percent improvement in functional capacity. Left ventricular cavity length was maintained, indicating that no pro-gression of CHF occurred. Additionally, blood pressure parameters were stable, patients felt better about themselves, and improved muscle strength were noted. The doctor added that since TRT also improves mood and cognition, it may benefit patients with CHF-related cachexia, or frailty. Importantly, there was no evidence of edema, or changes in BNP (B-type natriuretic peptide)—a lab mea-surement of worsening congestive heart failure. Lastly, no changes were noted for tumor necrosis factor, an inflammatory marker; PSA, a prostate disease marker; or hematocrit levels.

I welcomed this research for a number of reasons. First, the heart, being a mus-cle, *should* be expected to improve with TRT if T is indeed deficient. Second, replacing levels to the proper physiological levels as most newer research accom-plishes, usually results in more benefit with less side effects than the earlier stud-ies using improper dosing or supraphysiological levels. Those earlier studies gave TRT an undeserving bad reputation and scared many doctors and patients off, even though some remained true believers. Also, the newer research is important because most moderate-severe CHF patients are older men with many other ill-nesses that TRT incidentally improves. Lastly, I know of no other drug effective in *improving* CHF; there's only a few that only delay the worsening of CHF to some degree. These also have many potentially severe side effects. It's nice to see

---

160 According to Hugh Jones, MD, previous pilot findings published in *Heart* (2003) were confirmed. May, 2005. Noted then were significant improvements in functional capacity and treated patients were actually walking a mean 65 meters further at three months.

proper TRT is quite safe and actually *improves* many other accompanying illnesses in aging men with CHF.

Testosterone: A Case of Mistaken Identity?

Historically, laypeople and physicians alike have had the mistaken notion that it's probably the naturally higher level of T in men compared to women that puts us at higher risk for heart disease and an earlier death. Understandably, there would be a gut instinct never to use TRT if this was, in fact, the case. But it's not. This totally unfounded prejudice is saddening since decades of scientific research *don't* show TRT negatively affects heart disease and death. I've shown you data stating the exact opposite! TRT actually *improves* most risks for heart disease and prevents an early death. Commons sense would indicate it's really the *older* man who's at higher risk, right? The old geezer's T is much lower compared to when he was in his earlier prime. This lower T level accompanies increased disease rates.

Erectile dysfunction, or the mind-body-penis connection. Maybe we should use the term "penile attack" to parallel its shared vessel pathophysiology with brain attack and heart attack. That may be stretching things semantically. Basically, the same risk factors for heart attack and stroke also puts men at risk for ED—hypertension, hypercholesterolemia, diabetes, smoking, and obesity. The biggest risk factors happen to be smoking and obesity, when adjusted for other variables. Not surprisingly, age and depression also increase ED risk. And again, which came first (no pun intended)? Lastly, ED is very positively correlated with the risks for coronary artery disease. So much, in fact, that if a man presents with ED complaints, coronary risk assessment and even stress testing may be included in the workup.[162] This advice is based on the prospective results from the Massachusetts Male Aging Study (MMAS). Speaking of which, this study has a wealth of information concerning today's aging man and his health. I advise you get a copy of it and read it.

---

161 D. Simon, et al., "Association between plasma total testosterone and cardiovascular risk factors in healthy men: The telecom study," *JCEM* 82 (1997): 682–85.

162 This suggested also by Feldman et al. in *Preventative Medicine* April 2000 issue. There are many other authors that looked at the link of ED and CAD, diabetes, depression, etc.

To this end, it is also been shown that successfully treating the ED of depressed patients with Viagra© resulted in remission.[163] Quite impressive, I'd say. Mind you, Viagra is not classified as an antidepressant, as reflected by the nonresponders having no improvement in depressive symptoms. At the very least, this research reinforces what's presented above; improving a significant medical condition usually improves depression. ED is not yet classified as an illness, so Viagra is considered only a *lifestyle* drug—only thought to improve the quality of life. This is exactly what this book focuses on, the quality of midlife, and beyond! This correlation makes perfect sense to me; if you *physically* feel better, you *emotionally* feel better too. Sexuality is a reflection of how we feel about ourselves and our loved one. The mind and body are indeed intimately connected. This is not meant to insinuate in anyway that we guys think only with our penises. But according to the research, a healthy penis is a healthy mind and heart!

Of course, the urologists weren't going to let the cardiologists, endocrinologists, neurologist, and psychiatrists have all the fun with TRT; they have to have their say too. After all, this concerns men and their testes, right? Who knows this better than the urologists! In the *Journal of Urology* September 2005, Makhsita from Columbia University's Department of Urology concluded hypogonadism is likely a fundamental component of the metabolic syndrome. (I concur; I have yet to see a type 2 diabetic with a normal T level.) Besides treating hypogonadal symptoms, TRT may also have a tremendous potential to slow or to prevent progression to overt diabetes or cardiovascular disease via its beneficial effects on insulin regulation, lipid profile, and blood pressure. The MMAS identified obesity as the most important determinant of total T over time. T levels were 25 percent lower in the obese.[164] Additionally, TRT may also prevent age-related urinary complications such as neurogenic bladder and ED. He prudently advises testing for hypogonadism in those at risk for ED, with or without diabetes. I wholeheartedly agree and appreciate the research all these specialties are doing concerning testosterone's role in men's health. As a matter of interest, in Europe and elsewhere, it's much more common to treat hypogonadal diabetics with TRT. They have been seeing improvements in diabetic men's overall health for decades.

---

163 A twelve-week trial by Seidman published in *American Journal of Psychiatry* in 2001, showed 73 percent successfully treated depressed patients with ED, went into remission. The Beck's Depression Score, BDI, improved by 11 points compared with ED nonresponders' 4 points.

164 C. Allan, "Age-related changes in testosterone and the role of replacement therapy in older men," *Clinical Endocrinology* 60, no. 6 (2004): 653–70.

Some men walk into my office and ask for that free six-pack sample of Viagra they saw advertised on TV. Those ads are quite amusingly phallic-like, aren't they? I like the one from Cialis© with the guy throwing a football through the hole in the tire swing—what could be more suggestive? Well, given what you learned from above, it's not quite that simple. This guy may be suffering from diabetes, hypercholesterolemia, hypertension, vascular disease, depression, and more. He needs to be adequately worked up, as the same risks for *penile attack* puts him at risk for heart or brain attack. There is that strong correlation between ED and CAD we presented earlier, but this exists for emphysema and asthma too.

If a man doesn't favorably respond to the phosphodiesterase-5 inhibitors such as Viagra, Cialis, or Levitra, he may have vessel disease as explained above. In the healthier midlife man, I feel this lack of response commonly points to an androgen deficiency. Appropriate testing for testosterone levels should follow. Much research and my own clinical experience have shown such initial drug failures are improved with proper TRT. There's more on ED in the special topics chapter, too.

Dr. A. Morgentaler, the very well-respected associate professor of urologic surgery at Harvard Medical School relayed in a 2002 Review of Symposium Highlights that while most men undergo TRT for only complaints of sexual dysfunction, the majority of men go untreated simply because physicians are not comfortable with TRT. Probably doctors tend to err on the side of caution. He concluded by saying, "The risks of TRT are by and large known, and are really quite manageable with the proper monitoring. I think testosterone treatment is a very safe and valuable modality." He also encouraged knowledgeable physicians about proper TRT to become a resource for their local area because 95 percent of the affected deficient patients aren't taking the proper TRT needed. Many of the other guest speakers reiterated what I said previously, that TRT improves the myriad of systemic symptoms and diseases worsened by T deficiency. While it can help prevent the progression of such diseases in the younger male, TRT can also improve the multiple conditions I have previously stated for even the most aged and sick, i.e., those suffering from frailty, dementia, and depression issues.

For many men, suffering from erectile dysfunction, ED, is the last straw and finally gets them into the doctor's office. It's important to note that ED is a *late* symptom of having low testosterone. Before this, many other complications can arise—obesity, diabetes, depression, hypertension, high cholesterol, even vessel disease.

You've a great pair of lungs! Not to be outdone, the pulmonologists get to say their piece too. In 2004, the *American Journal of Respiratory and Critical Care Medicine* reviewed TRT effects in patients with COPD. This research is pertinent because emphysema is about the fourth biggest killer and increases in prevalence as we age. In the past, TRT has been believed by some to be contraindicated in those with COPD. The only *relative* contraindication I know of has to do with sleep apnea. (Again, that probably was related to the inappropriately high, supraphysiological dosing the earlier studies used resulting in subjects getting fluid retention and increasing hematocrit.) In the study, lean body mass increased in average of 2.3 kg with TRT alone and 3.3 kg with TRT and exercise.[165] They concluded the following:

> *This is the first demonstration that strength increases accompany androgenic steroid supplementation in COPD and raises the possibility that TRT may be appropriate therapy in conjunction with rehabilitative programs for patients with muscle weakness … another priority will be to conduct studies in women with COPD to determine whether gains in muscle mass and strength can be realized at T doses not yielding unacceptable virilizing side effects.*

---

165 R. Casaburi, *American Journal of Respiratory Care Medicine* 170 (2004): 870–78. In this study, forty-seven hypogonadal men, with what I would call moderate-severe COPD, an FEV1 of 40 percent predicted, underwent weekly T shots approaching physiological ranges. Four limbs of this study included one placebo with or without resistance training, or TRT with or without resistance training.

The *convergence of evidence* reveals the following when it comes to the benefit to risk ratio of TRT: First of all, the expansive symptoms of hypogonadism should be appreciated and T levels checked whenever suspected. Secondly, TRT benefits and risks should be clinically weighed and mutually agreed upon as any other treatment modality. There should be fully informed consent. Lastly—and this has only been alluded to in scant research—the *timing* of TRT is important. I believe TRT is overwhelmingly safer and probably more effective at disease prevention when started in middle age—when the deficiency would first occur. Getting healthy during this window *of opportunity*, as I've promoted many times earlier, is essential if we're to achieve optimal health in our later years. By maintaining a better body composition with TRT, many inflammatory and maladaptive metabolic changes are pre-empted. Concomitantly, age-related diseases such as diabetes, vessel disease, and the many other disabling outcomes we mentioned above are minimized or delayed. You're physiologically younger and healthier by preventing visceral fat from forming, and improving muscle and bone mass.

So why am I going through all this trouble talking about strokes, depression, metabolic syndrome, heart disease, dementia, and even ED? As promised earlier, I'm trying to establish some common ground all us guys should focus on. Rather than trying to separately treat all the *outcomes of aging*—each one—with many risky pills or surgery, there's a better, safer way. Isn't it far better to treat the *syndrome of aging*—the root cause—in the first place? Isn't middle age the last opportunity for us men to get our health in order? Gosh yes, as this book reveals! Lastly, just as risks for getting sick add up exponentially—i.e., one bad habit plus another equals three strikes against you—making the *right* lifestyle changes will synergistically improve your health. I'm just showing you the research to back all this up and then how you can put this plan into action. No one else is going to do this for you; you must connect the dots yourself.

E. Symptoms of Low Testosterone or Andropause. Most aren't aware of the vast beneficial effects TRT offers men suffering from low testosterone. The media has unfortunately fostered this confusion by lumping proper TRT with the recent sports scandals involving the obvious abuse of unnatural anabolic steroids—a totally different ballgame altogether. TRT maintains or improves bone and muscle mass, and decreases that unhealthy visceral fat. Libido and sexual ability, energy, sense of well-being, edge, and being—well, what a real man is really all

about—are restored. Emotional and cognitive improvements are noted. Here are the symptoms of low T:

Symptoms of Low Testosterone:

- Decline in muscle mass and strength. (Declines in muscle mass and strength are also correlated risk for falls and fractures, independent of bone density.)
- Increase in percentage body fat.
- Decrease in bone mineral density.
- Decrease in libido and frequency of sexual thoughts.
- Increase in frequency of erectile dysfunction. Less intense orgasms.
- Decline in scores on tests of well-being, mood, perception of overall health, and increase in irritability. These are frequently the first reported symptoms in associated with declining testosterone.
- Decline in aerobic capacity, VO_2 max, longer recovery time after exertion, decline in response to conditioning activities.
- Decline in cognitive skills, memory, and concentration. Increase likelihood of dementia.
- Increased risk of vessel disease, both coronary and peripheral. Dyslipidemia or high cholesterol.[169]

Figure 8.9. Low T, andropause symptoms. The many vague symptoms of andropause. Usually, the sexual complaints are a late manifestation. These improve with proper TRT. (Adapted Cenegenics©)

It's interesting to note the correlation of how low testosterone (gonadal insufficiency, failure or andropause) worsens the conditions listed above. Accordingly, once proper TRT is instituted, these are much improved. Lastly, you must remember about the *convergence of evidence* when it comes to understanding what the research out there *really* means. Once analyzed, it should make sense and be

166 Findings in patients are for a given reference age relative to other members of their cohort and are statistically normal subjects that are associated with age related longitudinal declines in testosterone levels. Findings for both groups are nearly identical, i.e., valid correlations exist for symptoms relative to age matched cohort or related to levels seen in individuals followed over time.

brought around full circle: T deficiency causes these symptoms. Proper replacement negates them.

As men age past thirty, T levels decrease about 1 percent each year. By age sixty, one-fourth of men clinically suffer from hypogonadism. That is, they get an F when it comes to possessing even the lowest range of what's considered *normal*. It's very important to appreciate these *normal* ranges greatly differ from *optimal* levels. The latter are the levels researchers have proven reduces your risks for getting many age-related diseases. Usually, these optimal ranges are in the upper quartiles, or one-fourth, of normal ranges. Many more men are suffering from what some researchers refer to as androgen deficiency of the aging male (ADAM), or *simply andropause.* These men are getting a C- or a D when it comes to their T levels. Shouldn't these be helped before they fail in life's many subjects? It's much better to prevent problems than to fix them, right? If TRT is then instituted, wouldn't it make sense to obtain T levels that correlate with the best health outcomes? Let's get them on the honor roll of life! Yet, for many reasons, conventional medicine hasn't grasped these concepts yet.

To see if you may suffer from andropause, or low testosterone, take the following quiz:

Male Andropause Test: Name_____Date_____

How you have felt overall the past few months, years?
Rank from: 0 - None 1 - Infrequently 2 - Somewhat 3 - Often 4 - Daily

1. Fatigue, tiredness, loss of energy.................0 1 2 3 4

2. Depression, low or negative mood 0 1 2 3 4

3. Irritability, anger, bad temper....................0 1 2 3 4

4. Loss of memory or concentration 0 1 2 3 4

5. Anxiety or nervousness 0 1 2 3 4

6. Relationship trouble 0 1 2 3 4

7. Loss of sex drive (libido) 0 1 2 3 4

8. Erection problems (hardness, lasting).........0 1 2 3 4

9. Loss of morning erections 0 1 2 3 4

10. Decreased intensity of orgasms 0 1 2 3 4

11. Stiff, painful joints, backache.....................0 1 2 3 4

12. Heavy drinking (past or present).................0 1 2 3 4

13. Loss of fitness 0 1 2 3 4

14. Feeling overstressed...................................0 1 2 3 4

(Add 4 if you had adult mumps, testicular problems,
prostate surgery) 4

CALCULATE TOTAL .... _____
(0–9 Unlikely, 10–19 Possible, 20–29 Probable, 30–39 Definite, >40 Advanced)
Chris Rao, MD, © 2007

Figure 8.10 Male andropause questionnaire. You may want to complete and bring this and the following to your doctor. If he's uncomfortable evaluating this, ask for a referral to someone else who's knowledgeable.

Concerning T levels, you should remember the following:

- As introduced earlier, not all the testosterone in the blood is in the active form. Only free testosterone (FT) is the true bioavailable form. This variably amounts to about 2 percent of total testosterone (TT). The other roughly 98 percent is bound to SHBG and albumin, as shown in diagram 8.5. This is important for a number of reasons. TT and FT should both be measured to get an accurate picture of T status. Many patients seen by other doctors were initially told their T was *normal*, when it fact it was in the gutter. The docs simply didn't know the right tests to order or how to interpret this to the clinical setting. More recent and valid, reproducible research concerning T levels routinely monitor and correlate symptoms to FT levels.

- Second, obesity, age, and illnesses can raise SHBG levels, thereby reducing FT levels. So it's good to check these levels if considering hormonal replacement. Routinely monitor both FT and TT. Check PSA levels and T metabolites such as estradiol and DHT for side effects and risks during therapy.[167] Digital prostate exams should be done every six months, or more often if clinically warranted. If your doctor doesn't follow these, you need to see one that does.

- Third, testosterone levels vary widely for each age group. As the below diagram shows, so-called normal levels for a sixty-year-old man can be anywhere from 275 to 1000, quite a variation. That would represent what I refer to going from the F to the A range. Further complicating matters is the variability in the *sensitivity* of the androgen receptors from individual to individual, much like all other hormonal receptors such as the thyroid, pancreas, etc. Because of this, it's harder to actually discern what the desired normal levels are for the specific individual. (Lab work really only helps us confirm or deny the probability of a diagnosis.) The only way to know for sure would be to measure one's T levels throughout their entire life span.

---

167 SHBG binds up the sex hormones, especially T. Estradiol is an estrogen metabolite of T. It can cause enlarged breasts. DHT is dihydrotestosterone and *may* worsen an enlarged prostate and cause hair loss. You should have these checked every three to six months, as clinically needed.

Testosterone Levels and Age.

Age	Total Test.	S.D.	10th %	33rd %	66th %
<25	692	158	468	534	850
25-29	669	206	438	463	875
30-34	621	194	388	427	815
35-39	597	189	388	408	786
40-44	597	198	378	399	795
45-49	546	163	358	383	709
50-54	544	187	348	357	731
55-59	552	174	338	378	726

Data are consistent with population and longitudinal studies

Figure 8.11. Declining T levels as we age. T levels vary greatly for each age group. Do you want to get a D or an A? (Adapted Cenegenics©)

For example, in seventh grade, there were boys in my class that were physiologically fully grown men. They had the height, muscle mass, fast cars, and all the foxes. They were great in sports, had to shave each day, and had enough body hair to make any "girly man" run and hide far away from Brokeback Mountain. These would be teenage males possessing the *upper levels* of baseline T. This would be represented at the sixty-sixth percentile, or upper-one third, levels for T, in the above figure. For further explanation, let's take a three-minute tour on one of the most favorite TV series ever created.

On the other end of the spectrum, is the more or less androgynous teenage male— slender, not much body hair, unaware yet of women, and would be … well, maybe more of the nerdy, klutzy, or artsy type, much like Gilligan on *Gilligan's Island*. Although all in TV land couldn't help but love this character, Gilligan would likely possess a lower baseline T level when young.

Hey, what happened to my "little buddy"? Later, the macho teen in this scenario—the Skipper, may start to experience some subtle changes as his T levels begin to drop in middle age. This *man's man* would then start to suffer from low

T symptoms such as irritability, obesity, lack of energy, and not being able to do it with Ginger or Mary Ann. (Face it, who wouldn't have if they could've.) Because of such, he's now relegated to often just beating on his "little' buddy." If measured though, Skipper's T level would probably *still* be within what's considered the *normal* range for his middle-aged cohorts, although now in the lower-tenth percentile. Yet, this T level would be relatively quite low compared to the optimum sixty-sixth percentile he enjoyed as a swashbuckling teenager. Simply put, Skipper's T level is in the low-normal range for his age group when taken as a whole; however, it's relatively *very* low for him as an individual. Optimizing his T levels now in midlife would certainly put back the "skip" in Skipper's step!

I'll take advantage of my poetic license and extend this analogy a little further. Let's take a gander at the professor. Well, he's smart, naturally thin, and practices a healthy lifestyle. He doesn't mope and keeps his mind and body active. He probably had a midrange baseline T while a teenager. His genes and healthy habits helped maintain this level during his midlife. Being a savvy scientist, he probably would be *up* on what proper TRT can do and, after studying all the data, had optimized his hormonal levels himself. (I really don't want to know how he accomplished that while on the island.)

How about Mr. Thurston Howell III? Being a millionaire, he can well afford to receive the latest in age-management modalities. He knows his health is his best asset, more so than even money. Given his age, he had to get all his hormones balanced, including HGH. Ergo, he has a youthful outlook and energy level—never expressing any health complaints. And, he's still quite romantic with his wife, whom he routinely refers to affectionately as lovey-dovey! (She must also be on bioidentical hormonal replacement in order to keep up with him.)

When you sit back and think about it, life is like one gigantic sitcom. It shouldn't be taken so seriously, and we should be allowed to laugh often at our inadequacies. There are many different men out there—all with different genes, lifestyles, goals, and responses to different therapies. Likewise, there is no *one* correct way to help prevent age-related diseases and optimize our sense of well-being. It must be a comprehensive and individualized approach. The facts are overwhelmingly supportive of this. If we don't follow this advice, we might feel at times as if we're stranded on a desert isle with no chance of a rescue. We may be left only to recall reruns of our virile, younger selves. Only, there would be no Mary Ann or Ginger to comfort us. After all, no man should be an island, should he?

The *convergence of evidence* focuses on more profound yet simpler and safer ways to optimize aging men's health by treating the root causes. More recent research uses free testosterone (FT) levels to diagnose andropause. Additionally, the monitoring of FT and its metabolites result in more proper physiological TRT. This results in more validity and agreement—all with less side effects and complications than many earlier problematic studies. Lastly, therapies have to be individualized to optimize outcomes.

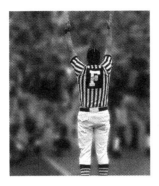

IX.

History of Testosterone Replacement in Aging Men: The Ups and Downs

After a few weeks, his reported aged symptoms of insomnia, fatigue, lack of energy and more improved ... feeling revitalized with increased physical strength and mental acuity, lastly adding he exhibited a remarkable increase in the length of his urine stream.
—Seguard

In ancient Egyptian and Roman times, it was quite common for the young pharaoh or emperor to have a harem, multiple wives, many concubines, or any combination thereof. Of course, this was long before any testosterone or any male enhancement methods were close to being identified. It's been shown nothing naturally increases testosterone levels more than having a new sex partner—although, I wouldn't try this at home if I were you.[168] Probably, this practice did increase testosterone production, thereby helping to maintain muscle mass, reducing fat mass, and outsmarting the competition. All these would be qualities demanded from such hierarchy. The longer these existed, the longer they could remain in power. The ancient Greeks, of course, appreciated the association between testes and masculinity; just look at the physique in their hard statues. Eunuchs, the

---

168 It would be best to spice things up and try new things with the partner you have—a new outfit, location, or different techniques. Maybe *you* can become a different, better partner instead?

castrated male servants, were some of the earliest men noted to display signs of andropause. Even Galen, the ingenious scientist, noted the similarities between young castrated men and old, frail, impotent men.

Throughout centuries, man has incessantly searched for the Fountain of Youth. Most have heard of the Spanish explorer Ponce de León and how he eventually landed on the shores of my home state, Florida. When you take a small tour of our oldest city, St. Augustine, you'll probably hear many historians theorize it may have been the sulfur content in the water that promulgated such curiosity and accounted for the increased longevity of the natives. Yes, that foul egg—smelling water coming from their fountains contained a low concentration of sulfur and probably did help the locals avoid infections to a degree. Back then, antibiotics, or even the idea of germs, weren't even close to being discovered. Common infections accounted for most illnesses and premature deaths.

Probably one of the first to consider testosterone replacement therapy as a secret to regaining younger health was Charles Brown-Sequard. The following revelations were reported in June 1889 in Paris. While apparently suffering the complications of old age, Seguard concocted a solution of seminal fluid, testicular blood, and extract from healthy dogs and guinea pigs and then injected himself subcutaneously. After a few weeks, his reported aged symptoms of insomnia, fatigue, lack of energy, and more improved. He further remarked of feeling *revitalized* with increased physical strength and mental acuity, lastly adding he exhibited a remarkable increase in the length of his urine stream. I can imagine his look when his partner exclaimed, "You ol' dog!"

Then in the 1920s, a few avant-garde surgeons began to implant monkey testicles into the scrotum or subcutaneous tissue of aging men. Frank Lydston, MD, even began implanting cadaver testes in men seeking improvement in senility, sexual power, or simply "rejuvenation." Another, named Serge Voronoff, apparently became quite famous treating wealthier elderly men worldwide. This may have been one of the first *antiaging* clinics! He noted patients exhibited "improvements in memory, greater aptitude for mental labor, and greater facility for intellectual effort." At the same time the genital functions became more active, and patients felt improved over all with a sensation of well-being. Meanwhile in Kansas, the Goat Gland Doctor, John Brinkley, would transplant goat's testicles for all about $750—a discount from the $5,000 for "death row prisoner" human testes. Because of his flamboyancy and unethical dealings, he eventually lost his license.

The search for more medically acceptable procedures ensued. Another procedure called *vasoligation* induced swelling of the testicles and supposedly increased testosterone levels. (This I find odd because similar operations today, such as a vasectomy, are considered to cause scarring, thereby decreasing T levels.) These dealings eventually caused more interest and media exposure. Some even claiming prevention of premature deaths, or advocating that everyone should receive these procedures as they age. Like today, only the most affluent would be privy to these options and able to afford such luxuries. William B. Yeats, the 1923 Nobel laureate in literature, reported, "It revived my creative power ... it revived also sexual desire and that, in all likelihood, will last until I die." Yet, the famous psychologist Sigmund Freud (and possibly his mother) denied any benefit. Regardless, such rejuvenation surgeries were quite popular with the aging affluent population. Testosterone replacement or drugs weren't an option at that time. The actual identification of testosterone will take about another forty years.

In about the mid-1930s, testosterone was purified. Much research was published in the 1940s in *JAMA*, describing the benefits of testosterone in treating the male climacteric—essentially the male menopause, or as we now call it, andropause. Thirty years later, research on testosterone levels and improvements in laboratory monitoring allowed better objective monitoring. In summary, TRT has been both praised and buried throughout the millennium. Probably, no other modality has been studied for such a long time. Yet, the debate continues today. So I say to testosterone, "You've come a long way, baby!"

A Personal Flashback. I would like to briefly review some research I did while an undergraduate at the University of New Orleans back in November 1987. Concerning the declining T levels in the aging man, the paper was entitled "Old Age Variation as a Developmental Stage in the Hypothalamic/Pituitary/ Testicular Axis and the Human Male." I presented then what was scarce data, and introduced some radical thoughts and hypothesis about decreasing testosterone levels and the role this plays in the aging male. My conservative female German endocrinology professor thought I was nuts; men don't have a *male* menopause—this is preposterous. She gave me a C!

I explained testosterone's pivotal role in determining sexual identity and preference in early fetal development. I presented pioneer research done in the early '80s that recognized lower androgen levels with advancing age and the correlation with increasing diseases. The diminished amplitude and frequency of LH pulses with advancing age were given as an explanation for diminished testosterone. I also pondered then what thousands more question nowadays, are these actually disorders or merely normal functions of aging? Should these neuroendocrine changes occurring in old age be taken as abnormal or just due to "wear and tear"? I summarized by purporting older age should be recognized and respected as a separate developmental stage. (This was before geriatrics was coined or even thought of being a specialty.) I ended with encouraging recognition of this evolutionary, significant, and beneficial maturing plateau in life.

My conclusion: "While these changes paralleled the declining sexual function that affects sexual activity, libido, and potency measures, such a decrease in typical male reproductive behavior may be advantageous in old age. Being less aggressive, competitive, and more gentle and caring of others would definitely be selected for successful traits developing in later years. Such an increase in androgyny is indeed observed in aging men. Also, androgynous old men were found to be happier, more competent, and possessing higher self-esteem. Changing gonadotropin levels have been demonstrated to have distinct effects on cognitive functioning. Changes in decision making occurring in old age may help older men arrive at a patient, contemporary, and thus 'wise' answer." I ended with, "So as a young man, if you find yourself rushing in traffic, late for a hot date, and being caught behind a slow-driving, cautious old man, relax; it's just a stage he's going through!" I wrote this roughly twenty years ago, yet today it's still considered cutting-edge thinking—so much for that C!

Chapter 9. MAG got his TT, FT, LH, and PSA[172] levels checked one morning. He found out his TT was normal, but his FT was moderately low. His score on the andropause questionnaire was okay. He wants to read more about options and discuss things with his wife. Granted, many of his symptoms have improved with his commitment to proper lifestyle interventions. He *still* has that visceral fat though. His main goals include lowering his risks of diabetes, osteoporosis, frailty, dementia, and cardiac disease. (He had signs of the metabolic syndrome already.)

---

169 TT—total testosterone, FT—free testosterone, LH—luteinizing hormone, PSA—prostate specific antigen, see text for descriptions. Metabolic syndrome is the collection of diabetes, hypertension, obesity, hypercholesterolemia, as described in text.

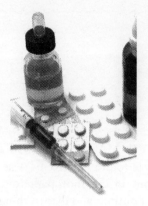

X.

Testosterone Replacement: The Ins and Outs

We age because our hormones decline; our hormones shouldn't decline just because we age. This is the paradigm shift of age-management.

According to the recent HIM (Health in Men) study, 34 percent of men aged forty-five to fifty-four years presenting to a primary care office were suffering from hypogonadism.[170] How do we determine if you are testosterone (T) deficient? First of all, you would be suffering from many of the vague symptoms presented earlier that are caused by low T levels. As mentioned before, the symptoms are quite varied and can affect many different systems in the body. Remember, erectile dysfunction is a late symptom of low T. (Please review the andropause quiz if needed [fig. 8.10].) Second, your lab work reflected a low free testosterone level (FT), and we ruled out the other many causes for similar symptoms and treated them without enough benefit.[171] Third, you're otherwise healthy and currently at no risk of having prostate cancer. We then fully reviewed the research on the benefits versus risks, and you finally decided to start TRT.

---

170 T. Mulligan et al., "Prevalence of hypogonadism in males aged at least 45 years: The HIM study," *International Journal of Clinical Practice.* 60, no. 7 (2006):762–69. Those with lower levels were more fat and more sick, overall.

171 I consider lab evidence for severe hypogonadism to be under 300 ng/dl TT and/or under 60 pg/ml FT.

> Even the most conservative doctors would say a total testosterone level below 300 ng/dl or a free testosterone level under 60 pg/ml objectively categorizes you as being hypogonadal, or having T in the "F" range. For every ten-year increase in age, your risk for hypogonadism is increased by 17 percent.

Congratulations, as only 5 percent of men with hypogonadism actually undergo treatment. This is mostly because patients and their doctors don't know the current facts concerning TRT safety, or when or how to even diagnose low T in the first place. If doctors don't know about it, how can they look for it? They may also be unfamiliar or uncomfortable with the necessary ongoing proper monitoring. Patients may also be confused by what they read or heard about various hormonal replacements. But you have now read the facts, done your homework, and are one smart, lucky dude. Where do we go from here? Well, there are many concerns and options. I will review them below, along with the most common benefits and risks of TRT. Notwithstanding, nothing replaces getting personalized advice from a physician having the expertise and qualifications in TRT. I find these are few and far between though.

First of all, **oral testosterone** shouldn't be taken by a man, as the dose typically used would be hepatotoxic (causes damage to the liver). So forget about taking any T pill. Second, some pharmacies tout *sublingual* testosterone as an option.[172] The problem here is a lot of the T is still swallowed and thereby still causing hepatotoxicity from what's known as the *first-pass effect*. This is caused by the oral form of T being ingested, *first* passing into the liver from the intestines, and *then* to the rest of the body (please see the below figure). This also taxes the liver to do more than its other normal duties. This route is not physiological, and that's what sets up many side effects. If you truly want to beat Mother Nature, remember you have to learn to beat her at her own game. It's not nice to fool Mother Nature; otherwise, she may bust out her ugly stick!

---

172 I have seen sublingual testosterone promoted more as an option for women with low libido, or sexual dysfunction. Although of a much lower dose, it's still quite risky because of the argument against any oral TRT in men. Since sublingual testosterone is shorter acting, it would also be difficult to obtain the longer-lasting, optimal levels that mimic the normal circadian rhythm. This route may increase the chances for symptoms such as agitation, hot flashes, and more. The physician would also find it quite difficult to interpret T levels in order to ensure they're not supraphysiological (abnormally, dangerously high) and not exposing you to many unnecessary risks and side effects.

The **first-pass effect** basically explains how a particular drug or hormone is absorbed into the body (see below). The first pass means the substance is ingested in the mouth, proceeds into the gastrointestinal system, and is then absorbed and passed on through the hepatic portal venous system into the liver first. There it is processed, stored for future use or metabolized (broken down) to less toxic substances, and released into the bloodstream. Now, if this is the way the compound was to be originally absorbed, as in food, it's well tolerated. If it's a toxin, there's trouble. If it's a synthetic drug or hormone, this can vary as far as the inflammation, workload, and subsequent damage to the liver is concerned. Making matters worse, to make up for the detoxifying effects of the liver on oral hormones, the typical doctor just gives an even higher dose. This only overworks the liver even more. It's like that famous *I Love Lucy* episode where Lucy has to keep packing up all the chocolate candies on that conveyer belt. Eventually, the increased amounts of candies overwhelm her to the point of having a nervous breakdown.

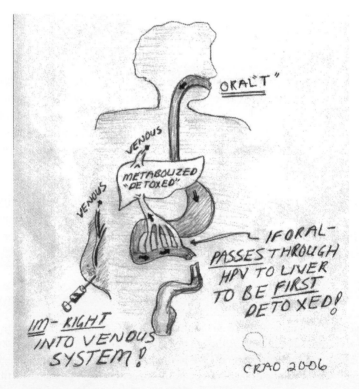

Figure10.1. First-pass effect of oral hormones. Oral hormones don't match what nature designed. Here, they're considered more of a toxin when presented in such high amounts to the liver via the hepatic portal vein (HPV). Intramuscular shots (IM) avoid this.

Hormones were originally designed by nature to be directly released into the bloodstream. When these are instead initially presented to the liver, the afore-mentioned problems arise and, even worse, can be additive. An example would be women on oral HRT (hormonal replacement therapy). If you read the *PDR* (*Physicians' Desk Reference*), you'll confirm that one of the most concerning side effects of taking oral sex hormones is liver damage. Additionally, the naturally detoxifying pathways in the liver are strained, resulting in impaired liver function. In men, because the dose is about ten times that for women, any oral TRT is *never* an option. When it comes to taking hormones orally, it's a simple case of being in the wrong place at the wrong time! Patients may also be taking statin drugs or other medications, which are metabolized through the liver and can further compromise function. The liver is intimately involved with the immune system and metabolic disorders; we should be extra careful what we present to it. For example, when patients have such multiple drugs metabolized through the cyto-chrome p450 system of the liver, we see lower IGF-1 conversion from HGH. This will increase your risk of suffering from adult growth hormone deficiency, as explained in the next chapter.

There are also **subcutaneous T pellets** that are inserted beneath the skin, releas-ing testosterone into the subcutaneous space, thereby escaping any *first-pass effect* to the liver. At least, this is more "bioidentical" meaning that, assuming the com-pound is identical to human testosterone, the hormone is being released directly into the bloodstream—as nature originally intended. The good thing about these implantable pellets is that after receiving a simple in-office procedure lasting only minutes, the patient will have worry-free TRT for about three months. No pills, or gels, or mixing it up and giving yourself shots, or dosing confusion. Of course, the downside includes going every three months for an in-office procedure with minimal risks and then paying any additional fees. Plus, you have more or less buried a set dose for three months beneath your skin, so you can't easily change it—be it too high or too low. This steady three-month dosing wouldn't remotely match the body's normal rhythmic release of T. Lastly, probably the biggest prob-lem I see would be the increased risk of supraphysiological dosing during the first month and a half, then decreasing to suboptimal levels the second month and a half. So the risks for feeling "over pumped up" initially or going through andro-pause symptoms (i.e., hot flashes, increase agitation, and such) in the later half are increased.

As stressed before, these regimens need to be individualized to the needs of the patient. Maybe a younger man doesn't have someone readily available to give him shots, or doesn't like shots in the first place. This route may be best for him. Or it may work for somebody always on the go with no time for gel or shots. An older man that may have compliancy issues because of depression or dementia may better fit this method of delivery. This may be most convenient for someone who travels a lot and doesn't want the hassles of explaining medication vials to airport security. These are all reasons why these modalities take much more time and expertise. It's because of the personalization that's indeed necessary—far from the contemporary one-size-fits-all approach.

The next application method would be **topical gels or patches.** For some reason, the latter is usually put on the scrotum, which I would consider quite a logistical problem. Topicals usually work well and are more convenient for those who doesn't like weekly shots or if such shots causes problems. Clinically though, the topical delivery methods may not increase the levels high enough if the patient is moderately to severely androgen deficient. The increased amount of gel needed, two or more packets, can create quite a mess on one's chest. Too much mousse on the old chest hairs! Also, the absorption depends a lot on when, where, and how it is applied. For example, if applied immediately after a shower on wet skin and then clothing is quickly put on, the amount absorbed into the skin is diminished. If the guy went right outside and sweated a lot, less gel is taken in too. Lastly, you must be careful not to expose your fertile female partner to topical testosterone because of possible effects on her or the developing fetus inside.

For many reasons, I just don't see consistency in T levels when patients use topical TRT. Additionally, there is research suggesting increased conversion of testosterone to dihydrotestosterone (DHT) and estrogens because of the higher exposure to converting enzymes found in the subcutaneous tissue and hair follicles (please see the diagram below). The former is associated with benign prostatic hypertrophy (BPH) and male pattern baldness. The latter is associated with enlarged breasts and possibly an increased risk for prostate enlargement. There is the incidence of allergic and local reaction to the gel, but I find it's less so than the patch. However, these remain a very favorable option because of the ease of use and because some insurances may reimburse for T gel. If not, topical gels can be really expensive. Again, it depends on what you and your physician are comfortable with and what works best for you.

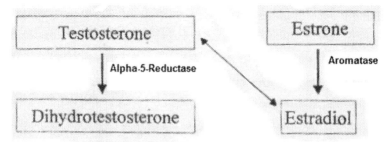

Increased coversion to DHT and Estrogens seen in hair and subcutaneous tissues

Figure 10.2. T conversion to estrogens and DHT.

> Oral testosterone is unsafe. Topical delivery systems as gels result in increased conversion of T to estrogens and dihydrotestosterone—not good. Additionally, it's hard for these to get you to optimal T levels

There is also **TRT via intramuscular (IM) shots.** These are usually given weekly; although it may depend on which specific testosterone compound is used. I usually prescribe testosterone cypionate, which has a half-life of about 8 ½ days.[173] An upside here is that T levels are quite consistent, which results in reaching optimal levels and, subsequently, optimal clinical results. The downside is it's a shot—best given by someone else. I can personally state the shot is virtually painless when given correctly, usually to the buttocks. Giving it yourself is quite difficult at first, but most master this easily. This is the route and T form I most often recommend to my patients.

In the past, TRT shots were usually given once a month by mostly urologists. This was really born out of convenience, but this dosing had all the bad effects of a supraphysiological dose. This method would initially result in an increased incidence of irritability, rage, anxiety, even psychosis. Also, this increased the risks of T's side effects as liver toxicity, worsening sleep apnea because of the increased hematocrit, and edema. As the level would wane toward the end of the month, the patient

---

173 The half-life is the time it takes for a drug or hormone to drop to 50 percent of its peak level.

would then go through hot flashes and all the bummers of andropause. This torture would ensue monthly. Today, with the backing up of a lot of research, proper physiological dosing is more approximated, thereby greatly diminishing these side effects and risks.

A vastly important decision factor in determining how T is replaced concerns the age of the patient and the functioning of the pituitary gland and testes. The latter is usually measured by lab work. As a rule of thumb, **if a male is below the age of sixty-five**, we assume his testes do work; they're a just a little bit, well … lazy. If you remember the feedback loop presented earlier, the pituitary increases LH levels in response to lower testosterone levels. As men age, this feedback loop becomes less sensitive. In early midlife, we may see this increased LH response in order to further stimulate the testes to make more T, but in later middle age, we see inappropriately low LH levels. The feedback loop has become less responsive or sensitive. Is this Mother Nature's design?

One point to make is we must first distinguish pituitary from testicular failure to make the proper diagnosis in order to decide on correct treatment options. This refers to the need to determine *secondary* from *primary failure,* respectively. For example, a young man may have undergone serious head trauma, thereby causing pituitary failure and no LH production. This is quite rare; but nonetheless, it happens and should be appropriately checked. Again, you don't find out what's wrong unless you look for it. For the most part, the testes in men below the age of sixty-five do function, but usually at a variable suboptimal level. See below:

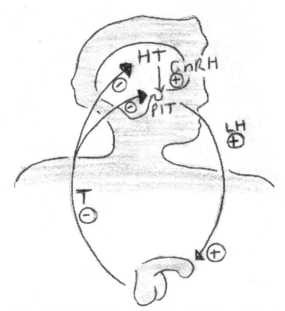

**In Primary Failure, there is no T, so LH goes up
trying to compensate. In age-related decline, both are
low because of burn-out and insensitivities.
In Secondary Failure, There is no LH, so no T either.**

Figure 10.3. Primary, or testicular failure. (HT-Hypothalamus, PIT-Pituitary, LH-Luteinizing Hormone, T-Testosterone.).

As I say, since the testes work, we should use them—the younger man's lab work usually shows the testes do work but are a bit lazy. Accordingly, we will then use a natural hormone to stimulate them to produce the optimal, yet physiological T levels. We have to basically crank them up a notch. The hormone is human chorionic gonadotropin, *hCG*, and is usually given in twice-per-week subcutaneous injections. It just so happens that it's is almost identical in composition to LH and fortunately has the same end-organ effect of stimulating the testes to produce more testosterone. I believe this is the best way to increase testosterone in a man younger than sixty-five years old, mainly because of fewer side effects. Usually, their baseline LH levels are in the *normal* range (which is actually suboptimal, or relatively low, since we would expect LH to be elevated in an attempt to whip the testes to make more testosterone). Again, the appropriate baseline lab work should be performed by a doctor who knows what to check and how to interpret these correctly.

Instead, if a younger man incorrectly uses *direct* TRT, be it topical or injection, the main side effects are testicular atrophy and infertility.[174] These effects can be permanent! Most guys enjoy having their *boys* around. It gives them something to play with and look at when no one is around. They wouldn't want these friends they've had since childhood to suddenly shrink and disappear. Therefore, using beta-hCG will achieve optimal T levels without your having to say, "Honey, I shrunk the kahuna!" The usual dosing is by subcutaneous injection, usually about 2000 to 3500 units divided twice per week. This is based on research comparing various dosages of hCG and its half-life in the body. This closely mimics the natural peaks and troughs in the most practical way. It doesn't have the *immediate bang* or *wow factor* that direct testosterone shots have the first week of initiation. *Indirect* TRT with hCG may take about six weeks to effectively stimulate the testes because of having to work through the body's own feedback-loop mechanism. This is usually no big deal. Even in men *above* sixty-five, I may use low-dose beta-hCG once per week to maintain testicular size. This is especially important for men that may model, wear tight clothes or beachwear, or participate in weight-lifting competitions. Mostly, this preservation of the testes is favorable to us guys who still want their boys around to hang with.

In men *over* sixty-five, we assume the testes don't function, or at only a fraction of what they used to, so direct TRT makes sense. To use hCG to stimulate the burnt out, older testes is like trying to whip a dead horse. Direct TRT can be with the options mentioned above: shots, pellets, or topical replacement methods.

> In men under sixty-five, it's usually better to use hCG to increase testosterone levels. Older men are best treated with direct TRT in the form of shots, gels, or topical routes. Shots give the best overall response. Any oral form is a no-no.

Interesting, quite new and promising for andropause treatment is a drug called Arimidex. This drug is an *aromatase inhibitor*—it blocks the conversion of T to estrogen (please see figure 8.2.) As mentioned before, the aging man generally produces less testosterone and more estrogen. This may account for them being more androgynous than during their younger macho years, but also carries the degen-

---

174 *Direct* would be *any* testosterone given directly from outside the body, be it intramuscular gel, patch, pellet, sublingual. This would include anything *besides* oral Arimidex or beta-hCG shots. Atrophy means shrinkage of the organ—in this case, the testes. Infertility means the inability to impregnate your mate or have kids.

eration and comorbidities associated with aging we have exhaustingly explained. (We do measure baseline estrogen levels as part of the andropause workup because of what follows.) Recall how T produced by the testes feeds back to the pituitary in order to regulate LH production. LH then stimulates the Leydig cells in the testes to make testosterone. (In the above diagram, if T levels were low, the pituitary would release more LH, thereby stimulating the testes to produce more T in order to achieve homeostasis.)

It appears that estradiol, as well as T, gives negative feedback to LH. Also, estradiol may decrease the sensitivity of androgen receptors, thereby decreasing testosterone's effects. Since Arimidex decreases estradiol levels in the T-deficient man, there would be less negative feedback, thereby increasing LH and T levels. Research since 2000 showed Arimidex increases LH production about two-fold and subsequently increases T about 50 percent—quite impressive![175] Also, DHT levels, suspected to be a player in undesirable prostate enlargement and hair loss, were unchanged. This last point I find surprisingly beneficial. Arimidex didn't cause the usual increase in estrogen and DHT seen with standard TRT. This would alleviate the need for additional medication to lower these T metabolites. Typically, an older middle-aged guy with *low* LH levels may be okay starting off with hCG shots and/or Arimidex. As you can see, which therapy to start takes some discussing; no two men have the same history, goals, or response.

Again, the expertise and the regular monitoring of treatment are key factors. As alluded to earlier, a combination of the above modalities may be used. I may have an older man on direct TRT via weekly intramuscular shots, who also does once-weekly hCG shots to preserve testicular size. He may also be on Arimidex to keep estrogen levels low and on Proscar to decrease DHT levels.[176] As you can also see, the physician must be very knowledgeable on the various treatment regimens and the specific monitoring of these hormonal metabolites in order to ensure the best efficacy and, more importantly, safety.

There are many options available when it comes to TRT. This personalized approach may include the aromatase inhibitor, Arimidex—an oral drug.

---

175 Mauras et al., *JCEM* 7/2000. Hayes, et al., *JCEM* 9/2000.

176 Proscar is an alpha-5 reductase inhibitor that blocks T conversion to DHT. This drug is also used to help shrink the prostate if enlarged. A lower dose pill called Propecia is used to help slow hair loss.

I must emphasize though, the necessity of individualized approaches in finding what is right for the patient. What specifically is the hormonal status? Is it primary or secondary failure? What are the patient's goals? Are they realistic and obtainable? What is he willing to do to obtain such? Is he fully aware of the benefits and the risks of TRT? And is he going to be compliant with the necessary follow-up lab work and prostate examinations? These matters and more need to be satisfactorily reviewed in order to ensure patient compliance and a good long-term, successful relationship.

We will now present some risks of TRT. Many of these have been introduced in prior discussions and diagrams. The many varied symptoms of andropause, as presented in the questionnaire, are improved with the proper replacement. As with most hormonal deficiencies, the symptoms of a specific deficiency are improved with the proper physiological replacement.

Possible Side Effects of TRT. Most side effects are due to the improper dosing of TRT, mainly being too high or too frequent. There wasn't the proper monitoring and adjustments made. In some, the delivery system wasn't ideal.

- **Abnormal liver function tests.** As mentioned, oral or sublingual T isn't recommended. Also, using the proper physiological dosing and proper routine follow-up testing for T levels and liver function tests should be performed. Baseline liver function tests should initially be performed as well to rule out preexisting liver disease. If a patient has existing liver disease such as hepatitis B or C, then extra counseling is necessary to ensure TRT benefits outweigh the risks. Others taking many drugs that are metabolized through the liver are at increased risk of liver inflammation. Minimizing drugs to the lowest dose necessary should be a goal anyway—especially the ones metabolized through the cytochrome p450 system. These include the cholesterol-lowering statin drugs. Lifestyle should be optimized as well. Patients should abstain from excessive alcohol or Tylenol use. (One of the supplements I recommend is milk thistle, the active ingredient of which being silymarin, which helps maintain liver health.) Liver tests should be repeated about every six months, three months after any increase in T dosing, or anytime clinically indicated. However, a man under sixty-five that's on hCG to increase T levels need not worry of these liver effects at all. This reinforces the need to have a doctor that knows what they're doing and keeps communication a two-way street.

- **Increased hemoglobin hematocrit (erythrocytosis), sleep apnea:** This was introduced in the last chapter, but we will explain things further. Historically, very supraphysiological T dosing was used to improve the anemia caused by *renal failure*. These doses were about ten times the physiological dosing we currently use. As an aside, even with such supraphysiological dosing, side effects were quite tolerable. More importantly, cachexia, osteoporosis, and sense of well-being were usually improved, something that today's erythro-poietin-based treatments don't offer. (Two or more such erythropoietin ana-logues, i.e., Epogen, Arenesp, are currently in the top ten costliest drugs.) Regardless, the proper diagnosis, treatment, and follow-up are necessary with any medical or hormonal replacement regimen. TRT in those with andro-pause symptoms has been shown to actually improve COPD parameters as well as exercise capacity and inflammation (please see the introduction to men's hormones chapter).[177] Again, baseline blood work should be performed, and if abnormal, proper medical workup and treatment should proceed.

For those with blood dyscrasias, such as polycythemia or similar diseases that exhibit increased hemoglobin and hematocrit, TRT should be used with extra caution and counseling. Smokers generally have increased baseline hemoglo-bin and hematocrit. Of course, cessation of smoking would be the best life-style change to attempt. But for smokers who can't quit, TRT helps prevents osteoporosis; and it may improve mood enough to help them quit smoking. For ones with benign increases in hematocrit, simply donating blood a few times per year should help keep blood levels from getting too high. I have yet to see elevated hemoglobin levels with TRT maintained at physiological levels. Those with hypertension and risks for coronary artery disease may add a daily baby aspirin to help prevent risks of clots. Lastly, obesity is the big-gest risk factor for sleep apnea. Proper TRT improves body composition—increases muscle mass and decreases visceral fat. Obesity also increases risks for diabetes, hypertension, restrictive lung disease, heart disease, and many more, besides just apnea. All were proven to have improved with proper TRT. So I find it hard to believe that TRT would significantly impair sleep apnea, especially if CBC (complete blood count) and T levels are properly correlated with the clinical picture. As stressed, TRT should be only part of a compre-hensive approach.

---

177 R. Casaburi, "Effects of testosterone and resistance training in men with chronic obstructive pulmonary disease," *Am J Resp Care Med* 170 (2004): 870–78.

- **BPH and prostate cancer:** Prostate cancer itself is the most common cancer of men when all ages are grouped together. As a killer, it runs third behind lung and colon. It's interesting to note that as a result of autopsies, a large percentage of men had cancer cells in the prostate gland, but didn't know it or suffered any reportable symptoms. These cancers earn the term *hidden* or *occult prostate cancer.* Worldwide, the incidence of hidden prostate cancer is relatively constant. However, American men suffer from more aggressive forms. Interestingly, all mammals have prostates; but only humans, dogs, and African lions get prostate disease. Are you a lion or a dog?

There's been a lot of research that's tried to find any link between TRT and an increased risk for new prostate cancer. This possible link has been suspected and studied for decades because of the fact that a standard treatment for metastatic prostate cancer has been surgical or medical castration. The bad part is that conclusions are variable because of different research design, the markers for BPH and cancer, the age and comorbidities of the subjects, the dosing of testosterone, the length of the study, and more. Overall, the convergence of evidence points toward proper TRT, not increasing the size of the prostate, elevating prostate specific antigen, (PSA) or even worsening the symptoms of BPH.[178] Additionally, there's virtually no increased risk of prostate cancer with TRT, according to the vast majority of scientific literature.[179] This does make common sense though. BPH and prostate cancer are both diseases of much older men, when testosterone levels are one-half to one-third compared to their younger years.

---

178 BPH stands for benign prostatic hypertrophy, a noncancerous enlargement of the prostate gland, which generally occurs as men age.

179 E. Rhoden and A. Morgentaler of Beth Israel Deaconess Medical Center in a comprehensive review of seventy-two studies. "Risks of testosterone replacement therapy and recommendations for monitoring," *New England Journal of Medicine* 350, no. 5 (2004): 1533–4406; L. Marks, The Journal of the American Medical Association 296 (2006): 2351–61. News release, American Medical Association.

The *New England Journal of Medicine* (January 29, 2004), presented a good review article, entitled "Risks of Testosterone Replacement Therapy and Recommendations for Monitoring" by E. Rhoden and A. Morgentaler, both highly respected in the field of TRT. Most of the risks mentioned are based on earlier supraphysiological TRT dosing and are minimized with proper TRT dosing. They reviewed much research and concluded, "Thus, there appears to be no compelling evidence at present to suggest that men with higher testosterone levels are at greater risk of prostate cancer or that treating men who have hypogonadism with exogenous androgens increases this risk … in fact, it should be recognized that prostate cancer becomes more prevalent exactly at the time of the man's life when testosterone levels declined." This basically parallels what I've stated above.

Even PSA, as a prostate cancer screening test, has its challenges and limitations. Unfortunately, I can get into all the particulars in this book but will try to surmise my take on things. Screening tests generally are designed to have high sensitivity, resulting in low specificity though. Therefore, an increase in PSA may not be due to prostate cancer. It may be *prostatitis,* an infection or inflammation of the prostate gland, which is simply treated with antibiotics. PSA levels correlate the best with prostate size—somewhat high, yet stable PSA levels are likely due to simply a larger-sized prostate, BPH, not cancer.

PSA levels must be correlated with the *digital rectal examination* (DRE), family history, risk factors for prostate cancer, and the overall clinical picture. Routine annual PSA levels and DRE should be performed on all men, starting at forty years old if at increased risk. Often, the interpretation of the result is complicated. In a younger man at risk, a baseline PSA level above 4 may warrant additional monitoring or workup. On the other hand—no pun intended—a large percentage of urologists don't recommend checking PSA levels in a man once over eighty. This may be because by the time such a prostate cancer would typically cause any symptoms or problems, the man would probably die from something else first. (This would make going through such workup and treatment unnecessary and possibly unethical.) In the earlier case of the younger man, who has quite a lot more life expected, aggressive diagnosing and treatment should ensue.

So on one side, we have that prostate cancer is so common in sickly elderly men; it may not even make much sense to check a PSA. On the other, it's still a big killer, thereby demanding a definitive diagnosis and aggressive treatment in younger, healthier men. PSA levels themselves are not the whole story, but must be taken into the context of the complete clinical picture. Additionally, I find that the *velocity* of serial PSA lab results is more important as a cancer marker. For example, if somebody had a baseline PSA around 3.0 ng/ml for years that suddenly jumps above 5.0.

> If PSA levels increase 1.5 ng/ml within one year, or 0.75 each year for two to three years, I would initiate a workup or refer to a urologist for the proper evaluation.[183]

So, proper monitoring is not as simple as measuring only PSA levels. The clinical picture, routine examinations, and a trusting, long-term patient-physician relationship are just as important. Getting back to our discussion, we must remember about the *window of opportunity* middle age presents us guys. Granted, the earlier age-management modalities are started, the better and safer the gain. If started later, we probably can't obtain the optimal health or as long a health span we could've, as represented in figure 1.5. Nonetheless, *any time* beats *no time* when it comes to taking a more proactive, natural approach to your health. By combining a healthy lifestyle with TRT, we will probably achieve better and safer outcomes, the best of both worlds. The integrative approach we use emphasizes an anti-inflammatory diet, much like the one Dr. Dean Ornish found reversed and treated prostate cancer.[181] Other studies have tied inflammation with poor prostate cancer prognosis.[182] This helps prevent prostate carcinogenesis in the first place. And remember, preventing carcinogenesis—the formation of cancer—and disease should be one of our primary goals.

---

180 In men on TRT, these values may be more aggressive, as hypogonadal men are a special population at increased risks for prostate cancer given their low T and relatively higher estrogen levels.

181 D. Ornish, AUA 98th Annual Meeting: Abstract 105681, presented April 27, 2003.

182 *Journal of Urology* 176 (2006):1012–16. J. R. Stark, "Data from the Physician's Health Study," 2006, as presented to the American Association for Cancer Research's Frontiers in Cancer Prevention Research Meeting in Boston, Nov 12. Higher CRP and IL-6 in normal weight men gave 77 percent more risk of prostate cancer.

As mentioned earlier, adding *anabolic* modalities in an older person has inherent risks. Again, there must be a balance. On one hand, we want to improve, or at least preserve bone and muscle mass yet decrease visceral fat. We want to fight off frailty. We desire less inflammation and an optimized immune system—all these are great things. On the other hand, such senescence, or *catabolic state*, in old age is what Mother Nature designed for us to experience. This was reviewed earlier in the introduction. She intends for us to become weak, frail, degenerate, and eventually die; that's truly natural, right? We have to make room for the younger generation. Times have changed though. People are living longer lives now, thanks to medical innovation. Many old patients I interview each day are surprised they've lived this long. Many even wonder why. Thanks to modern medications and various surgeries, we are generally living a longer time, but are generally more disabled toward life's end. These have also greatly increased personal and society's costs. In a way, current *reactive* medical innovations have interfered with Mother Nature's intentions in an unnatural way and have increased the suffering in our older years. You can't have it both ways … or can you?

It's a fact that older men are at increased risk of possessing prostate cancer—even the hidden, undetectable kind. That raises the risks of TRT in them, since doctors shouldn't prescribe sex hormones for somebody with a known sex-hormone sensitive cancer, i.e., prostate or breast cancer. TRT in elderly men may *unmask* such occult prostate cancers. Hopefully, this would be identified by an increased PSA velocity that would warrant the appropriate dialogue between the patient and physician. But a more proactive, comprehensive approach with proper hormonal therapy during middle age would have prevented many of the risk factors for prostate cancer by lowering inflammation, obesity, toxicities, and more.

You must pair the proper hormonal anabolism with preventative anticarcinogenic modalities. The proper diet, exercise, and antioxidants help accomplish this goal. The earlier you apply these, the better your chances are to prevent cancer.

Yet the older man is who benefits the most from TRT. Their testosterone is usually in the gutter, and they probably suffer from most of the morbidities proven to improve with TRT—dementia, depression, osteoporosis, frailty, CHF, COPD, and more. This was explained in the introduction to men's hormones chapter. I believe the *convergence of evidence* will parallel in men what I feel about HRT in healthy, younger menopausal women. TRT has less side effects, risks, and better long-term preventative outcomes when used by healthier middle-aged men. To start anabolic methods late in life has its own set of problems. Remember, the old man's testosterone has been deficient for decades. At the very least, this somewhat contributed to most of his illnesses. To suddenly try to reverse the clock and start hormonal replacement at such a late stage may initially confuse the body. This may be like suddenly waking a guy up from a deep sleep.

Biologically though, this can be partially explained by the upregulation of T receptors in an attempt to compensate for lower testosterone production in the aging male. This adaptation may predispose them to some side effects when initiating TRT. So I am not surprised that TRT may have some increased risks in the older man—again, the very same one who benefits the most from TRT. This mandates good communication of the benefits and risks by a doctor who has the experience, expertise, and qualifications to practice age-management medicine. As recommended by the *Journal of Urology*, August 2005, by Gaylis et al., "Prostate cancer may become clinically apparent within months to a few years after the initiation of TRT. DRE is particularly important in the detection of these cancers. Physicians prescribing testosterone, and patients receiving it, should be cognizant of risks and serum PSA testing and DRE should be performed *frequently* during treatment." It also appeared to them that non-urologist physicians may not follow serial PSA labs and perform the DRE frequently enough. I wholeheartedly agree and recommend these be performed three months after any initiation or change in T dosing, and then every six months thereafter. We doctors do want to pick up any *hidden* prostate cancers that TRT may *uncover*.

Lastly, men are indeed different from women; and TRT in the older man probably presents a better benefit-risk ratio than does HRT in the older women. This would match my hypothesis for natural selection and Mother Nature's role in all this. Men are able to produce viable sperm and father children their whole lives; therefore, there is no distinct *change of life* or two populations of men as there are in women. I would assume many young men died in battle, thereby necessitating the preservation of reproduction in the older man for the overall survival of the human species. High T in an older man would offer a selective advantage—he's stronger, more virile, and still mentally in the game. He probably has another good twenty years ahead. A lower T in an older, sicker man with ED would make natural sense—he won't be around long enough to help raise any offspring. No sex for him!

In women, there is the younger sex kitten whose job it is to bear children. However, menopause was selected, to ensure a "grandmother pool" was around to take care of the cave, husband, and kids just in case the mother died during childbirth. Granny's more … well, let's just say, she's not a tigress. Ideally, one woman has two distinct roles in her lifetime, a wonderful conservation of effort and resources by nature. In men, TRT is not as much of a stretch as HRT is for women. Trying to reverse aging after decades of the natural degeneration and progression of age-related complications will have its inherent risks, but still offers much hope. What are the other options?

> TRT in men may wind up being not as much of a controversy as hormonal replacement therapy in women. Many healthy older men without supplementation still possess testosterone in the upper one-fourth of normal levels. They also happen to be healthier and not as overweight as their cohorts with lower levels.

- **Skin/Acne:** Likewise, with puberty and its increased incidence of acne, replacing testosterone to optimal physiological levels can increase sebum production and the resulting acne. If TRT is done correctly, I usually don't see any increase in acne. I find the degree of increased acne to be a good indication of androgen levels; if acne is increased, the T level is getting pretty close to the upper high limits of normal to supraphysiological levels. Often, the patient may be inadvertently taking too much T. Lab values are very helpful here but must be correlated to the clinical picture. I use lab values as only one facet of evaluating a very complex, dynamic system. For example, if a patient has an initial concern about acne, I may not shoot for the upper normal level. If there's some beneficial clinical response, I may be happy to obtain middle-ranged levels. (I find that a good skin regimen, fish oil, and an anti-inflammatory diet also help limit acne eruptions.)

- **Fluid Retention:** As mentioned earlier, most problems with edema were noted when supraphysiological TRT dosing was instituted. I haven't seen this in the past seven years of my clinical practice of age management. You have seen the research stating TRT helps coronary artery disease, hypertension, and even congestive heart failure—the pathological causes of edema in aging men. If somebody has increased edema while on TRT, they need their levels checked and should undergo a basic workup for edema and avail of the proper nonmedical and medical therapies offered.

- **Gynecomastia:** As presented earlier, T is aromatized into estrogen metabolites; and even the untreated older male is apt to have relatively higher estrogen levels, resulting in increased breast size and peripheral abdominal fat. At any rate, men on TRT should have testosterone metabolites regularly checked. If clinically warranted—i.e., when estrogen levels are increased with gynecomastia—then an aromatase inhibitor such as Femara or Arimidex may be used to counteract this. More commonly though, simply decreasing the TRT dosing a bit helps this without any additional medication or any appreciable decrease in clinical gains. Lastly, breast cancer does occur in men. Although rare, it demands an immediate evaluation by your doctor, as TRT would be absolutely contraindicated.

- **Hair Loss:** As mentioned above, this can be a combination of genetic factors and the effects of increased dihydrotestosterone (DHT). Likewise, as a metabolite of testosterone, these levels should be routinely checked and correlated with the clinical picture. Proper lifestyle, hygiene, and the complete hormonal picture—including thyroid testing and replenishment if indicated—should be undertaken. As alluded to, I treat the patient. If he has a fear of hair loss, I may not initially push the T levels as high. As opposed to these being in the upper one-fourth, it may be fine to be in the upper one-third.

If higher, though still physiological, levels of T dosing is needed to achieve the optimal health and goals of the patient, and DHT levels have substantially increased from baseline levels, then decreasing the conversion from testosterone to DHT is an option. If you recall, T through the action of alpha-5 reductase, is converted to DHT. Thus, we simply add an alpha-5 reductase inhibitor, commonly known as finasteride. Trade names for these are Proscar or Propecia. There's also a newer variety, Avodart© that may have less side effects. I must reemphasize the importance of having a qualified physician with the expertise and knowledge to be able to routinely monitor and adjust hormonal levels and their many metabolites. There are many potential side effects and risks.

The above are the most common side effects of TRT. There may be many others pertaining to you and your treatment that warrant addressing. Age-management medicine prefers a more individualized, proactive approach, emphasizing prevention of diseases. It uses integrative modalities that empower the patient to accept responsibility for his optimal health. The physician is a learned advisor and confidant. As I routinely explain, my main goal is to present you with the research and facts in order to allow you to connect the dots and decide which path in life you wish to proceed. If you are currently going in the wrong direction—say, toward getting degeneration and disabilities—then you will eventually get there. The only way *not* to arrive there is, of course, to change direction. You lead a healthier life and become more proactive. This is quite different than the one-size-fits-all and reactive view of contemporary medicine, the health-insurance industry, and lay public. Don't get caught in the (perfect) storm!

Chapter 10. MAG reviewed all the research and decided to try low-dose subcutaneous hCG shots twice per week to increase his testosterone levels. His baseline dihydrotestosterone (DHT) and estrogen levels were fine. His digital rectal exam and PSA lab work were normal. He realizes he needs to get these checked more often while on TRT.

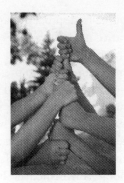

XI.

Pregnenolone and DHEA: The Testosterone Precursors

Each precursor has its own role and a supportive one, much like the cheerleaders in a pyramid formation.

A. Pregnenolone. If you recall from Chapter 8, pregnenolone itself is a sex steroid hormone, as well as a precursor to testosterone, see figure 11.1. These synthetic pathways ultimately lead to estrogen and progesterone production. As such, pregnenolone also declines with age. Most of what I read about pregnenolone suggests it's quite benign and has been suggested to *help balance immune and mood function.* Reflecting that, I generally recommend all midlifers take 25 mg in the morning. Typically, checking pregnenolone level doesn't have any clinical significance and, therefore, is a moot point. I'm unaware of any drug interactions; however, as with anything else, if there are undesirable side effects, stop it. There are many other options explained in this book that help boost immune and mood function. Some tidbits below:

Pregnenolone

1. A neurosteroid that positively affects learning and memory.

2. Initiates memory storage process through stimulating adenylate cyclase in neurons. It probably regulates processing and encoding though calcium pump (ion exchange) in the neuronal membrane.

3. Modulates intacellular calcium-binding proteins and, thus, gene expression, protein turnover, and metabolism in cell.

4. Pregnenolone stores do deplete with age and consequently exhibit less optimal synchronization for mental functioning.

5. Research shows influence in the brain's limbic system, including the hippocampus. An increase in concentration of acetylcholine with pregnenolone treatment is seen in the amygdala and cortical areas of the brain.

6. Probably increases DHEA levels and offers those associated benefits (see DHEA topic).

7. Acts as a GABA agonist in low doses and used in generalized anxiety disorder treatments.

8. Mostly believed to help memory, cognition, and emotional balance.

9. Easily replaceable; usually 25 mg orally per day and is affordable with no real adverse effects.

B. DHEA. Dehydroepiandrosterone is a sex hormone and a precursor to T (please see below figure). Besides being a precursor—a building block to testosterone, each metabolite in this synthesis pathway plays many other roles in optimizing health. As mentioned before, pregnenolone, besides being a precursor to T, also plays an important role in proper immune and mood functioning. It's important to realize these metabolites are indeed hormones with distinct benefits, as well as some risks if used improperly.

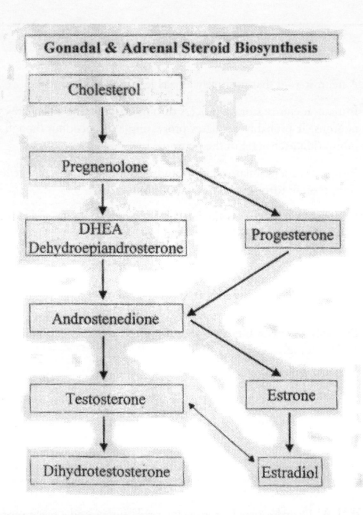

Figure 11.1. DHEA and pregnenolone synthesis.

DHEA levels variably start to decrease in our thirties (please see below diagram). If you're symptomatic from low DHEA, age-management doctors would say you're going through *adrenopause* (adrenal glands are slacking off). As you will read, the symptoms are similar to andropause. When restored to optimal DHEA levels, your symptoms generally improve.

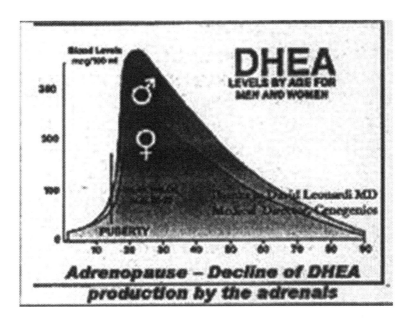

Figure 11.2 DHEA levels decline as we age, starting in our early thirties. (Adapted D. Leonardi, Cenegenics©)

Again, I refer to the Massachusetts Male Aging Study, MMAS, which found an inverse correlation of DHEA and incidence of ED.[183] This prompted an investigation on the efficacy of DHEA replacement and research by the Department of Urology, University of Vienna in Austria. This concluded that 50 mg DHEA for six months was associated with a significantly improved erectile score compared to baseline and placebo for those with ED, having hypertension but without organic pathology.

The MMAS also found that the prevalence of complete impotence tripled between forty and seventy years old. Old age was the most strongly associated with ED. After adjustment for age, a higher probability of ED was found with heart disease, hypertension, diabetes, and their associated medications. Also, ED was seen more in those with higher indexes of anger and depression, and *inversely* correlated with a serum DHEA, HDL, and index of dominant personality. "Cigarette smoking was associated with the greater probability of complete impotence in men with heart disease

---

183 *MMAS* 1994; W. Reiter, "DHEA in the treatment of ED in patients with different organic etiologies," *Urological Research* (August 29, 2001): 278–81.

and hypertension."[184] So if you smoke, in fact, you *can't* poke. As mentioned below, testosterone and SHBG also play roles in the development of insulin resistance, diabetes type 2, and the resulting vascular disease that predisposes men to ED.[185] Findings from MMAS also confirmed prior evidence that low DHEA can indeed predict ischemic heart disease in men. As recommended before, a complaint of ED should at least prompt an investigation into coronary disease risk factors.

DHEA's role in disturbed mind and mood disorders is also found in the *American Journal of Psychiatry*, January 2006. Here, Dr. Rabkin et al. found DHEA to be superior to placebo in reducing nonmajor but persistent depression symptoms, which is quite common yet difficult to treat in patients with HIV/AIDS. There were no adverse effects reported, and amazingly the number needed to treat was a nominal four. Many of the symptoms of AIDS mirror the frailty and immune system decline seen with advanced age.

One of my favorite review articles on DHEA was done in 2003 by the Endocrine Research Unit of the Mayo Clinic. If indeed interested and great references desired, you should get a copy and review it yourself.[186] It is quite lengthy, but is chock-full of useful, trusted information. Succinct points will be presented below.

- DHEA is mostly found to have positive effects on *skeletal* as well as *heart muscle*.

- Also, *immune function* is thought to be improved by the associated increase in interleukin-2 production. Most investigators argue that replacement therapy with DHEA restores the normal immunocompetence that tends to be lost with aging. So states Daynes in the *Journal of Immunotherapy* (1992) issue 12. This also touts the beneficial effects of DHEA seen on immune function and increased natural killer cells noted by other researchers. This research and the potential enhancement of the immune system by DHEA have led to studies using DHEA as a vaccine adjuvant. Even patients with dysfunctional immune systems, rheumato-logical or inflammatory disorders have seen benefits with DHEA. Since it's been shown to help reduce glucocorticoid dose and symptom scores without an increase in disease activity, DHEA use could effectively lower

---

184 H. A. Feldman, "Impotence and its medical and psychosocial correlates: results of the MMAS," *Journal of Urology* 151(1) (1994): 54–61.

185 Feldman, in the January 2001 *American Journal of Epidemiology*.

186 S. Nair, "DHEA: Is there a role for replacement.," *Mayo Clinical Proceedings* 78 (2003): 1257–73.

the substantial toxicity and morbidity of the chronic glucocorticoid treatment typically used in these debilitating conditions.

• DHEA levels are usually higher in humans and primates exhibiting *longevity*, but this may be another case of "which came first, the chicken or the egg?"

• Decreased DHEA levels are also found in *sarcopenia and osteopenia*, the age-related loss in muscle and bone mass, respectively. This would give rise to the *frailty syndrome* mentioned earlier. Many other disorders of aging such as reduced immune competence, obesity, diabetes, and cancers have been attributed to such changes in DHEA. This is based on animal and human epidemiological data. Open label studies have shown DHEA administration to make a significant difference in bone mineral density in healthy elderly subjects, thereby helping to prevent progression to the frailty syndrome.

• Through its beneficial effects on GABA and serotonin pathways, DHEA has been found by most studies to also improve *mood* and *sense of well-being.* It was also found effective for midlife-onset minor and major depression, according to the results of a placebo-controlled, randomized trial published in the *Archives of General Psychiatry* (2005).[187] Hey, not many legally prescribed pills help you feel good. It's important to note most of the studies indicating a positive influence of DHEA on mood, well-being, cognition, and memory studied both men *and* women that were healthy *or* sick. They were also midlife to elderly. So the whole spectrum was covered in one way or another. There were also suggestions of improved REM sleep and its potential as a memory enhancer. Some of the research I reviewed having conflicting results on DHEA suffered from a small sample size, either negligible or supraphysiological DHEA dosing, or basic, good experimental design.

• DHEA may also modulate the pathologically higher neurotoxic glucocorticoid levels seen in *acute distress* and *other psychological disturbances.* Though the exact mechanism is unknown, it is theorized that DHEA works synergistically together with pregnenolone, and DHEA may lower the cortisol/DHEA ratio, thereby improving cognitive decline. I have generally found DHEA supplementation to be beneficial in lowering high-normal cortisol levels in mildly depressed patients undergoing acute stress. Also, I may use DHEA to improve older patients' mind or mood

---

187 Peter J. Schmidt, MD, from the National Institute of Mental Health in Rockville, Maryland, and colleagues. *Arch Gen Psych.* 62 (2005):154–62. Doses used were quite high and improvements were noted at six weeks.

disorders. As a bonus, it helps their physical conditioning, thereby preventing further mental, as well as physical, decline. This being done in the proper clinical setting, of course.

- *A decline in sexual functioning*—a common complaint I hear from both middle-aged men and women. For both pre- and postmenopausal healthy women, the best-designed studies show improvement in sexual desire, arousal, and well-being. Some studies with conflicting results only used a single 300 mg dose of DHEA, which is totally ridiculous. Others never required a baseline DHEA level drawn to even determine if DHEA replacement was medically necessary. Some had no follow-up levels drawn to ensure proper physiological replacement. It certainly wouldn't be the standard of care or even ethical to give all subjects, no matter what their baseline levels were, a supraphysiological dose of thyroid hormone, for example. The vast majority, having normal thyroid function, would suffer many severe side effects as anxiety progresses to even psychosis, increased blood pressure and heart rate, palpitations or congestive heart failure, insomnia, and more. Why the researchers would do this with DHEA and expect a favorable outcome is beyond my comprehension.

- Concerning *Alzheimer's disease*, there is also evidence that suggests DHEA reduces free radical damage and thereby decreases the cognitive decline seen in AD. The hypothesis for the association between low DHEA levels and AD concerns the risk of people carrying a specific gene, the apolipoprotein E allele. People having this allele are more vulnerable to AD at an earlier age. Additionally, higher levels of both *beta-amyloid* protein and the pathological *tau* protein seen in postmortem AD patients' brains also exhibited lower DHEA levels. Other research also found inverse relationships between DHEA levels in the presence of either AD or multi-infarct dementia. Additionally, lower DHEA levels are found in those most severely debilitated by AD and patients in nursing homes. Lastly, restricted caloric intake, as in the CRAN diet, may delay or help prevent AD by extending the availability of DHEA.

- Many animal studies have shown DHEA supplementation *reduces insulin* and *atherosclerotic plaque formation*. This result may be directly due to the manner it decreases insulin—a big inflammatory mediator. However, the lowered incidence of diabetes would benefit vessel disease risks too. Interestingly enough, DHEA has been shown to lower HDL levels, yet like testosterone, it may lower total cholesterol and thereby not adversely affect the cholesterol/HDL ratio.

Other DHEA effects mostly parallel testosterone's—*increased muscle strength* and *improved body composition*—although not as impressive or always as convincing as TRT. The most-quoted data on this come from studies by Morales, et al.[188] Clinically, I see DHEA as a minor player, not a magic bullet, to completing proper hormonal replacement in men and women. When total testosterone is minimally low, or when free testosterone needs some improvement, DHEA replacement may be helpful. This would only be part of a total integrative approach that includes the proper diet, exercise, other supplements, and hormonal replacements in order to synergistically optimize things. I find it quite safe and most effective in basically healthy but stressed or mildly depressed middle-aged persons. As a bonus, it's easily replaced in pill form, costs little, and there's no drug interaction. I take 50 mg per day.

A more recent study by Nair looked at elderly men and women who were replaced with DHEA for two years and found no improvement in muscle mass or quality of life.[192] Only the men received additional T. The media and the researchers of this one study then proclaimed that replacing DHEA and TRT has no role in "antiaging" therapies. It's odd they chose to overshadow many decades of research showing better results on these parameters. So what's the *convergence of evidence?* One of the main questions they set out to answer was if replacing DHEA and T had any ill effects. Their answer, "It didn't." That's good to know; and unlike most drugs, there was an improvement in bone mineral density noted, which would help decrease risks for frailty and fractures in this elderly group. This would be quite a large benefit. The dosing of T used was quite low, and there was no attempt to individually adjust any levels of T or DHEA to optimal physiological ranges.

Contrary to the above, I feel this more recent study actually makes many good arguments *supporting* what I preach, as well as practice. First, these therapies are quite safe. Second, to really affect the ravages of aging, it's best to *prevent* disease earlier, as in midlife, as opposed to treating these later. But it's never ever too late. Third, there are no magic pills or potions; it's better to have a more integrative

---

188 A. J. Morales et al., "Effects of replacement dose of dehydroepiandrosterone in men and women of advancing age," *J Clin Endocrinol Metab.* 78 (1994):1360–7. A. J. Morales et al., "The effect of six months treatment with a 100 mg daily dose of dehydroepiandrosterone (DHEA) on circulating sex steroids, body composition and muscle strength in age-advanced men and women," *Clin Endocrinol.* 49 (1998):421–32.

189 K. Nair et al., "DHEA in elderly women and DHEA or testosterone in elderly men," *N Engl J Med* 355 (2006):1647–59, 1724–26.

approach that uses diet, exercise, and other modalities mentioned in this book. Remember 1 + 1 + 1 = 4? Fourth, hormonal therapies should be individualized and adjusted to the upper physiological levels the majority of scientific literature shows benefit. The doctor has to know what he's doing and rely on patient feedback. When you really look at it, the above researchers may have unintentionally praised the age-management paradigm, not buried it.

DHEA Summary

- Raises T and Free T in women
- Usually No change in T men
- Increases libido in women
- May or may not improve body composition in women
- Improves body composition in men
- Reverses osteoporosis
- Raises IGF-1?
- Improves Depression
- Reduced CV risk

DHEA Summary

- DHEA enhances immune response
- Patients on corticosteroids benefit by DHEA
- Autoimmune diseases benefit from DHEA RT
- Since aging is a state of cortisol excess, patients with adrenopause should have DHEA RT to balance Cortisol
- No significant adverse effects

Figure 11.3. DHEA Summary—probable DHEA benefits.

When you review the studies done on humans with DHEA, the *convergence of evidence* points to the improved parameters mentioned above. The lengthy review article from the Mayo Clinic in 2003 mostly confirmed the many vast beneficial effects and relative safety of DHEA. Yet, it concluded with a very valid point but then a somewhat unfair recommendation *against* widespread use of DHEA by doctors. The valid point made was that DHEA is, in fact, a hormone that should be regulated and prescribed as any other hormone. I wholeheartedly agree. DHEA, as any other hormone, has a definite benefit-risk ratio that should be objectively and subjectively clinically followed by a doctor who's knowledgeable in these modalities. Currently, DHEA is available OTC in most drugstores and so-called wellness or vitamin shops—being pushed by mere salesclerks. Clearly, this practice is improper and a danger to the public.

As a precursor to testosterone, DHEA poses real risks similar to testosterone. (I will not go into these here because of unneeded redundancy [please see TRT risks mentioned in chap. 8].) Mainly though, it can worsen any hormonally sensitive cancer, as in breast or prostate. Of course, DHEA levels and the patient's clinical picture should be routinely monitored. But we shouldn't throw out the baby with the bath water. The contemporary medical establishment is probably partly biased against DHEA because we doctors weren't originally taught about DHEA and many other such potentially beneficial, safe, natural modalities. Therefore, the traditionalists feel these simply can't be any good and proceed to bury their head in the sand.

The main point I would like to make is that DHEA replacement in the right clinical setting is quite beneficial and safe when performed correctly. The doctor should make sure to only prescribe *pharmaceutical-grade* or *GMP-certified* DHEA supplements. In the United States, food supplements are not required to undergo strict safety and third-party testing, so there are inherent problems with quality control. One study published by *JAMA* in 1998 revealed the actual DHEA content in OTC varieties ranged from 0 to 150 percent from the amount stated on the label. You get what you pay for. Don't trust your health—your most valuable asset—to some kid behind the counter or some manufacturer in a faraway land.

Chapter 11. MAG's DHEA level was low, so he started taking 50 mg in the morning with 25 mg of pregnenolone. Wanting to ensure the proper dose and safety, he made sure these were GMP-certified or of pharmaceutical-grade quality.

XII.

Stress and Sleep: Cortisol and Melatonin's Role

Love is like Oxygen … you get too much, you get too high … not enough and you're gonna' die.…

—Sweet

Well, cortisol is similar.

A. Anxiety affects the part of the brain that helps control creative expression and complex communication. It can become more difficult to express yourself, be creative, or even function effectively in relationships. If left unchecked, these can snowball and cause greater emotional and physical harm.

Emotional symptoms of anxiety include:

Restlessness, irritability, and on-edge feeling
Excessive worrying
Fearing that something bad is going to happen, sense of impending doom
Inability to concentrate, "blanking out"
Excessive startle reflex
Constant feelings of sadness or inadequacy
Trouble sleeping

Chronic stress can wear down the body's natural defenses, leading to a variety of *physical symptoms,* including the following:

Dizziness or a general feeling of "being out of it"
General aches and pains
Grinding teeth, clenching jaw
Shortness of breath, or worsening asthma
Headaches
Indigestion
Increase in or loss of appetite
Muscle tension in neck, face, or shoulders
Sleeping problems
Racing heart
Cold and sweaty palms
Tiredness, exhaustion
Trembling/shaking
Weight gain or loss
Upset stomach
Sexual difficulties
Immune system decline[193]

Do you, or anyone you know, suffer from any of these vague, elusive symptoms? These probably account for most visits to the doctor's office and usually result in an extensive workup and referrals to multiple specialists. Initially, it's important to rule out other serious causes for the above symptoms. Often, in the case of a younger, healthier individual, the diagnosis is usually stress related. Given today's hectic lifestyle, toxic environment, and the tendency of increased mood disturbances in midlife, it's no wonder. Let's get a better understanding of what else may be going on.

If you remember the earlier chapters on midlife hormonal changes such as andropause and thyroid dysfunction, it's understandable there's usually no single cause for these symptoms. Complicating matters is the fact that most physicians are trained to diagnose and treat only pathological diseases, not these annoying "normal" age-related conditions. Usually, these are casually dismissed with, "Thank god, nothing is wrong; you'll just have to learn to live with it. Here's a prescription to treat the symptoms … just don't read the *PDR,* or you'll get every side effect listed." But

---

190 Even modest stress can reduce antibody formation after getting the flu shot. G. Miller, *Health Psychol.* 24, no. 3 (2005): 297–306.

inside, you have the good sense to know you're not feeling right, or feel like you used to. There *must* be something wrong. You want to do something before this gets any worse. This attitude should be commended and welcomed by the doctor instead. You just need to find one that's properly trained in these newer modalities.

This gets back to what I said earlier. A healthier lifestyle combined with optimal hormonal replacements work synergistically together. Part of this lifestyle change is adopting healthier ways to better cope with stress. It's much part of that profound, integral mind-body interaction. For example, if your hormones aren't balanced, your mind and body starts to get bent out of shape too. This can start a spiraling, downward course. This usually includes many of the symptoms listed above. You have to look at the *complete* picture. Anything less, and you'll never feel the best you can. This is nothing you should attempt halfway.

Let's try to understand a little bit more about stress. First of all, stress is a normal part of everyday life. As a matter of fact, one of the very definitions of being alive is the ability to respond to stressors. Even if you were a protozoan, you'd respond to a bright light by squirming to a darker spot. This *stress response* Mother Nature has provided for us has evolved from these single-celled organisms throughout the millennium. The stress response is supposed to help our chances for survival so that we can live long enough to pass on our genes. Let's gain insight in this phenomenon, so we could eventually have it (life) *made in the shade.*

What exactly is this stress response? Biologically, it's the stimulation of the sympathetic autonomic nervous system. This neurological adaptation basically gets our body pumped up for the "fight or flight" response. It stimulates the release of epinephrine, adrenaline, cortisol, insulin, inflammatory mediators, and more. If you can recall how you felt the last time you almost got in a serious accident or had a police car with lights flashing behind you, that's the feeling! Your heart pounds, blood pressure spikes, hands get cold, and you become jumpy. This is a good thing—if you were one of our earlier caveman ancestors being chased by a saber-toothed tiger! If your stress response is prolonged or exaggerated, you may feel dizzy or may even faint. Some animals have adapted catatonic responses to fear. Others simply bury their head in the sand. Know anyone like that? As you can see, a lot of these selected beneficial adaptations parallel the above symptoms of chronic stress in humans.

Furthermore, there are subtle things going on of which you're not consciously aware. Inflammatory mediators are released, which more likely causes your blood to clot and vessels to constrict. This is considered by nature to be a successful adaptation in acute stressful conditions—in case you were cut, your blood loss would be limited. Glucose is released into your bloodstream to provide extra energy. Cortisol is also raised, causing a myriad of compounding effects.

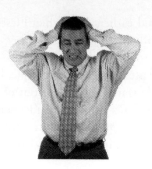

The typical stress response was designed to be beneficial. But how can that be? Well, look at it this way. These biological mechanisms adapted mainly from *acute* or short-term-like *stressful situations* in a more primitive "eat or be eaten" scenario, like the case with the tiger. In that environment and time, these responses were good for overall animal survival. It was selected by natural design. However, it's very important for the sympathetic nervous system to remain in balance with our *parasympathetic* system. This represents the *calming* side of the emotional equation. It's how you feel after a massage, sex, or a warm bath. Have you ever noticed the lion in the zoo? He spends most of his time relaxing. Together, these two opposing autonomic systems represent the yin and yang of our complicated neurological, physical, emotional, and mental balance.

What happened? The short answer is we moved too quickly from this primitive jungle to the *concrete jungle* we live in today. The survival mechanisms remained the same, but it's a whole different board game now. Sure, we still have acute stressful situations; and the typical stress response is beneficial in these instances. But there has been an overwhelming increase in *chronic* stress. The saber-toothed tiger has now been replaced by the ungrateful boss, mounting bills, increased unrealistic expectations, and more. In these modern times, the stress response in such a daily, long-term fashion is *detrimental*. All the above-mentioned systems get out of balance. You have poor sleep, lack of energy; and you eventually burn out or freak out. You may get irritable and display emotional outbursts about the smallest things, or cry over nothing at times. You may bury your head in the sand in an effort to become comfortably numb to things, unknowingly going about the same boring routine week after week without smelling the so-called roses in life. What are you to do?

In the 1960s, there were a lot of different behavioral and personality theories postulated. Remember the introvert versus the extrovert? Another was the type A versus type B personality? The introvert was the one that kept his feelings in, be it good or bad, for long term. Type A personality was the boisterous, stressed out, get'er-done bossy guy. Research at that time revealed he had increased risks for heart attack and other stress-related health conditions. Wouldn't it be nice if our personalities were so simply black-and-white?

Later research into further understanding these complicated issues resulted in a slightly different angle of looking at this. It winds up it's not so much the *amount or type* of stressors you get that determines how well you do, rather it's how well you *deal* with the stressors that matters most. Read that again slowly and make sure it sinks in.

Let me give an example. You may be a top executive in charge of dozens of employees and make hundreds of decisions a day that affect the lives of thousands. But you grew up in a stable, loving home; did sports; and learned good coping mechanisms in the meantime. You can probably deal with stressors in a successful way, trying your best to maintain balance between work, home, and play. Or you may be working in an automobile factory, screwing in lug nuts all day. You feel this is a very redundant, unrewarding work with little opportunity for advancement, but you have to do this in order to pay the bills for your family. Feeling trapped, you start to resent your family, to feel guilty, or to feel as if you're a failure. You may then start drinking too much alcohol or doing drugs to help relieve the pain. These behaviors only make matters worse. So it's not so much of the actual stressors, it's more of the perceived amount of stress and how you deal with it that determines how well you'll survive.

In today's society, with all its unrealistic expectations, it's no wonder a lot of things are going awry. There is increased anger and violence in the media spilling into the homes, or vice versa. We have what I consider a pandemic of childhood and adolescent mood disorders including anxiety, depression, ADHD, and others. We even have adult ADHD now. (I wonder just how much of this behavior has been learned by our kids.) The divorce rate and number of single-parent homes are on the rise. Homes and jobs change repeatedly. We supposedly have the best communication systems ever—satellite and Web-based phones, yet we hardly get together at dinnertime to see how each other's day went. Couples don't communicate as

well as they should. They're too busy playing head games or on the Internet looking for love in all the wrong places. Parents don't communicate with the kids, and
vice versa. It's called *paying* attention, right? That means you have to *willingly
give or donate* your time and yourself to listen. Remember the last line the Beatles
sang on their very last album, *Abbey Road*? "And in the end … the love you take is
equal to the love … you make."

Well, I sort of digressed a bit there. The point is the primitive, reactive ways of dealing
with the chronic stress we encounter in today's concrete jungle simply won't work and
are even counterproductive and unhealthy. We humans, we can understand and are
intelligent. We love! We shouldn't react with the anger-related defense mechanisms of
lower animals; we should *proact*, or choose love and understanding instead.

When I interview patients, one of the basic things I ask is, "What are your goals in life?"
Surprisingly, I usually get a deer-in-the-headlights look, and they usually need some assis-
tance in arriving at an answer. Almost invariably, it comes down to peace, or happiness
and good health. We all know we have to die one day, although we may not think about
it. What concerns us midlifers more is how debilitated and how dependent on others we
may become when older. Notwithstanding that, peace of mind comes first.

Then I will follow up with, "Well, what do you do during the day to help accom-
plish that?"
"Well, I'm too busy to think about it or do anything about it," they'll answer.
"Busy doing what?"
"Busy getting *ready* for work."
"Then what?"
"Well … then, I'm busy *at* work." They'll say with a "duh" look.
"How about during lunchtime? …"
"I'm usually catching up on work, making phone calls, or surfin' the net, checking
e-mails, or blogging … then, it's back to work for the rest of the day; so don't ask
about after lunch."
"Okay, so what do you do *after* work … to accomplish your main goal of obtain-
ing peace?" I'll continue.

"Probably, grabbing a quick bite for me and the kids, straightening up the house, or
catching up. A little TV or Internet. Then, it's time for bed.…" (Many may express
a similar routine. By then, it usually sinks in, although not exactly like a light bulb
going off above their head. Usually it's a combination of that "hmmmppphhh …
now I see" look combined with some disillusionment or embarrassment.)

I'll usually conclude with, "If your main goal is peace, then why aren't you spending any time of your day trying to obtain it?

I believe the main cause for the stress and our improper responses stems from our *ambivalency*. Ambivalence is not the *lack* of feeling. On the contrary, *ambi* comes from a Latin word meaning "either sides or ends." *Valence* means "strong affinity." Thus, *ambivalence* means feeling strongly about both ends and thus not knowing what to choose or do. In lab animals, we create and study stress with such ambivalence. In animal behavior experiments, we may offer treats (positive reinforcement) to hungry rats for pressing on a bar. Yet, they are variably shocked (negatively reinforcement) at random times. If the hunger gets worse, they'll risk getting shock in order to eat. You may feel at times you're in a rat race; the only problem is that the rats are always winning! Some crooked CEOs and politicians are prime examples.

Society has fooled us into believing we need rewards such as a bigger house and fancier cars than our neighbors'—many of whom we don't even know. We make sure our kids have the latest designer clothes and are the best in after-school activities. Think about it, there will always be somebody with more toys than you. Toys wear out, get lost, or can be stolen. Remember, you can't take it with you! So you really can't buy your way out of this one. Look at the enormous amount of energy and time some have wasted, literally a lifetime, on such foolery. Don't be like a naïve, impressionable kid and fall for such silly Saturday morning advertisements. We are smarter than that. I've never heard a dying person wish they worked more or saved more money. Usually it's more like he wishes he had taken more time off, went on that dream vacation, or expressed his love to his family more often. He may hope he forgave more often and didn't always put money ahead of more important matters. Bottom line, spend the time you've got left on what's really important.

I guess what I'm trying to point out is that a lot of the stressors are self-induced, and you do have a choice in how you react to them. Don't react, proact instead. The old-fashioned advice of counting to ten, taking a few deep breaths, or getting away for a walk or a ride makes good sense. Try it. I find writing down your thoughts and feelings helps you express more heartfelt responses, as opposed to reactive verbal volleying. I only discuss relationships and finances because a lot of stress comes from strained relationships, most of these concerning money. Here are some more communicating tips to hopefully obtain some peace.

Using *you* when talking to your loved one may make her feel attacked. This usually results in her firing back and pressing all the wrong buttons in defense, thereby escalating fear and anger. Same thing with finger-pointing; you'll have three fingers always pointing back at you, right? Example, "*You* don't listen to me. *You* don't care about me. *You* always …" Remember, you don't fight fire with fire; you fight fire with water. Instead, try to express your true feelings inside without accusing her of anything. Say, "I feel frustrated at times when I feel you're not listening to me" or "I feel insecure when I feel you may not care about me." This opens up the truth and welcomes constructive dialogue.

At times, you may need to get to the next level of effective communication. That is, when something makes you upset or angry, just sit back and think about why it does? Is it because you feel inadequate? Are you scared? Why are you so insecure in the relationship to reveal your true inner self, thoughts, or background? I find most people become angry because of two things. One is they don't know how or are uncomfortable with expressing love. They may not have been exposed much to love or learned how to love in the first place. They may come from a dysfunctional family. When faced with a challenging situation demanding love and understanding, they paradoxically revert to a simpler, reactive survival-like response—anger or hate. Two, these feelings are derived mostly from underlying fear. They are scared, but may be trying their best to hide it. Scared because of deeply hidden feelings they may be afraid of sharing for fear of losing you and your trust, support, dependence, or whatever. This vastly varies from person to person. Only some introspection may reveal this.

If you think your relationships may suffer from this, two more thoughts may help. One, you're far from being alone. The other, you've got to get some help. This may be from many different books, from the library, support groups, friends and family, church, or from a professional. You shouldn't feel embarrassed about this; you should feel good about your strength and courage. Didn't you have professionals to help you learn about the *outer* world? Well, use professionals again to help learn about your *inner* world, a vastly more important, complex system. Besides your health, your next most important assets are your closest relationships—spouse, kids, extended family, and friends. Who else is going to help you enjoy that fancy house or car, anyway? Who's going to love you when you're old and wrinkled? Remember the saying, "Count your age by friends, not years"?

Changing themes a bit to round out the discussion, we must recall the important role hormonal balance plays in helping maintain the proper emotional milieu. The chapters on testosterone, DHEA, and HGH cover this in detail. Remember, hormones are the chemical messengers, or the directors, of the body that Mother Nature gave us. As you will read, cortisol is either with you or against you. Lifestyle and age affect this balance. Melatonin helps you get the needed quality sleep. The bottom line—all the proper diet, exercise, pills and psychotherapy in the world won't get you feeling 100 percent mentally and physically well if your hormones aren't happening. It's all integrated.

B. Cortisol. We introduced cortisol above, but let's give a more hormonal background. Cortisol has a normal *bell-shaped* response curve. In those acutely stressful situations mentioned above, it normally should sharply rise and fall back to baseline levels much in the shape of a bell. Cortisol normally has a diurnal baseline rhythm consisting of an early morning peak (please see the figure below). This cortisol peak is when HGH (human growth hormone) production naturally diminishes.

It is an accepted endocrinological principal that cortisol and insulin are in a *yin-yang* relationship with HGH. Meaning, when insulin or cortisol goes up, HGH levels go down. To fight this, we promote a diet consisting of complex carbs which possess a lower glycemic index. You can increase your HGH naturally, without any shots. Lowering insulin and cortisol levels through proper dieting will up your HGH levels. We also mentioned earlier that insulin and cortisol levels unhealthily increase as a byproduct of aging. This relationship also help promotes the age-related decline we see in HGH production and the resulting frailty syndrome.

Insulin is mainly *pro-inflammatory* and sets us up for the metabolic syndrome. Cortisol contributes to most the conditions mentioned above, including osteoporosis, decreased immune function, and glucose intolerance. Indeed, these programmed hormonal changes are the very effective weapons of war that nature will use to whack out us middle aged guys. Remember what I said earlier? As we age, the hormones you wish would go up, go down and vice versa! Well this is how she does it.

> Higher insulin and cortisol levels mean lower HGH.

There are a few more very important aspects you need to know about cortisol. As a review, you should appreciate that cortisol levels have a diurnal rhythm that generally spikes in the early morning (please see fig. 12.1, curve C). During times of acute stress, there is normally a bell-shaped curve that returns back to baseline. But in the concrete jungle, there are those grossly, abnormally high, lengthy physical and emotional stressors we simply haven't had time to adapt. How does this affect the levels in the blood? Basically, in two ways:

In exaggerated, acutely stressful scenarios, we see startling cortisol responses—a higher peak combined with a much longer time to return to normal. Mathematically, these add up to a greater *area under the curve,* or AUC. Physiologically, these result in the abnormally longer and more intense sympathetic symptoms mentioned above. The unhealthy metabolic changes alluded above ensue also. The more frequent these episodes occur, the more physical and emotional erosion happen, much as the waves on the seashore. See figure 12.1, curve A.

What happens then if this continues? Well, it's like hearing that alarm clock you can't shut off. Initially, you'll jump, right? If it keeps on ringing, you'll progressively jump less. After a while, you won't jump at all. You're desensitized now. Eventually, you'll get really aggravated and try to mentally block it out until the alarm clock stops or you throw it against the wall. Well, your body basically does the same thing. The adrenal glands essentially burn out from all the intense, chronic stimulation. This eventually results in an abnormally low, nonpulsatile cortisol level (see curve B).[191]

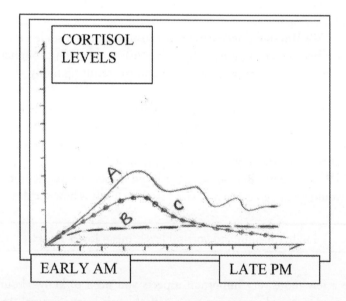

Figure 12.1 Acute versus chronic stress effects on cortisol secretion. Adrenal glands can burn out as in B and not give the needed diurnal and nocturnal cues the body needs.

---

191 This is similar to what happens in the beta islet cells of the pancreas in type 2 diabetes. Initially, the pancreas has to produce higher amounts of insulin to deal with the increasing amount of serum glucose. As the disease progresses, the pancreas must make increasingly higher amounts of insulin. Eventually, it burns out, necessitating that the diabetic patient now be placed on insulin therapy.

The above two abnormal curves can be usually diagnosed by blood work. If the patient expresses elusive stress-related complaints and is undergoing a good deal of stress, be it acute or chronic, we'll draw early-morning serum cortisol level. If it's *high-normal*, as in A, it is indicative of an exaggerated *acute* stress response by the adrenals. If *low-normal*, as in B, it suggests *chronic* adrenal burnout. I may also check a serum cortisol level around 2 p.m. if clinically indicated or when monitoring cortisol replacement therapy.[192]

In both instances, *sleep disturbance*s are common as the normal diurnal and nocturnal rhythms are out of synch. Commonly, physicians would only prescribe a potentially addictive and dangerous narcotic, which only treats the symptoms at most and actually may compound problems long term. So what do we do?

If the morning cortisol is *high-normal*, then an integrative, personalized approach is taken to lower stress levels. Of course, diet and exercise is a big player. Replacing DHEA, especially if low, may help out (K. Nair, 2003). This improvement probably occurs because of DHEA's direct effects and feedback mechanisms to the adrenal glands. I have seen some clinical improvement in insomnia with DHEA, although I add a more integrative, holistic approach, as will be explained.

If the morning cortisol is *low-normal*, then I may restore levels with some Cortef, of which the amount and dosing throughout the day depend on the entire clinical picture and response. The above represents how I generally approach *nonoptimized* adrenal-gland functioning commonly referred to as *adrenopause*. Any suspicion of pathologically abnormal adrenal functioning warrants a thorough medical evaluation including additional lab work and imaging studies, as this can be deadly. Notwithstanding that, clinical response and follow-up levels need to be routinely monitored with any replacement therapy by someone who's qualified.

> If chronic stress continues, the adrenal glands will burn out. This causes fatigue during the day and poor rest at night. These are symptoms of adrenopause.

---

192 Some non-MDs may use saliva tests for serial cortisol measurements; they can't legally order blood work. Although this may be convenient, I've not seen the scientific evidence to back this method of testing. There are just too many variables involved. It's paramount to get the proper diagnosis and safe, proven treatment.

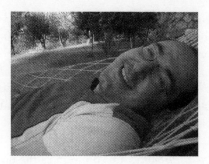

C. Melatonin is a hormone secreted by the pineal gland—what the wondrous Greeks called the third eye. Increased levels are produced by darkness, and levels generally decline with advancing age at rate of about 10–15 percent per year (see the figure below). Additional points are bulleted:

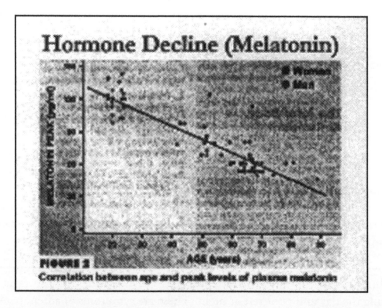

Figure 12.3. Melatonin levels decline as we age. Many believe this contributes to the increased sleep complaints expressed with aging.

- Manages "inner clock," temperature, and other diurnal and nocturnal rhythms, allowing for proper pulsing of hormones. With hormones, it's not just the absolute levels that are important, but also the number of pulses. If you remember my analogy of all the hormones working as the musicians in an orchestra, you will see that melatonin helps set the tempo and rhythm, or the optimal pulsatile nature, of other important chemical messengers. For example, melatonin generally helps improve stage 3 and 4 sleep. This in turn improves the pulsatile nature of those critical four-to-five-early-morning HGH spikes we spoke about earlier. Improved quality of sleep is one of the best ways to naturally raise IGF-1 levels—the serum marker for HGH.

- One of most effective free radical scavengers, protecting DNA and mitochondria, more than vitamin E or glutathione, although E concentrates better in the tissues of the body.

- Enhances the immune system and inhibits tumor growth though multiple effects. Used in treatment of brain and breast cancers.[193] Recently shown to decrease side effects, especially nausea, of chemotherapy allowing higher and longer dosing, but more importantly more nourishment and overall energy.

- According to an Israeli team of researchers, 2 mg of melatonin before bedtime can improve nocturnal blood pressure control by an average of 7 points and prevent early-morning pressure surges in hypertensive patients who don't show the typical nighttime pressure drop. These patients, who are actually at increased risk of target organ damage, reported no adverse effects; and the compliance rate was high. That's quite unlike any prescription medication for hypertension.[194]

- Treats jet lag and helps in shift work the so-called delayed sleep phase syndrome in children and adults. The way I advise this is as follows: If you're going to be three hours earlier, say going from a pacific standard time to an eastern standard time zone, you would dose your melatonin three hours earlier the night before to help *reset* your inner clock. So, instead of taking it at 9 p.m. the night before, you would take it at 6 p.m. and continue this as long as needed. In one study, melatonin improved the total sleep time the same as Ambien.

- Less is more! Most people do better with smaller doses of melatonin, so it's better to start out taking 1 mg as opposed to 3 mg. I've never recommended taking more than 3 mg, although the literature and some studies went up to 10 mg. Some people may have a mild hangover the next

---

193 Nelson, Ann *N Y Academy of Sciences* 917 (2000): 404–17; J. Kreigfeld, *Pineal Research* 30 (2001):193–8.

194 Y. Sharobi re-presented this to the annual meeting of the European Society of Hypertension in 2006. Taken from Erik Goldman, August 15, 2006, *Family Practice News.*

morning. For these, I'll recommend taking it two to three hours before bedtime, or simply take a smaller dose. Again, I must emphasize getting only pharmaceutical-grade supplements to ensure you're getting the right ingredients in the right amounts without any bogus fillers or other potentially dangerous ingredients. We don't want another L-tryptophan-like problem happening again.

Melatonin Replacement: No serious adverse effects.

Usually produces drowsiness and improved sleep onset and maintenance.
Occasional paradoxical stimulation in some.
Can produce vivid dreams which are interesting to some, disturbing to others.
Can produce a "hangover" the next morning, although this usually resolves over the next few days.
Some just don't feel good taking it.
Most though are "wild eyed and bushy tailed" and well rested.

NEJM review

Figure 12.4. Melatonin replacement therapy summary. Results from a NEJM review.

Measuring melatonin levels in the body are usually not done; this has no practical significance, as far as I'm concerned. It has an established, universal age-related decline, which parallels with poorer sleep patterns in the aged; and individual dosing is usually based on the clinical response. Because of the aforementioned benefits of melatonin, including improving the quality of sleep and possibly increasing HGH release, I routinely recommend replacing it in virtually every middle-aged or over. It's very safe and usually well tolerated. There are saliva tests available for melatonin; however, I find these to be of no real practical use.

We have spoken about how proper diet and exercise greatly influence the hormonal balance. The diet will help keep insulin and cortisol in their optimal groove. More stable sugar levels will help stop the crash-and-burn mood cycles caused by higher glycemic foods. Exercise will help keep your diurnal rhythm normal. Being more active during the day and getting that runners' high will make you more tired at night, resulting in improved sleep. No drug or hormone is going to do it all for you.

Today's convenient lifestyle simply doesn't have the manually laborious component in which we evolved. I can recall when I was a kid, my quite elderly grandma would still wring clothes out of the washer, hang them up outside to dry, and then fold them, and put them all away. There were lots of singing and smiling. All meals were painstakingly hand made with love. Grandpa would be using his push mower and hand clippers in the yard. He'd walk to the corner store later on. Fast forward thirty years—nowadays, we have remotes and all the modern conveniences. Somehow, we must make up for this lazier lifestyle by substituting in some recreational exercise, at least a half hour to an hour per day. That's good for the mind and body; it's a win-win situation! Increasing your physical activity and eating right during the day, along with adding optimum hormonal replacement, will synergistically result in a stress-free individual.

> We're basically combining the lifestyle of our wise forefathers with optimal hormonal balance as designed by Mother Nature in order to obtain a healthier, longer life. This is the best from both worlds—the past and present!

Chapter 12. MAG has many of the symptoms of anxiety, fatigue, and poor sleep. His morning cortisol level was on the low-normal side, so he began taking Cortef, 5 mg in the morning. Taking DHEA will also help normalize his insulin and cortisol levels. MAG also takes 1 mg of melatonin before bedtime. He and his wife notice his sleep and mood are improved. They're both glad he was able to nix his prescribed sleeping medication. As a closer couple, they both enjoy the local yoga classes in order to help relieve stress.

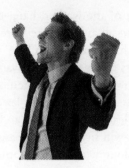

XIII.

Human Growth Hormone: The Fountain of Youth?

The overall deterioration of the body that comes with growing old is not inevitable....
We now realize that some aspects of it can be prevented or reversed.

—D. Rudman, MD

Well, here we are—human growth hormone, HGH, the miracle elixir. Finally, the *fountain of youth* we've all been trying to discover for hundreds of years! Is it, really? If anything I've said has sunken in, you would know HGH is no panacea either. You're more educated now and skeptical of such proclamations. You want to learn the real science on the efficacy and safety before drawing any conclusions. Right on, man! More power to you!

A. The History of HGH. As a preface, let me say that probably no other hormone has received such an undeserving reputation—both good and bad. The very name, human *growth* hormone, may lead some to conjure mental images of freakish height disorders such as gigantism, or acromegaly. They may believe it causes growths or tumors to suddenly sprout out all over them like a well-watered *chia pet*. Yet to others, HGH may be the one magical potion that helps them become faster than a speeding bullet, more powerful than a locomotive, and able to leap tall buildings in a single bound and at the same time reverses twenty years of aging. The fact of the matter is HGH works as any other hormone. When in upper physiological levels, it has benefits and works synergistically with all the other hormones and the proper lifestyle to help ensure optimal health. Conversely, when deficient, it creates a well-defined syndrome and a cascade of problems mirroring age-related complications. When appropriately replaced, these symptoms are then abated in the safest, most natural way. Lastly, if used inappropriately, HGH can cause serious problems. Indeed, HGH has received both extreme praise and criticism from the scientific community, as well as the media. However, once we look fairly upon adult HGH deficiency as a true medical illness with well-established symptoms and proven treatment options, we should arrive with solid scientific knowledge to back up our opinions. That's exactly what we'll do.

HGH has a suspect reputation that needs to be properly addressed. *Acromegaly* is the specific disease defined as the "abnormal supraphysiological production of HGH throughout one's entire life span." When most lay persons and physicians think of replacing HGH, they recall those textbook pictures of freaky, grotesque circus giants. As you will read, this doesn't happen with appropriate HGH replacement. On the other end of the spectrum, *somatopause*—the age-related HGH decline in adults—and its appropriate treatment aren't generally taught in medical school. It should be of no surprise most physicians believe somatopause simply doesn't exist. Therefore, HGH replacement can't offer any benefit. Remember what I said earlier, we physicians can only diagnose what we've learned. Unless we spent some elective time with an advanced-thinking endocrinologist, the only education on HGH we got were those few hellacious textbook cases of acromegaly. Heck, who's not scared of a giant! You run far away and don't easily forget that encounter.

Most early research done on HGH was based on this abnormal *lifelong overproduction* of HGH and its deleterious associations. These ranged from the obvious physical malformations to joint problems, heart disease, and possible increased risks for colon cancer. You must appreciate that acromegaly is the complete opposite of what we're introducing here—the appropriate physiological replacement in older adults who suffer from deficient HGH production. To deny HGH therapy to these deserving individuals would be like denying appropriate thyroid hormone replacement in those with *hypo*thyroid simply because of the many severe consequences of *hyper*thyroidism.[195] The latter can be caused by disease or induced by overdosing on thyroid medication. H*yper*thyroidism can cause a myriad of symptoms such as abnormal physical appearance, extreme psychotic behavior, and

---

195 *Hypo*thyroidism is caused by an *underactive* thyroid and *low* thyroid hormone. *Hyper*thyroidism is caused from an *overactive* thyroid gland, or *high* levels of thyroid hormone. This will be covered in the thyroid chapter later.

deadly heart failure. *Hypo*thyroidism—a whole different disease altogether—can cause loss of hair, abnormalities of skin, nonresponsive depression, coma, and a different kind of heart failure. Any decent physician out there wouldn't think twice about replacing thyroid hormone in a symptomatic individual possessing low thyroid hormone levels. Only the most inept physician would have second thoughts about restoring these levels. It wouldn't be logical, scientific, or ethical to deny the appropriate therapy to a symptomatic patient with *hypo*thyroidism because of the risks and symptoms associated with *hyper*thyroidism—an entirely different disease entity altogether. In fact, his *not* doing this would be considered malpractice. Unfortunately, the medical community—generally a very conservative, hardheaded bunch—have unfairly lumped appropriate adult growth hormone deficiency (AGHD) treatment and acromegaly together. To the average physician, just the mere mention of HGH treatment may warrant him to make a sign of the cross like he's trying to ward off vampires. Because the very name contains the word *growth,* it causes doctors and patients alike to unfairly associate it with promoting *tumor* or *cancer growth.* We may all be running from the giant again. Let's not throw out the baby giant with the bath water.

> Unfortunately, the proper diagnosis of adult growth hormone deficiency and its treatment have been unfairly lumped together with acromegaly—the lifelong pathological *over*secretion of HGH. These are, in fact, two opposite disease entities.

HGH replacement got off to a rough start. In the 1950s, before it was synthesized and became commercially available, it could only be obtained from human cadavers. I know that sounds pretty gross, but follow along with me here. If you heat cadaver-derived HGH enough to destroy all contaminants and potentially infectious agents, you would also denature the molecule, making it totally ineffective. This hindered early purification methods. Apparently, this resulted in a few recipients becoming afflicted with a rare disorder called Creutzfeldt-Jakob disease from unknown but infected HGH donors. This is like a human variety of mad cow disease, which progressively affects the nervous system and has no current cure. Even its causative agent is largely unknown; small particles called *prions* may play a role. But, thanks to the advancing scientific research in the 1980s, *recombinant DNA* technology allowed us to then sequence the HGH gene. This discovery eventually allowed the mass production of the safe, pure synthetic *recombinant* HGH we use today. Historically, HGH was only second to insulin to be mass-produced using these novel DNA-cloning methods by Genentech Corp.

In the late 1980s, both Genentech and the movie *Cocoon,* a story about octogenarians obtaining the fountain of youth from space aliens, raked in millions of dollars. Remember the swimming pool scene? Now fast forward to 2007, when a video copy of *Cocoon* is going for a measly $2.95. Depressingly, despite the expiration of the HGH patent status, it still remains quite expensive. Pricing starts at about $500 per month! The FDA has been quite vigilant in fighting generic HGH, even to the point of shutting down pharmacies and revoking licenses from doctors prescribing non-FDA-approved HGH varieties. These mostly come from overseas or local *compounding* pharmacies. The effectiveness and safety of these aren't proven; avoid them. I believe this discouragement is a good thing because there is a lot of bogus bootleg HGH out there today, preying upon the unsuspecting and improperly educated.

On the other hand, major drug firms such as Genentech, Eli Lilly, Upjohn, Savient, Serono, and Novo Nordisk have long enjoyed a cash cow that is grazing on an estimated $1 billion annually since 1995. Not bad, especially considering mostly all HGH research and development was paid by the government because of its orphan-drug status. Looking at all the battling for HGH rights and lawsuits settled by the major drug firms over the years, it makes me wonder how much of this is for patient safety and just how much is about corporate profits? Add to this the increasingly aging U.S. population now enjoying a government-sponsored drug plan. Eventually, almost all the sick elderly population would be found symptomatic of HGH deficiency and therefore demand replacement.[196] Lawyers would line up to sue those denying therapy. So, even if HGH cost much less from approved generic manufacturers and we replaced it in most all Medicare beneficiaries, the added expense would break the system. You can begin to see how HGH replacement has many political and financial hurdles to jump before its widespread acceptance into mainstream medicine.

At any rate, HGH replacement has been controversial since Dr. Daniel Rudman published his landmark, age-reversing results in the *New England Journal of Medicine* back in 1990.[197] He injected twelve elderly patients with HGH for six months and noted that they basically got younger. Among the benefits was roughly a 9 percent increase in lean body mass, 15 percent decrease in fat mass, 2 percent increase in bone density, and 7 percent increase in skin thickness. He esti-

---

196 Granted, according to Savin in *Hormone Research* (2000): 53, almost all adults over forty have some IGF-1 deficiency.

197 D. Rudman, "Effects of human growth hormone in men over 60 years old," *NEJM* 323 (1990):1–6.

mated HGH replacement reversed about ten to twenty years of age-related degeneration. The doctor famously quoted in conclusion, "The overall deterioration of the body that comes with growing old is not inevitable.... We now realize that some aspects of it can be prevented or reversed." This groundbreaking research sent sparks, igniting further research for decades that's still trying to vindicate or repudiate this statement.

Let's get a little background on HGH. If you look at figure 8.3, you'll see HGH is produced in the pituitary, released into the bloodstream, and then converted to intrinsic growth factor-1 (IGF-1), by the liver. This is mostly through the organ's cytochrome p450 system. Although the relationship of HGH and IGF-1 is more complex, it's suffice to say IGF-1 is considered an "active metabolite" of HGH. Thus, it's obviously helpful to have a healthy liver and to limit drugs that can strain this pathway. These include not only many prescription drugs, but also ones such as acetaminophen, as well as alcohol. As you can appreciate in the below diagram, HGH levels variably decrease as we age, some of us age worse and subsequently are more symptomatic from low HGH than others.

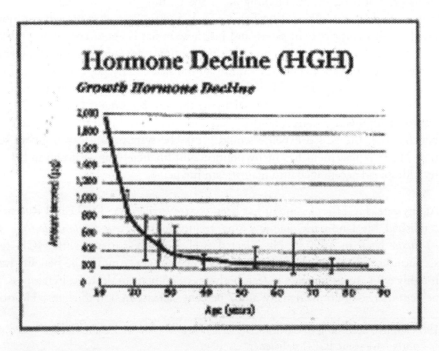

Figure 13.1. HGH levels variably decline as we age and are affected by many other factors.

A lot can affect HGH levels. There are actually only about four to five HGH pulses daily that occur in the early morning, during deep sleep. Thus is the importance of getting quality sleep. The diet and stress and sleep chapters discussed how higher insulin and cortisol levels diminish HGH production in a yin-yang fashion.

If we look at the symptoms of HGH deficiency and compare it to the conditions we get with advancing age, we see striking parallelism. The *paradigm shift* in thinking occurs when we look at aging itself as a *clinical syndrome* that can be treated, even slowed or somewhat reversed. I could keep on singing the same old blues tune we docs were originally taught to give patients, "As we age, such hormonal decline and these symptoms are inevitable and normal. Get used to it." But I had an epiphany and, instead, wail the more rocking anthem, "Many of the progressive symptoms of aging can be attributed to decreasing key hormonal levels. These conditions can be improved once the hormones are restored. Let's correct what's really ailing you deep inside." While this may not sound very poetic or even rhyme, when orchestrated right, it'll rock your world!

Conventional medicine: We can treat most of the symptoms of age-related diseases.

Age Management Medicine: We can favorably affect the process of premature aging in the first place.

This has been the standard of practice with other deficient hormones such as thyroid, women's sex hormones, and more recently, testosterone in men. Proponents of HGH replacement ask why HGH should be any different. On the other hand, you could just follow the advice of your regular, out-of-shape, impotent doctor, "All your lab tests are normal. You're just getting older. Hey, join the club!"

B. How HGH Works and Doesn't Work.

To further understand how HGH works, you'll need to review the introduction to men's hormonal changes chapter and figure 8.3. Remember, our hormone system is best understood as a cascade with the brain being at the top, followed by the pituitary gland, then target organs (i.e., ovaries, thyroid, testicles), and finally physical and mental functions (i.e., skin thickness, menstrual periods, sex characteristics, aggression, hair distribution).

As with any feedback loop, it's hard to say where things actually begin, but we'll start in the brain. The hypothalamus is the part of the brain where various hormone releases originate, starting off the cascade by secreting "releasing hormones," which then help stimulate and direct the pituitary. Here, growth hormone—releasing factor (GHRF) is released. In the hypothalamus, emotional or physical stressors are balanced with advanced reasoning from the cerebral cortex, yet have to also satisfy basic urges from our more reptilian-like mid- and hindbrain. No wonder there's a lot of conflict.

The pituitary is known as the "master gland." It sits at the base of our brain and communicates directly with the hypothalamus by special nerves and blood vessels. Releasing hormones travel from the hypothalamus to the pituitary and stimulate the formation and release of pituitary hormones into our circulatory system. Here, GHRF causes the release of HGH. The pituitary hormones exert their effects on many of our organs such as the thyroid, adrenal glands, testicles, ovaries, and breasts. Specifically, HGH has more than one target organ, but its primary target is the liver, where it causes the formation and release of insulin-like growth factor-1 (IGF-1, a.k.a. somatomedin C).

HGH has many metabolic effects, the most predominant of which is protein synthesis. It is released in bursts, most of which occur during deep sleep. After we stop growing and become adults, there is a significant decrease in the amount produced. IGF-1 is a by-product of growth hormone and is thought to be responsible for most of the anabolic (building) effects of the hormone itself. Fortunately, IGF-1 levels are fairly constant in the blood and can be measured more easily than HGH. We, therefore, measure blood levels of IGF-1 to assess the amount of circulating HGH in the body.

HGH is essential for bone and organ growth in our youth. Too little of it causes short stature; too much causes gigantism, as mentioned earlier. It is very clear that HGH and IGF start to decrease in our late teens and continue to do so quite rapidly. Although it's no longer needed for "growth" after adulthood, HGH is essential for many other vital functions, and the significantly lowered levels seen as we age are thought to be correlated with everything from diminished energy to weight gain (fat) and decreased muscle mass.

In the past, if a pituitary gland was removed or destroyed due to a tumor in an adult, HGH was not replaced even though the more "essential" hormones such as thyroid, hydrocortisone, and testosterone or estrogen/progesterone were replaced.

It wasn't until the work of Dr. B. Bengtsson and Dr. Rudman that the value of HGH in adults was recognized. It was found that deficient patients had an almost 50 percent higher rate of death from heart disease than expected.[198] Bengtsson then replaced HGH in pituitary-deficient patients and achieved excellent results. This led to Dr. Rudman's research in 1990 mentioned above. Today, there have been over one hundred clinical trials studying AGHD.

In 1999, the National Institute on Aging (NIA) completed another landmark study that was designed to either refute or substantiate the results of Dr. Rudman. It also measured some other parameters. This was a double-blind, placebo-controlled, multicenter trial that studied a large number of men and women. It used not only HGH, but sex hormones too. This study not only confirmed the benefits of HGH that Dr. Rudman had asserted, but also demonstrated that the addition of sex steroids improved the effectiveness in both men and women. Although the NIA study showed HGH alone didn't increase muscle strength, it did substantially improve lean muscle and aerobic capacity. The addition of testosterone did increase muscle strength substantially, thus reinforcing the importance of hormonal synergy.

In November 2002, most cutting-edge doctors were waiting for a form of vindication from Dr. Mark Blackman's latest HGH trial, as he is widely considered a long-standing supporter of replacing HGH in deficient adults. If anyone knew HGH, it would have to be him and coauthor Mitchell Harmon, although they're both solely academians. You're more than welcome to look at the article yourself and come to your own conclusions, but I'll give you my two-minute spiel.[199]

Incredibly, the HGH dosing used didn't closely mimic the physiological dosing we suggest, nor as recommended by the *PDR* and the drug's manufacturers. Basically, they gave unusually large doses three times per week, as opposed to the lower dosed daily shots we've instructed for years. Starting off with that high a dose usually results in more side effects. More importantly, the subjects weren't necessarily HGH deficient but are healthy, normal adults; and they were only studied for six months. Most times, side effects diminish in the first few months, while the full benefits can take a few more months or more. As stated before about these therapies, no two people respond at the same rate. Lastly, I certainly wouldn't expose

---

198 T. Rosen, B. A. Bengtsson, "Premature mortality due to cardiovascular disease in hypopituitarism," *Lancet.* 4, no. 336 (1990): 285–88.

199 M. Blackman, "Growth hormone and sex steroid administration in healthy aged women and men," *JAMA* 288 (2002): 2282–92.

the risks of HGH therapy to someone that wasn't the appropriate candidate; they would have to be symptomatic from AGHD. I would consider this somewhat unethical.

It's of no real surprise that their conclusions paralleled many earlier, similarly flawed trials on HGH therapy, the results of which include worsening of glucose intolerance, joint or muscle aches, and edema. These undesired effects are greatly diminished by starting off with the lower-dosed daily injections we typically recommend and then adjusting according to the clinical picture and follow-up lab work.[200] When you review most research, there is a tendency for insulin to go up the first few months of HGH use; however, this typically reverses and improves after about six months. When replaced for over six months, HGH replacement invariably shows loss of visceral and peripheral fat, which would, in fact, improve metabolic parameters and the risk for diabetes. Additionally, there are volumes of research showing decreased inflammatory markers and improved cardiovascular risks with proper HGH replacement.[201] Going back to 1994, research done by Stephen Grinspoon published in *Neuroendocrine Clinical Center Bulletin* confirmed the aforementioned benefits and the lower risk of side effects when lower doses were used in HGH-deficient but healthy aging adults.

Lastly, Blackman had a subset of men and women on what most would consider grossly improper sex hormone replacement. This included nonphysiological, infrequent testosterone dosing and even some women being put on supraphysiological dosing of synthetic progesterone and estrogen. Subjects weren't allowed to exercise! Needless to say, most of my colleagues were quite disappointed about the above study design and could've easily predicted the unfavorable outcomes. In the end, Blackman's study revealed nothing new to those who are up-to-date on appropriate hormonal replacement research. It's a shame that the media, as well as the medical community, let this single paper overshadow many volumes proving the relative benefits and safety of appropriate HGH replacement in deficient, symptomatic adults.

---

200 Reinforcing this was research by Bengtsson published in the *Journal of Clinical Endocrinology and Metabolism* 76 (1993): 309–17 (there were only minor side effects that improved by lowering the HGH dose), and by Lewis Blevins, *The Endocrinologist* 12 (200): 405–11.

201 These points are reflected in an excellent meta-analysis study published in the *New England Journal of Medicine* (1999): 1206 and in the *Journal of Clinical Endocrinology and Metabolism* (2002): 87.

HGH therapy for those suffering from AGHD has been shown by most studies to be overwhelmingly safe and beneficial. I feel M. Blackman's study in 2002 that questioned HGH use had suffered from poor design and therefore resulted in some expectedly poor outcomes.

C. The Safety of Human Growth Hormone Replacement. Taking HGH does raise IGF-1 levels in the blood. It is believed this higher IGF-1 mediates most of the effects attributed to growth hormone. Most studies in adults and children fail to show any risk of cancer related to the use of growth hormone or higher levels of IGF-1. In fact, an extensive review article published in the *New England Journal of Medicine* October 14, 1999, by Drs. Mary Vance and Nellie Mauras concluded, "There is at present no evidence that Growth Hormone modulation affects the risk of cancer." All patients should be aware there are other reports that do indicate there may be an increased risk.

In 1998, two published studies claimed a higher incidence of prostate cancer among men who had higher IGF-1 levels years before the onset of the cancer; but a number of experts agree that these studies are inconclusive and may be flawed. Problems cited with these studies include the method of statistical analysis, the several year intervals between the drawing of the blood and the onset of cancer, and the absence of any IGF measurement at the time of diagnosis of the cancer. Several other studies show no difference in IGF-1 levels between normal healthy men and those with prostate cancer at the time of diagnosis and beyond. The addition of any anabolic-like hormone may *uncover* a *masked* prostate cancer, allowing its detection to be picked up earlier, which would favor a better prognosis. This was discussed in the chapter on testosterone.

There is a lot of research to suggest IGFBP-3 (insulin-like growth factor binding protein 3, part of the IGF *superfamily*, actually promotes apoptosis, or cancer-cell death. As a matter of fact, if there is a marked increase with initiation of HGH treatment, we may consider the possibility of uncovering a masked cancer. It is believed that the p53, or the tumor suppressor gene, increases production of IGFBP-3. Though according to *JCEM* May 2001, "There is no data to suggest that IGF-1 and IGFBP-3 modulate cancer risk in HGH treated patients." Still, current labeling for HGH states that active malignancy is a strong contraindication; and given the data as it stands now, I certainly agree. There has also been research, albeit in young kids, that HGH treatment didn't increase any chances of cancer recurrence.[202] Lastly in *JCEM* 2002, Molitch concluded that HGH treatment of adults is quite safe adding, "although there has been some concern about an increased risk of cancer, reviews of existing, well-maintained databases of treated patients have shown this theoretical risk to be nonexistent." HGH also treats the cachexia, or the wasting-away syndrome, of AIDS. As you probably know, this end stage of HIV infection causes severe immune system failure, which results in the increased appearance of cancers—much more so than advanced aging. Yet, HGH therapy has proven to be quite safe and beneficial. In the future, many other chronic, debilitated disease states, like CHF, may be commonly helped by HGH.

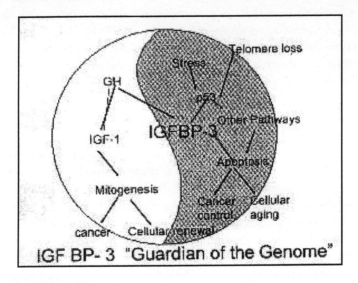

Figure 13.2. The IGF *superfamily* helps to balance apoptosis and mitosis. Confusingly, many times the research doesn't state which subtype was measured. We expect to see higher IGFBP-3 with cancers.

What about the safety of *long-term* HGH use? It would be important to not just look at studies with HGH-treated children and then extrapolate these to older adults, an entirely different population. Furthermore, if we plan to use HGH long term, we need to look at relatively long-term studies. This task is compromised by the fact that recombinant HGH has only been widely used since the 1990s. Svenssson, in the July 2004 *Journal of Clinical Endocrinology and Metabolism*, revealed the results of a ten-year prospective study, looking at deficient men and women treated with HGH. The average IGF-1 at baseline was 125 ng/ml—an adequate level to *diagnose* HGH deficiency. Important to also note is that the average replacement levels were 290 ng/ml for men and 210 for women—about the levels many shoot for when *replacing* HGH.

Outcomes were most favorable. The *treated* deficient group had the same relative risk for total mortality, stroke, all cancers, and cancer deaths, including colon types, as the *normal* population. There was remarkably a 0.27 risk reduction observed in heart attack though. The *untreated deficient* group had *increases* in relative risks ranging from 1.4 to 5.33 for all those conditions. Besides the safety of proper HGH replacement observed, the latter point reinforces the healthier outcomes expected when treating HGH-deficient patients.

My treatment goal for HGH in deficient men ranges from 250 to 320 ng/ml, which falls within the average level for a forty-year-old man. Note that this range isn't supraphysiological for *any* age group, even for a seventy-five-year-old! I reached that bar by not just trying to mimic the average level seen in the overall population, but by looking at the actual risk reduction of age-related diseases with different HGH levels, as indicated by scientific literature. (Please see the afore-mentioned research by Svensson.) Again, it must be stressed, we aren't just aiming for mere *normal* ranges; rather, we want to approximate optimal levels. In the end, it has to all come full circle by the following: We first must see the increase in the mortality and morbidity in age-related diseases with lower levels of IGF-1. We then *must* couple this with the subsequent improvement or risk reduction in these diseases with HGH replenishment that's proven in scientific literature. This way we establish a cause-and-effect relationship and the benefits of replacing HGH. (It's not enough to establish just an *association* of increasing age and its many diseases with diminishing HGH levels.) It was previously explained how treating AGHD improves obesity, metabolic disorders, osteoporosis, and other such age-related diseases. More evidence follows below.

Roubenoff and colleagues in the October 15, 2003, issue of the *American Journal of Medicine* found that lower IGF-1 levels in subjects from the Framingham Heart Study predicted a higher *cardiovascular mortality* rate. Additionally, those possessing the upper-fiftieth percentile of IGF-1 levels had 13 percent lower *total* mortality. He concluded, "Decrease in IGF-1 levels is a risk factor for mortality in the elderly." This research helped establish IGF-1 as an independent disease marker. Along those lines, Denti et al., in the September 1, 2004, issue of the *American Journal of Medicine*, found lower IGF-1 levels predicted poorer *stroke* outcomes.

If you've been listening to some rats at the gym, you may have heard about "cycling on and off" various synthetic, nonhuman-based anabolic steroids. I strongly advise against using these—they're illegal. If you're in pretty good shape, usually no hormones are that deficient to begin with. The levels weren't appropriately checked via lab work or even evaluated by a properly trained, experienced MD. Supraphysiological, improper dosing is typically used, which can then cause a myriad of serious health and mental problems, both acute and long-term. This causes the need to *cycle off* in a haphazard way, which has its own set of serious consequences. This is a far cry from normal physiological homeostasis. You can die from endocrine gland shutdown, as in the case of an *Addisonian crisis.*[203]

It's not so hard to believe that there a lot of quacks out there who think that they're capable of providing medical care after reading a few magazine ads or by following unscrupulous practices. That's right—all with no degree, certification, or formal education. On the other extreme, I occasionally get calls from people who just want a simple Rx for HGH or those who may put cost above quality and expertise. They may say, "I can get this from others for a lot less." This reply really scares me. You should be wise enough to know the cheapest always costs more in the long run. It's not the hormones; it's the doctor behind the hormones that matters most. This is your health; don't mess around with it!

---

203 The adrenal glands have suppressed their natural production of hormones because of the body getting so much of fake ones from an outside source. When these endogenous steroids are stopped suddenly, the adrenal glands can't restart production that quickly; and the body basically shuts down from the lack of the needed hormonal stimulation and support.

Although the majority of studies overwhelmingly point toward the safety of human growth hormone, as in virtually any area of medical science, there is always some conflicting data. This is true because of the complex nature of the human body, its physiology, and the truism that medicine is not an exact science. As in all aspects of medical therapeutics, each of us must evaluate the information that is available along with our needs and goals, and measure these against potential risks. A well-trained physician in age-management medicine can help you understand and evaluate all the information available. However, only you and your doctor can make the final judgment call.

> HGH is not for everyone.
> HGH is not for anti-aging purposes or sports enhancement!

To put it into context, similar controversy has surrounded the use of estrogen in postmenopausal women for the past thirty years. We now know that artificial estrogen replacement in women may increase the risk of breast and endometrial cancer in older women with family histories of breast cancer, and other risk factors. However, because of estrogen's mostly proven protective effects against many other diseases (heart disease, osteoporosis, and colon cancer), *overall* mortality is lower in younger, healthier women who take estrogen. It will be many years before we have as much data on HGH, but I feel that for most symptomatic people with low IGF-1 levels, replacing HGH to optimal, physiological levels represents a viable option.

D. How to Know if You're HGH Deficient. As mentioned before, it seems to be the *modus operandi* of nature—as you age, the hormones you wish would go up, go down. Conversely and equally unfortunate, the hormones you wish would go down, in fact, go up. As alluded before, both advanced aging and HGH deficiency mirror the symptoms of insulin and cortisol excess. This reflects the yin-yang of the hormonal system. It was mentioned in the diet chapter and in the introduction that as we age, insulin and cortisol tend to increase. Some prefer to call these the "aging hormones." These cause the age-related increased inflammation, frailty, immune decline, degeneration, and more. As men age, T, DHEA, pregnenolone, melatonin, thyroid, and HGH all variably diminish.

The below symptoms of HGH deficiency overlap those of many other hormone deficiencies. This lends support to their synergism when all hormones are optimally balanced:

- Sarcopenia and osteopenia—loss of muscle and bone mass, respectively
- Less strength and endurance
- Increased visceral and peripheral fat
- Glucose intolerance to diabetes
- Hypertriglyceridemia and other lipid disorders
- Loss of soft tissue padding and skin elasticity
- Decreased immune function with increased inflammation
- Overall decreased sense of well-being, quality of life, and mood.

Adapted and modified from M. R. Blackman, 2000. Age-related alterations in sleep quality and neuroendocrine function: interrelationships and implications. *JAMA* Aug 16; 284(7). Dr. Stephen McKenna of the Galen Research Center in the UK also developed the Qol-AGHDA, a quality-of-life questionnaire that can be helpful in diagnosing AGHD and HGH replacement. It's only part of my comprehensive clinical assessment, though. You can visit their Web site at www.galen-research.com.

Accordingly, proven benefits of proper HGH replacement include the following:

- increase in libido
- decrease in body and bad visceral fat
- increase in lean muscle
- increase in bone density
- increase in skin thickness
- decrease in skin wrinkling
- improved cholesterol profile
- faster wound healing with lower infection rate
- decrease in hospitalization rate by 50 percent
- decrease in sick days from work
- increase in exercise capacity
- decrease in diastolic blood pressure
- decrease in waist/hip ratio
- increase in renal blood blow
- increase in feeling of well-being, improved socialization
- strengthened immune system
- improved cardiac function, decreased coronary inflammation, and normalized intima media thickness (IMT) of carotid artery.**

**Journal of Clinical Endocrinology Metabolism* 84 (1999) and 86 (2001); *Annals of Internal Medicine*, July 18, 2000; *Clinical Endocrinology* 59, no. 6 (2003) with excellent resources and background information previously given.

Anecdotally claimed benefits include the below:

- improved memory and mood
- improved cognitive function
- hair regrowth, less gray
- reduced spider veins

Just how low an IGF-1 level helps determine if you're HGH deficient? Again, we must look at the research. In 1997, HGH-treated subjects with initial IGF-1 levels under 120 ng/ml demonstrated a 50 percent lower risk for hospitalization and 45 percent fewer workdays missed.[204] That same year, Johansson, in the *Journal of Clinical Endocrinology and Metabolism (JCEM)*, found treating patients with initial levels below 160 ng/ml had significant improvements in abdominal fat mass, waste/hip ratio, improved glucose metabolism, and reduced diastolic blood pressure.[205] Trying to put a lot of this together were Carroll and colleagues in 1998. They correlated the signs and symptoms of HGH deficiency and defined these as a *clinical syndrome*, with particular lab values of IGF-1. The authors even described a *partial* deficiency of HGH as a separate syndrome.[206] In 2003, researchers calculated that approximately 95 percent of adequately replaced HGH-deficient patients possessed an obtained level of 194 ng/ml. This means 5 percent of these would still be missed if this was the cut-off level.[207] Furthermore, these levels remained relatively consistent from ages forty-one through seventy. So, over the past decade, the cutoff of HGH deficiency has been raised some. Based on the above, many progressive proponents of HGH therapy believe it's both reasonable and scientifically based to diagnose a male with HGH deficiency if he's symptomatic and possesses a baseline IGF-1 level below 190 ng/ml.

A most interesting study, the Rancho Bernardo Study, is a large ongoing, prospective, community-based study of relatively healthy aging middle- and upper-middle-class Caucasian adults *since 1988*.[208] After adjusting for known coronary

---

204 J. Verhelst, "Two years of replacement therapy in adults with growth hormone deficiency," *Clinical Endocrinology* 47 (1997): 485–94.

205 G. Johansson et al., "Growth hormone treatment of abdominally obese men reduces abdominal fat mass, improves glucose and lipoprotein metabolism, and reduces diastolic blood pressure," *Journal of Clinical Endocrinology and Metabolism* 82 (1997): 727–34.

206 P. V. Carroll et al. and Growth Hormone Research Society Scientific Committee, "Growth hormone deficiency in adulthood and the effects of growth hormone replacement: A review," *J Clin Endocrinol Metab* 83, no. 2 (1998): 382–95.

207 A. Mukherjee, "Seeking the optimal target range for insulin-like growth factor I during the treatment of adult growth hormone disorders," *J Clin Endocrinol Metab* 88, no. 12 (2003):5865–70. (For women, it may be more around 140 ng/dl.)

208 Laughlin et al., "The prospective association of serum insulin like growth factor I (IGF-1) and IGF binding protein-1 levels with all cause and cardiovascular disease mortality in older adults: The Rancho Bernardo study," *JCEM* 89, no. 1 (2004):114–20 looked at the relationship of IGF-1 and IGFBP-1 on "all cause" and cardiovascular mortality.

risk factors, researchers found that for every 40 ng/ml decrease in IGF-1 there was a 38 percent higher relative risk of death from ischemic heart disease. Those subjects in the lowest 25 percent of baseline IGF levels had over *three times* the relative risk.

In my practice, about one forth of patients were symptomatic from AGHD and needed to replace HGH. Yet, for that minority, it made a dramatic difference. For the majority though, proper lifestyle changes and all the other hormonal replacements we discussed earlier made enough of a difference to obtain their goals of feeling better overall and risk reduction for future disease. With such comprehensive changes in effect, IGF-1 levels substantially improve without having to resort to direct HGH replacement. We should expect this because of the synergism of all these other modalities. However, if these modalities didn't substantially improve the symptoms of HGH deficiency and there were still low IGF-1 levels, then HGH replacement may then be reconsidered. Also, HGH has been shown to help those plagued with overlying symptoms of fibromyalgia, myofascial pain syndrome, chronic fatigue syndrome, and related painful syndromes. As clinically indicated, any chances of an active cancer should be reasonably ruled out, and the benefits and risks fully reviewed. Proper HGH replacement in those deficient has no known drug interactions.

> Determining if you need HGH is based on the severity and number of symptoms that should be then correlated with IGF-1 levels. If symptomatic and baseline levels are below 190 ng/ml, it's reasonable to undergo a therapeutic trial. Replacing to levels around 290 ng/ml in a male is reasonable and backed by scientific research to reduce many disease risks. Proper HGH replacement should be only *one aspect* of a comprehensive approach to one's health.

Other problems I would have prescribing HGH besides those previously mentioned include the following:

- Pulmonary fibrosis or Prader-Willi syndrome, which are both very rare and clinically apparent.
- Uncontrolled diabetes, CHF, or unexplained swelling, which would initiate a comprehensive workup and definitive treatment. However, if controlled and indicated, HGH therapy may be considered because of the benefits mentioned.

- Somebody wanting a magic bullet and not really desirous of needed life-style changes. It's basically doomed to failure from the get-go because of the synergy and proactivity needed for things to work.

- Somebody not willing to do age-appropriate routine cancer screenings, as in colonoscopy, GYN exams, prostate screenings with PSA levels.

E. How's HGH Dosed? Here are some tidbits about HGH dosing. Keep in mind, these all depend on your particular situation. As mentioned, we generally start you on a low dose, about 7.35 units subcutaneously per week or about 0.2 mg daily. This helps limit side effects when starting off. Yes, yes, yes, it's a *daily* shot, but it goes just beneath the skin; it's given subcutaneously like insulin, not intramuscular. With today's 32-gauge needles available, you barely feel it. Don't be scared like a little girly man.

It's most important your HGH come only from U.S. FDA—approved drug manufacturers such as Genentech, Eli Lilly, Upjohn, Savient, Sorono, and Novo Nordisk. There's also the first follow-on version approved called Omnitrope by Sandoz. Novartis is also working on one, I believe. (Although still investigating the research on this, I've not found these to cost any less yet.) Don't trust any *compounded HGH*; you're running worse risks than getting bogus Botox©. HGH shouldn't come in prepackaged containers. These products appear to be misbranded, adulterated, and are legally unapproved drugs.[209]

On the Internet, in the magazines, and in gyms, there are also many flashy ads touting *HGH sprays*. Don't waste your money, these are totally bogus! Only God knows what's really in that spray bottle—anabolic steroids or speed? That's even scarier. HGH is a very complex, sensitive molecule; it's not easily replicated. Some of these fraudulent ads even quote references; these won't check out and will be biased or inapplicable to what they're selling. With real HGH, it's often imitated but never duplicated. *Secretagogues* are also big snake oil sellers. These variations of *protein stacks* may help somewhat in children but are useless in adults.[210]

Granted, a lower glycemic meal, as in eating more proteins, may theoretically raise HGH, but it's a much better argument that a high-glycemic meal lowers HGH

---

209 T. Perls, *JAMA* 294 (2005): 2086–90.

210 Growth hormone releasing peptides, i.e., secretagogues, have shown some success in research trials, only. None of these are OTC or available to the public. Hopefully, the development of these could lower costs and ease delivery.

by causing the rise in insulin and cortisol levels. (We presented earlier how the CRAN diet, or calorie restriction, raises HGH levels.) As mentioned in the exercise chapter, simply exercising causes an extra HGH spike. Quality sleep is also a big player. Both of these are fully natural, proven means to boost HGH. You access my Web site (http://www.cenegenics-drrao.com/) and link up to the dangers of fake HGH. Run from any quack that recommends compounded HGH from a non-FDA-approved manufacturer. Better, yet, report them to the State Board of Medicine. Remember, even with FDA-approved HGH, it's the doctor behind the hormones that matters most.

> Don't trust any compounded, prepackaged HGH or the quack doctor that recommended it. Avoid any sprays or secretagogues; they're bogus. It's dangerous and a waste of money.

Another important question I get asked often is, "Once I start HGH, am I obligated to stay on it for the rest of my life?" The answer is not so simple. It really depends on your particular clinical situation, response, and, because of the high cost, your wallet. It's not necessarily true that once you start HGH, you have to continue it indefinitely. Two examples will help illustrate this.

Let's say a middle-aged guy comes in, complaining of being fat with loss in muscle mass, is achy, depressed with poor sleep, has erectile dysfunction, and is on a few drugs for hypertension, cholesterol, mood, sleep and pain pills, even Viagra. This scenario is quite common, actually. Anyway, he's become more serious about his health. He starts the diet and proper exercise we recommended and is receiving appropriate replacements for thyroid, DHEA, pregnenolone, melatonin, T, and HGH. He then proceeds the next few months to shave off fifty pounds of fat, gains muscle mass and strength, now sleeps well, has improved mood, and is now free of pain. He feels as he did twenty years ago and has weaned off all his drugs. His body is much better *in sync* now. Because of the loss in visceral fat, there's less inflammation and metabolic deranges which, in turn, corrected most of his medical conditions. In this case, once he obtained his goals and achieved proper risk reduction, it may be okay to wean off HGH but to continue the other therapies and follow things clinically. Often, we see IGF-1 levels remaining about the same for months, even a year or so. This probably occurs because the body is back in sync, and the synergism of all the improved lifestyle changes. Doing the HGH appreciably helped him obtain his goals and optimal shape, allowing his body to get back on the right path and perform as originally intended. The follow-up clinical picture and lab work will help determine if he needs to go back on HGH.

For the other example, there may be a guy with a more complicated clinical picture. He may have a degenerative disorder as Parkinson's and has mild osteoporosis. Not exercising as he should, he also suffers from fibromyalgia with resulting sarcopenic obesity. Additionally, he may have food allergies that necessitates he avoid various foods such as fish, most vegetables and fruits. He suffers from the clinical syndrome of adult HGH deficiency, and this is verified by lab work. He similarly receives appropriate supplements and hormonal replacements and takes these with his other necessary prescriptions, most of which are metabolized by the liver. His heavy metal burden was then treated. After a few months, he reported he feels 50 percent better, weaned off some medications, and is quite satisfied with his progress. This would probably represent somebody that needs HGH replacement for the rest of his life. Although an attempt to titrate his dose downward and observe for worsening symptoms still may be appropriate after a year or two of treatment.

> Once you start HGH replacement therapy, it's a mutually derived clinical decision as to the ideal dosing and how long you may need to continue treatment.

There are many more studies on the topics presented above. You can easily do a search, now that you're armed with some knowledge about HGH and know how to better interpret research. You can go to my HGH link on my Web site, http://www.cenegenics-drrao.com. Please keep in mind what I presented above. In the May 1, 2006, issue of the *Journal of Clinical Endocrinology in Metabolism*, the Endocrine Society published guidelines for the evaluation and treatment of adult growth hormone deficiency (GHD), which mirrors what I've recommend for years. They added, "GH therapy has been shown to benefit many adults with GHD. Confirmation of GHD before beginning therapy is crucial and usually involves biochemical testing. The demonstrated benefits of GH therapy include improvements in body composition, exercise capacity, skeletal integrity, lipids, and quality of life."

As you can see, it's often difficult to interpret scientific data and then apply this to the clinical setting or the *real* world. In research, we must control as many variables as we can so that we can isolate only one measured effect. For example, to measure *only* the effects of one cholesterol-lowering drug, we need to limit or control all other the variables, like the beneficial effects of improved diet and exercise. In M. Blackman's study in 2002, the treated group wasn't even allowed to exercise! The *real* world is much more complicated. We typically recommend a more realistic approach including diet, exercise, and possibly some supplements to drugs in order to obtain better, safer results. We always recommend such an integrative, comprehensive approach in age-management medicine. The literature and logic should always be able to back up what we're proposing. We're intending to keep *all* of your aging body as when younger—strong with plenty reserve. Ergo, we must include the *prevention* of carcinogenesis, dementia, inflammation, and immune decline for all of this to work safely and be worthwhile.

F. My Personal HGH Story.

To what extent these benefits reduce mortality and whether or not they add *quantity* to life won't be determined for many years. We *do* know that the *quality* of life for those deficient and symptomatic is substantially improved by the use of growth hormone. *Personally*, I began using HGH off and on over the past few years as I suffered from a lack of energy, increase in fat, and loss in what little muscle mass I ever had. I also had high cholesterol and risks for hypertension and early heart disease. Completing the picture of symptomatic HGH deficiency, I also was concerned about my mood. Starting off with DHEA, pregnenolone, and thyroid replacements, I was mostly compliant with the diet I recommend and exercised a balanced program *twice* per week. Initially, I weighed a little over 170 pounds at almost 5 feet 8 inches and had a waist over 33 inches. I still felt I was above par when compared to my middle-aged cohorts. Yet, I wasn't as I felt ten to fifteen years before when I used to jog regularly and had overall better conditioning. I didn't feel right *for me*, if you get my drift. After a few months on this regimen, I felt like my old self again. (You know what I mean.) I was down to between 150 to 155 pounds and had a waist size of about 31 inches. I continued on this similar regimen for about another six months. At that time, I noticed I wasn't gaining any more of the good stuff or losing any more of the bad stuff. Since my only other initial abnormality was a low IGF-1 level of 117, I decided to see if adding HGH would make any difference.

I proceeded to add a relatively small dose of HGH six days per week for about three or four months. At the end of that time, I probably gained a little more muscle mass and experienced some additional losses in visceral and peripheral fat. I felt at the time that adding the HGH didn't do much more than possibly adding another day per week at the gym. So I stopped the HGH and began just that. I did this for another few months and felt quite satisfied, feeling no better or worse than when I was on the low dose HGH.

Then in 2005 came two *bad muthas* back-to-back named Jean and Francis. No, I didn't have any women troubles—these were hurricanes! With all the difficulties they brought, my regimen then got all messed up. Yes, I admit it. I fell off the proverbial health wagon. It took months, but eventually I got back on track doing the diet and exercise and all the hormonal replacements except HGH again. I got back to feeling okay again. Nonetheless, I wondered at this point what adding HGH would do. I was still pathologically low in my lab work according to most endocrinological literature.

So I added 7.35 units of HGH per week. Within the first few weeks, I noted a marked difference. I could lift more weight with more repetitions and could jog faster and longer. I could actually sprint the last few blocks! That high hadn't been felt in about fifteen years! I was skipping and jumping around like a kid. People at the gym noticed I was more defined. Now my waist is less than 30 inches with a six pack, and I weigh 145 pounds. I had some hair growth, although it's still quite thin. Despite being lots thinner, I noticed the skin on my hands was much less wrinkled. The benefits didn't stop here. I began going to art class and painted a portrait of my son for his Christmas present. This and another piece was on display in a local art gallery. I haven't had a piece in an art show since I was twelve and this was my best piece yet! My drum playing reached another level. I'm finishing three books. Sex, well … it takes two, of course. Suffice to say, we're both satisfied as newlyweds. Austin Powers would say, "Yeah, baby!"

Objectively, my blood pressure remains normal, which is remarkable because both my parents have high blood pressure. My cholesterol went from 285 to 205 with lower triglycerides, LDL decreased from 163 to 105, and HDL went from 58 to 85. Of course, I don't attribute all this solely to HGH. As I've always stressed, it's the combination of the diet, exercise, and proper supplements. I take fish oil and niacin too. If anything, I am even less careful about my diet than I used to be, eating ice cream a few times per week and a little rice, cake, and bread. Again, there is no magic potion, yet adding HGH has made a noticeable difference in many important parameters. I got my mojo back!

This basically reflects what I see in my patients as well. It all depends on *your* goals though. Some may be quite happy feeling how I was with the diet and exercise, yet without HGH. They may not want the shots, unknown risks, and expense.

I can thoroughly appreciate this and is precisely why we individualize our treatments to fit the patient, not the other way around. There are no two patients on the same regimen for there are no two patients with the same physiology, deficiencies, or goals. Lastly, they all don't react the same way to the same interventions. It's quite complex to say the least, but this is what makes it challenging, as well as rewarding.

Chapter 13. MAG originally had low normal IGF-1 levels and most the symptoms of low human growth hormone. However, he wanted to raise his HGH levels without shots by first trying all the many other nonmedical modalities we mentioned. Exercise, better sleep, and a diet that normalize insulin and cortisol levels will all help in this regard. He's lowered his alcohol intake to help his liver too. Upon rechecking his IGF-1 level three months into the program, he found it was up by 30 percent, and many of the deficient symptoms are better. His physician and he decide to hold off HGH, as he is doing quite well and in line with his goals.

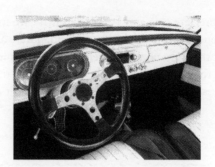

XIV.

Thyroid: The Gas Pedal of the Body

If you optimally age, you'll still eventually die; but think of how great you'll feel and look!

The thyroid, located in the middle of the neck, is indeed quite an amazing gland. *Hypo*thyroidism, or an *underactive* thyroid gland, is probably the most common hormonal deficiencies recognized by modern medicine. Because of such, I find it quite ironic that in many cases it still remains undiagnosed or appropriately treated. As we age past twenty, especially if female, there's an increased risk of getting a thyroid abnormality. The high prevalence of such in women usually results in men being underdiagnosed. If there's a family history of thyroid disorders, Asian ancestry, or autoimmune diseases, the risk is even higher. Ten percent of women and 2 percent of males over sixty have *pathologically* low thyroid functioning.[211] It's even estimated one in five patients over sixty-five years old have a minimally underactive thyroid and doesn't even know it.[212]

---

211 U.S. Department of Health and Human Services, *Put Prevention Into Practice: Clinician's Handbook of Preventive Services.* 2nd ed. (Washington: U.S. Government Printing Office, 1998).

212 S. R. Gambert, "Atypical presentation of thyroid disease in elderly," *Geriatrics* 40 (1985): 63–9; G. S. Meneilly, "Should subclinical hypothyroidism in elderly patients be treated?" *CMAT* 172 (2005): 633.

The thyroid hormone is generally considered *the* major hormone in the body, playing many integral roles throughout the body and throughout one's lifetime. It's like the "gas pedal" to the body's hormonal engine. Well-known, important effects of the thyroid hormone include the following:

1. Regulating other important hormones at important developmental stages, as in working with HGH and prolactin in producing secondary sexual characteristics at puberty.

2. Helping maintain healthy skin, nails, and hair.

3. Maintaining proper mood and energy. Many with undiagnosed hypo-thyroid may be given a psychiatric diagnosis ranging from dysthymia to psychotic depression, or other elusive conditions such as fibromyalgia, chronic fatigue syndrome, and others. If severe, it can even progress to myxedema coma and death.

4. Maintaining proper heart function. An underactive thyroid can cause anywhere from mild edema to acute, severe CHF.

5. Helping regulate body composition including keeping fat mass down (for example, if a patient is really trying but has difficulty losing weight).

6. Keeping optimal immune function. All people with suspected allergic problems, diminished immune function, or repeated infections, should be checked.

7. Maintaining proper bowel function. A hypoactive thyroid causes consti-pation or a "bilious" feeling.

8. Regulating temperature. Hypothyroidism typically causes "cold intoler-ance" or simply "cold hands."

9. Assisting cholesterol metabolism. Hypothyroidism typically causes hypercholesterolemia.

If anything, proper thyroid replacement begs the physician to truly *listen* to the patient expressing the abnormal symptoms above and then secondly, use the *appropriate* lab work as a *guide* to properly *treat* the individual. Wow, just like we were taught in medical school. Can you imagine? The doctor must remember to treat the person first, the lab work second; not the other way around. Believe it or not, this unfortunately represents somewhat of a paradigm shift, in and of itself, in modern medicine where the focus is usually on lab work and expensive, fancy imaging studies such as CT scans and MRIs.

I can't begin to tell you the countless number of overweight, tired, depressed midlife patients I've seen who also suffered from hypertension, glucose intolerance, and high cholesterol. Almost invariably, it will be relayed they've already had multiple normal thyroid tests elsewhere, yet they could've sworn they had an underactive thyroid. Their bodies and conditions were literally screaming, "Replace the thyroid!" You can almost just look at them and get the diagnosis. Again, part of the problem is that most doctors are trained to treat only truly *pathological* diseases. In defense, how *can* we know something we're never taught? Simple, by us listening to the patient—the *best* teacher, as we doctors were taught by our wisest mentors back in medical school. Alas, the majority isn't aware of the nuances needed to adequately diagnose and then optimally treat the individual with these subtle yet varied presentations of hypothyroidism. Most will screen with a blood test called TSH (thyroid stimulating hormone). If this comes back any level but pathological, they assume there isn't any hypothyroidism and thus, the end of the story on that one. To understand this further, we must learn about the thyroid and its hormones.

Basically the hypothalamus and pituitary gland, located in the base of the brain, release TRH (thyrotropin-releasing hormone) and TSH respectively, according to the thyroid hormone levels. This system, as the other hormones' explained earlier, operates in a *feedback loop*. If lower thyroid hormone is detected, more TRH and TSH are released in order to stimulate the thyroid to make more. This is similar to the thermostat in your home that regulates the inside temperature. When it gets warm inside, the thermostat turns on, giving *positive* feedback to the AC to cool the house back to the preset level. It then turns off the unit, giving *negative* feedback, once the desired temperature is reached. That way, *homeostasis* is maintained. See the below diagram.

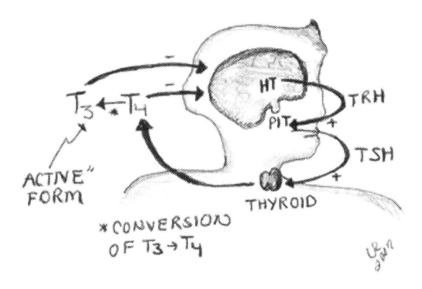

Figure 14.1. Thyroid feedback and the importance of T3. Many factors as age, D1 and D2, diseases, medications, and vitamin deficiencies effect the conversion of T4 (thyroxine) to T3 (triiodothyronine).

As nature would have it, any step along the way is subject to abnormalities. Problems occur when the feedback loop gets sluggishlike, or less responsive, as things generally do with aging. Generally, I consider any TSH above 2.0 mIU/L to suggest an abnormality and be clinically correlated. Secondly, T4 is more of a prohormone and must be converted to the more active T3 form. *It's actually T3 that does most of the work.* Older people, or those on many medications, or ones deficient in zinc or selenium, may not convert T4 to T3 that well. Lastly, a person's thyroid hormone receptors may not be as responsive as they should and require a relatively higher T3 level. Again, treat the patient, not the lab value.

Those patients with suboptimal thyroid function via lab work, yet possess the symptoms of more pathological hypothyroidism are considered *euthyroid* or having *subclinical hypothyroidism.* (You won't even find this listed in the ICD-9 code book that doctors use for insurance and Medicare billing.) There are volumes of research indicating better clinical outcomes when you focus on the patient and individualize T3 and T4 replacement. Studies show improvements in cardiovascular disease, CHF, arrhythmias, and even fibromyalgia and chronic fatigue syndrome.[213] When added to SSRIs (selective serotonin reuptake inhibitors), prob-

213 The latter was presented in *Rheumatology* (1998): 57.

ably the most common class of antidepressants used today, T3 improved depression in patients with posttraumatic stress disorder.[214]

Proper replacement of the thyroid *does not* cause osteoporosis or any of the other symptoms of *hyper*thyroidism, basically an *overactive* thyroid, producing *excessive* amounts of thyroid hormone. Symptoms include tremor, insomnia, nervousness, excess sweating, palpitations, and similar hyperactive-like symptoms. If you experience these while on thyroid replacement, call your doctor for advice and get your levels checked. Remember to take thyroid replacements in the morning on an empty stomach, as many drugs and food interfere with its absorption.

Most forms of T4 come as Synthroid or various generic names as levothyroxine. T3 comes in the name of Cytomel. There are combination pills containing various percentages of T3 and T4, called Armour thyroid (derived from pig thyroids) or synthetic Thyrolar.[215] There are others; these are just the ones I am most familiar with and usually prescribe. Which one, or which combination, I use depends on the clinical situation; it's highly individualized. Additionally, regular follow-up comprising of feedback from the patient and its correlation with repeat lab work is crucial to obtaining optimal thyroid replacement.

In summary, proper individualized thyroid testing and replacement is critical to one's optimal health. It's still only one facet to a very complex equation for health, energy, and weight—there is, again, no one magic pill. Rather, it's the *holistic* approach as explained in this book. Unfortunately, fine-tuning thyroid functioning usually demands a patient insisting there is something wrong and then finding a doctor willing to spend the time, listen, and then obtain the best remedy. Don't give up! This does take a little more work by the well-experienced physician, but I find it highly rewarding to see so many of the above abnormalities easily improve with one small pill. For some, it's enough to get the ball rolling in the right direction.

---

214 This according to the *Journal of Clinical Psychiatry* March 2001: 62 (3).
215 T4—Synthroid, generics. 25 mcg on up. T-3—Cytomel 5 mcg, 25 mcg on up. T-3/T-4 combinations: Armour (pig) 15 mg, 30 mg, 60 mg (1 grain)= 38 mcg T4 and 9 mcg T3. Thyrolar (synthetic) 1 Grain= 50 mcg T4 and 12.5 mcg T3.

Chapter 14. Despite being told by his prior doctor his thyroid was fine, it really wasn't. His TSH was above 2.0 mIU/L. MAG always thought his thyroid was underactive. He found it really hard to lose sufficient weight despite being aggressive with diet and exercise. Plus, he was embarrassed to shake hands with his cold palms; and he had dry skin and dandruff. Once six weeks on a combination of T3 and T4, he felt all warm and fuzzy inside. He concluded this was the best money he ever spent.

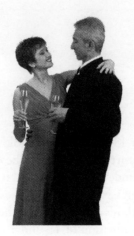

XV.

The Heart and Brain in MidLife

A. The Midlife Heart

Heart disease is the number one man killer. This can be delayed or improved with proper lifestyle modification.

Now we come to the so-called *heart of the matter*. Since the dawn of man—and woman, the heart has certainly enjoyed being the focus of attention, in both a physical and emotional sense. Likewise, it's good to have a *totally healthy* heart in midlife. After having great health, I believe having fulfilling relationships—marriage or being close with family and friends—comes a very close second. As you heard many times before, "Money can't buy you happiness." Certainly money helps—no one can deny that. But happiness usually comes from *trying* to obtain inner peace and *developing* loving relationships. I've stressed many times before that you have to regularly invest in your health in order to obtain your optimal shape. The same can be said for a marriage and our relationships. You must also take time out to make those closest to you feel special. This doesn't demand much time or money—a simple phone call or heartfelt note will do. According to behavioral theorists, when you behave in a more loving way, you will feel more loved and become a more loving person. As you act, you do so become. Simply, choose to react with love. Less anger puts you at less risk of heart disease—both physically and emotionally.

How one cares for one's heart is analogous to the above. Although integral, we tend to take it for granted, yet it keeps up dutifully beating. For even decades, we may just keep overindulging in not-so-healthy habits. Usually, we don't pay much mind to it, until something goes awry. Your heart skips a few beats or you may get chest pain and have to go to the ER. It's similar to when you're away from your wife or kids. You sort of take them for granted too—until you're separated for a weekend. Anyway, with this small digression of an introduction, I hope to have illuminated what's really important in life and likewise demands attention. Midlife is a great time to evaluate and reenergize things. Without further adieu, as they say, more tidbits on obtaining and maintaining a healthy heart throughout your life span follows.

A lot of this has been covered in earlier chapters, but I will add some caveats and tidbits about cardiovascular health during our midlife. In the chapters on diet, exercise, and hormones, we covered a lot about disease risks and the pro-active things that you can do to reduce sickness and death from heart disease. Remember, it's how *well* you are during midlife that mostly determines how well you do in your older age. Let's make the golden years truly golden!

Not only does having an increased body mass index (BMI) correlate strongly with diabetes, this increases your cardiovascular disease risks too. That should come as no surprise to well-learned doctors, as well as laypersons. According to a thirty-two-year study published in the January 11, 2006, issue of *JAMA*, healthy middle-aged persons who are overweight are at higher risks of hospitalization and mortality later in life when compared to their peers of normal weight, regardless of other risk factors. Along the same lines, it showed that older people having a normal BMI in young adulthood and midlife provided health benefits at all levels of conventional risk factors. This reinforces two points I made earlier. One is that midlife health determines how well you do in the later years. Two, that today's unhealthy kids have a bad head start in life. That's the skinny on these matters.

Another long-term study done in Finland studied over three thousand healthy Caucasian males for thirty-nine years. They found that having lower cholesterol levels at middle age predicted lower total mortality and better physical quality of life in older age. Postponed physical disability was also noted. This parallels many other studies such as the MRFIT (Multiple Risk Factor Intervention Trial) study.

This further supports my push for a proactive approach during this window of opportunity, including aggressively lowering cholesterol levels and blood pressure. However, I recommend first maximizing nonmedical approaches because of their many other far-reaching benefits. Besides the side effects and cautions to be used with statin drug therapies, reports published in *JAMA* revealed these drugs had no effect on lowering risks of developing or dying from any form of cancers. As presented earlier, cancers are the biggest killer of people aged less than eighty-five years. A healthy lifestyle, as presented many times earlier, *does* help prevent cancer *and* cardiovascular disease further down the road. Mother Nature knows best!

As a partial review, I remind you that it is not just the LDL (bad) cholesterol that we are concerned about, it's also the HDL and triglyceride levels—the good and ugly types respectively. These are all independent risk factors. It's important to note that most statin drugs have minimal effect on improving HDL and triglyceride levels. In the VA-HIT (Veterans Affairs High-Density Lipoprotein Intervention Trial) involving over 250 patients, a minimal 6 percent increase in HDL resulted in a 34 percent decrease of cardiovascular-related disease and deaths. Additionally, a Norwegian study looked at about two thousand men and women with preexisting carotid atherosclerosis for over seven years and found HDL was independently and inversely related to plaque growth. Therefore, a higher HDL means having less carotid artery plaque and less risk for stroke.[216] The regressed lesions and patients with higher HDL were more fibrotic (more scarred down and healed) and contained less macrophages and foam cells (less inflamed and likely to rupture). We were taught in medical school that basically HDL particles scavenge the LDL particles and bring them back to the liver to be metabolized, thereby lowering LDL levels. This research reinforces that HDL probably reduces this plaque growth by decreasing inflammation and lipid component, resulting in a more stable plaque.

Recently, there has been more research and subsequent understanding about how these inflamed, fibrofatty plaques progress. Granted, the *inflamed* plaque is more unstable and likely to rupture, causing a *thrombus,* which leads to a locally blocked vessel; or it can embolize, traveling further down and ultimately leading to a more distant blockage. If this occurs in a coronary vessel, it leads to heart attack; if in a carotid artery, it leads to a brain attack, or stroke. The pathology is the same, regardless. Because the role a particular white blood cell, the macrophage, has in this entire inflammatory milieu, it has been theorized that infectious components may also be involved. Cytomegalovirus particles have been isolated

---

216 S. Johnsen et al., "Elevated HDL cholesterol and carotid atherosclerosis," *Cardiology Review* 23, no. 5 (2006): 20–24.

in these plaques and proven to increase risk for strokes. Even *Helicobacter pylori*, the bacteria causing many stomach ulcers, have been identified. Some chlamydial bacterial forms have been isolated too. However, trials studying some antibiotics as azithromycin for the possible prevention of coronary disease have not exhibited any appreciable benefit. On the other hand, a Canadian study that reviewed over thirty thousand health records of hypertensives from 1982 to 1995 found that current penicillin use was associated with a 50 percent decrease in risk for stroke. To date, I find no convergence of evidence to suggest taking an antibiotic helps prevent stroke or heart attack in the so-called normal individual. I do strongly recommend antibiotic prophylaxis for those clinically indicated who are undergoing a procedure. Along these same lines, a healthy mouth including teeth and gums free of infection and inflammation is paramount to having a healthy body.

As presented earlier, there aren't many drugs that lower triglycerides and raise HDL levels. Of course, diet and exercise are the best ways. Fish oil, with its anti-inflammatory effect, and niacin probably help the most. (Please see these topics in the supplements and the diet chapter, especially the information on "good versus bad" fats.) Interestingly enough, a study published back in October 2003, studied Ashkenazi Jews aged over ninety-eight and found they more frequently possessed a genetic mutation that caused their HDL and LDL cholesterol particles to be larger than normal. They also exhibited higher HDL levels. Theoretically, this would offer some protective effect by limiting the penetration of these lipid particles into the vessel wall and causing less plaque formation. Researchers suggested that such a gene that determines cholesterol molecule size may also promote longevity by protecting people from cardiovascular disease, diabetes, and other age-related diseases. Recently Pfizer had to pull their investigational drug that was supposed to raise HDL levels. There were too many bad side effects noted.

Medical therapy may be additionally warranted to achieve the desired risk reduction. These may include metformin, Lopid, Zetia, and others. Basically, you want your fasting total cholesterol to be under 200 mg/dl, with an LDL under 70, an HDL above 50, and triglycerides under 75. The cholesterol/HDL ratio should be under 3.5. These drugs can have severe side effects and need routine monitoring, so talk to your doctor. If at increase risk of heart attack, i.e., a male over fifty, you may one to add taking a daily baby aspirin. Of course, per my and the American Heart Association's recommendation since 2004, you should be on a gram of fish oil per day. As stated before, this can decrease your risk of sudden cardiac death by up to 45 percent. That effect beats any drug out there, with basically no side effects or need for routine monitoring. As mentioned, fish also helps mood, so that you also can have a happier, healthier heart.

According to recommendations by the National Screening for Heart Attack Prevention and Education Program (SHAPE), every one over age thirty-five should know their long-term risk of having a heart attack. This is usually obtained by an assessment of traditional risk factors such as high cholesterol, using the Framingham Risk Score, as well as testing CRP-hs—a specific marker of vessel inflammation. Additionally, noninvasive imaging should be done in those considered high risk. This would include undergoing a heart scan for imaging coronary vessels or calcium scoring. If these were positive, then the person should undergo intravascular ultrasound to identify vulnerable coronary arteries. The Association for Eradication of Heart Attacks believes the aforementioned routine heart attack screening protocol could prevent hundreds of thousands of heart attacks each year. I agree with this emphasis on screening because a large number of "healthy" people unexpectedly suffer heart attacks each year yet have relatively good cholesterol levels based on the guidelines set by the National Cholesterol Education Program (NCEP).

As I stressed many times before, low LDL levels are only *one* parameter of a healthy cardiovascular system. Inflammation, as measured by CRP-hs, has long been known to a be a better independent risk factor for heart attack, yet is not included under the current NCEP guidelines. Focusing on all known risk markers with proper screening, as well as identifying risk factors, would help identify and prevent these additional unsuspecting, yet vulnerable individuals. The president of AHEA, Dr. Naghavi, stated in a March 2004 article that such aggressive screening for heart attacks in high-risk subjects is absolutely necessary because in more than 50 percent of coronary heart disease cases, the first symptom is sudden death. If you get *this* symptom, as the Cornelius Brothers sang back in the '60s, it's truly "too late to turn back now."

Based on the overwhelming research, I wholeheartedly agree and have been measuring CRP-hs as well as recommending calcium scoring and ultrasound imaging for coronary vessels for many years now in patients at unknown or more-than-moderate to high risk. I shoot for a CRP under 2.0[217] Even the American Heart Association and the Centers for Disease Control and Prevention recommend

---

217 Dr. Paul Ridker suggested in *Circulation* 109 (2004): 1955. In *NEJM* 336 (1997): 973 and 342 (2000): 836. Ridker also exposed how subjects with a *high* CRP and *low* LDL levels may have overall survival then those with *low* CRP and *high* LDL levels. *NEJM* 347 (2002): 1557.

measuring CRP in adults *without* known coronary disease. Inflammation indeed plays a big role and I typically compare CRP-hs with the cholesterol/HDL ratio to arrive at an individual's cardiac risk. High CRP is also associated with increased risk for developing stroke, metabolic syndrome, diabetes, and hypertension. I have never seen a diabetic patient that didn't correspondingly possess a high CRP level. Yet, in another reflection of the current health-care system being upside-down, most insurance plans, including Medicare and Medicaid, don't reimburse for checking a CRP-hs unless there is a diagnosis of *established* coronary artery disease. So according to them, we have to wait until you first *get* heart disease to find out your risks, as opposed to checking your risks and trying to *prevent* the number 1 biggest killer! Quite *reactive* as opposed to *proactive* prevention, I would say. Yet, that's where we are today—smart enough to know *what* to check for, but too dumb to use it.

We additionally may check homocysteine, uric acid levels, vitamin D, and clotting factors such as fibrinogen, or various lipoprotein particles (lipoprotein-a or apoprotein-b), depending on the clinical picture. CRP-hs is a simple blood test that probably costs less than fifty bucks and calcium scoring of the coronary vessels, about $350. Both are quick and noninvasive. These costs are quite miniscule compared with the costs of an early, preventable heart attack or stroke. Factors that can contribute to the toxic blood syndrome, according to an esteemed colleague and cardiologist, Dr. Stephen Sinatra, are homocysteine, CRP-hs, fibrinogen (a clotting factor), oxidized LDL, lipoprotein (a), and ferritin. His favorite herbs for keeping the young at heart follows what we also preach:

1. Garlic
2. Onions
3. Hawthorn
4. Ginkgo biloba
5. Green tea
6. Guggulipid
7. Phytosterols
8. Flax lignans (sesame seeds)
9. Soy isoflavones
10. Grapeseed (What? ... No CoQ_{10} or fish oil?)

Of course, proper diet and exercise also helps lower your risk for diabetes and hypertension during midlife and then the myriad of subsequent complications during older age. Hypertension is nicknamed the *silent killer*, and if you are genetically predisposed, you will probably get it sometime during your life depending on how proactive you are. If you're like me, having *both* parents with hypertension and high cholesterol, you're at even more risk. Yet, at almost fifty and on no prescription drugs, I have great blood pressure and cholesterol levels. Additionally, as hammered many times, adult-onset diabetes is on the rise and is about the worst disease you can get yet ironically almost totally preventable, in my view. I succinctly defined diabetes as *premature aging of the body*. Instead of getting all these serious diseases at seventy, you start to get them in your forties.

In the introduction we reviewed how, with the proper lifestyle, your good genes are expressed and the bad ones repressed. So be a healthy geneticist—no stem cells needed here! Even more so than hypertension, unknown but advancing complications of diabetes are usually well underway before the clinical diagnosis is made in the doctor's office. Today, you have to get an *F* first or "fall off a cliff" for today's health-care system to recognize what's wrong. This underscores the importance of early prevention, or at least, early diagnosis and successful, aggressive treatment options. *You* have to take the initiative and be responsible for yourself. According to *Diabetes Care* 26 (2003), younger adults aged eighteen to forty-four newly diagnosed with type 2 diabetes were much more likely to require insulin therapy, were at a greater risk of kidney failure, and had a marked increased risk of myocardial infarction and stroke compared to new diabetics aged forty-five or older. Such young diabetics had a shocking thirtyfold higher risk of cerebrovascular disease and a fourteenfold increase risk of myocardial infarction. Studying almost eight thousand patients, the author suggests that early-onset adult diabetes appears to be a more aggressive disease than usual-onset types. This is quite unfortunate because common sense would've placed the younger diabetics at increased protection based solely on their youth. I guess, unlike the older diabetics, they had a less-healthy head start. This research further emphasizes the importance of proactively avoiding diabetes or becoming overweight in midlife.

Blood pressure should run under 120/80 mmHg and resting heart rates 85 per minute or below. For proven optimal risk reduction, we recommend a *fasting blood sugar* in a nondiabetic individual of 86 mg/dl or less, and a *hemoglobin A1c* under 4.6 percent. A *fasting insulin* level under 10 is desirable. This effectively lowers the amount of *glycosylation* and subsequent production of advanced glycation end products presented earlier. Although these are our age-management *opti-*

mal guidelines, much current research also recommends lowering the threshold for diagnosing and subsequent treatment of diabetes.[218]

As far as the supplements that help the heart is concerned, please review the supplements section and the references given there. Again, there is no one magic herb; and any supplement will have a minor effect, if any, at most. Diet, exercise, and proper hormonal balance overwhelmingly play the major roles. However, for completeness sake, I will mention that probably fish oil, coenzyme Q_{10}, melatonin, and a few others may have some blood pressure lowering effects. Cholesterol fractions, as presented elsewhere, may be helped by the oil of fish and niacin, but less so by the other omega-3 fatty acids, green tea, garlic, soy, and by some others too numerous to mention. I promote the mainstay of a healthy lifestyle foremost, obtaining most of the antioxidants and vitamins naturally from fresh vegetables, fruits, herbs, and spices. Further information can be found at the http://www.familydoctor.org, the Web site for information from the trusted American Academy of Family Physicians. Stick with America's Heartland!

B. Brains

Because the mind is a terrible thing to waste.

—NAACP

Let's go back to the example I gave earlier of the young *whippersnapper* being asked to imitate an *old geezer*. Of course, the young actor would stoop over, becoming a quite frail and shaky unfortunate soul having trouble hearing, seeing, and remembering recent events. Such is the look of *normal* aging. You may add to that a wheelchair, trouble with bowel and bladder control, or worse yet, being stuck in a nursing home fully dependent on others and merely existing with end-stage dementia, CHF, osteoporosis, and more. It is estimated 70 percent of those living over a hundred will have Alzheimer's disease. The modern health-care system has developed many innovations that improve mostly quantity as opposed to the

---

218 According to Osei et al. in the *Journal of Clinical Endocrinology and Metabolism* (2003): 88, higher-risk siblings of African American diabetics possessing A1c levels 5.7 to 6.4 percent, although still within the *normal* range, should be considered as having metabolic syndrome and undergo preventative treatment. Other studies, as the one by Lorenzo in *Diabetes Care* (2003): 26 suggest lowering the cutoff to a *fasting glucose* of 97 mg/dl when diagnosing diabetes.

quality of life. These have allowed people to live longer than before; however, further age-related decline has become a lot more complex than we ever imagined.

Do we really know where we are going with all this? The current system is a reactive one, treating the later, more severe outcomes as opposed to being more proactive in treating the root causes of aging. This has led to increased costs as well and will certainly break the system. Most elderly patients desire to be as independent as possible and not to become a burden to others. They additionally wish to have some quality of life—to be pain free. What they fear most is getting dementia, or losing their mind. We all must eventually face this challenge headfirst! Similar to the argument I gave for preventing carcinogenesis before progressing to cancer; let's find ways to *prevent* dementia instead of trying to delay it some once it starts. Things don't merely happen. We just aren't doing a good job today of picking up abnormalities early and preventing these from worsening. Instead of succumbing to the disabilities of *normal* aging, let's opt for *optimal* aging. The brain should be no different.

It's essentially an organ of the body, though it is by far the most complex. The mind is only as healthy as the body, and vice versa. This is referred to as the *mind-body connection*. Anything that would make the body more disposed to inflammation and degeneration would likewise negatively influence the brain and its many functions. Glycosylation makes the neurons more apt to degenerate and malfunction. Pro-inflammatory fats would only add to this monstrous milieu. Lastly, toxins and heavy metal exposure pollute the pondering pons. All the things we have spoken about, the proper diet, exercise, fluid intake, proper rest, and so on have been shown to help maintain one's cognitive ability into later life. Additionally, proper hormonal replacement has been shown to improve the mind as well as the body. Having DHEA, pregnenolone, testosterone, thyroid, HGH, (estrogen and progesterone for women) at optimal levels have overwhelmingly been proven to improve many mind and mood qualities. A lot of this had been reviewed in the previous chapters. Although this makes perfect sense, I will present and review some additional supporting literature below.

When talking to midlifers, mood disorders and memory concerns frequently come up; so I will focus on these. An article in the September 15, 2004, issue of *Family Practice News* entitled "Healthy Lifestyle Benefits Patients Brains, Too" supports much of the above. Basically, eat more veggies. Eat less saturated fat. Turn off the TV. Keep your brain, body, and social life active. Those following this advice exhibited half the relative risk for dementia. Don't become a *vidiot*! Hey, that's deja vu. Isn't this what your parents preached? Think of all the memory storage you used up for those reruns of *I Love Lucy, Gilligan's Island, Bugs Bunny, Road Runner, Pink Panther*, etc.

Researchers using data from almost nine thousand members aged forty to forty-five years from the Kaiser Permanente health plan have found that fatter people, as measured by skin-fold thickness, were almost four times more likely to develop Alzheimer's disease. This was reinforced by previous research presented in the March 2003 *Archives of Internal Medicine.* Here, overweight and obesity in *middle age* as measured by BMI, increased the risk of dementia and Alzheimer's disease.[219] Besides animal studies showing that long-term low-calorie diets extends life span, a study reported in the *Proceedings of the National Academy of Sciences* suggested such could also lessen the effects of Parkinson's disease. Increased dietary intake of fruits and vegetables has been known to lower risk of ischemic stroke. Investigators from the Physician's Health Study looked at over twenty-two thousand healthy male physicians beginning in 1982 and followed them for about thirteen years. Docs having higher antioxidant levels were at a 40 percent lower risk of developing such brain attacks. Of the antioxidants studied, carotenoids had the biggest role in prevention. That's food for thought.

As presented earlier, as we age, inflammation goes up and immune function goes down. Additionally, risks for depression and dementia increase as well as the usual increasing onslaught of debilitating diseases. Some evidence pointing to the association between inflammation and depression was revealed in the *New England Journal of Medicine* (2001).[220] Therefore, besides the negative way that inflammation plays in cardiovascular disease, diabetes, metabolic syndrome, and cancer, it also plays a role in depression. Indeed, inflammatory mediators are mostly produced by glial and microglial cells (the fatty insulation layer), but neurons themselves can also produce these sinister cytokines. These cause anhedonia (the hallmark of depression), fatigue, cognitive dysfunction, and other flu-like symp-

---

219 R. Whitmer, *BMJ* 330 (2005): 1360. Others Too, *Arch Intern Med* 163 (2003):1524–8.

220 Dr. Miller and associates, *New England Journal of Medicine* 344 (2001): 961–6. Depressed patients are noted to have elevated inflammatory mediators as interleukin-6 and CRP in accord with the severity of their illness and that stress or depression affects the hypothalamic pituitary adrenal axis, a.k.a. the neuroendocrine system we've spoken so much about.

toms in sick patients. Even the administration of these cytokines, as in interferon, induced depressive symptoms in human and animal studies.[221]

On the improvement side of things, I have often found anti-inflammatory treatments such as fish oil and SAM-E as well as most medications to help mild depression, but with no side effects. (The research on this was presented in the supplements chapter.) For mild, uncomplicated depression, I also may suggest a trial of pharmaceutical-grade St. John's wort or lithium orotate, if appropriate. For treatment or prevention of dementia, there is some evidence phosphatidylcholine, phosphatidylserine, alpha lipoic acid, and ginkgo biloba may offer benefit.[222] I take these in a brain support formula every day. St. John's wort and ginkgo are *not* without some side effects and can have serious herb-drug interactions, especially with blood thinners. Further information may be found from the Web site http://www.nim.nih.gov.

Alzheimer's and lapses in episodic memory were twice as common in those who experience negative emotions such as depression and anxiety. According to December 2003 *Neurology*, chronic stress had previously been associated with changes in the hippocampal area of the brain that's seen with learning and memory problems. Dutch and Japanese researchers have previously found that stress hormones and the associated impaired function of naturally occurring protective proteins both appear to play a role in susceptibility to Alzheimer's. It makes perfect sense to find ways to healthfully deal with acute and chronic stress. We reviewed this in the hormonal chapter concerning insulin, DHEA, and cortisol. As mentioned, I find most people desire both inner peace and avoidance of any form of dementia in their older years. Why wait until then? Additionally, avoiding toxins and getting the proper rest are important aspects that are commonly overlooked.

There are numerous studies that overwhelmingly suggest proper TRT in men and women improves many mind and mood abnormalities. Noted brain researcher Dr. Patrick Braverman suggests that low levels of HGH were associated with Alzheimer's-based memory loss in fifteen hundred patients, and may provide evidence for early detection of the disease possibly twenty years before the onset of traditional symptoms. This could result in more effective diagnosis and treatment options. Alzheimer's is a tremendously humiliating and debilitating disease,

---

221 One of the best-known cytokine drug used to treat hepatitis C and malignant melanoma, Interferon-, can cause depression in up to 60 percent of treated patients according to *Neuropsychopharmacology* (2002): 26.

222 M. Katzman, "Herbs for mental illness: effectiveness and interaction with conventional medications," *Journal of Family Physicians* 54, no. 9 (2005): 789–99.

which will only exponentially increase in incidence given our aging population. Currently, up to half of people eighty-five years or older have appreciable dementia; and current costs run at about $100 billion per year for the estimated 4.5 million Americans affected. Most believe that about 70 percent of people who live to be a hundred will develop AD, and more than 13 million will be afflicted by the year 2050. Unfortunately, there is no current cure. As presented in *Lancet* (June 26, 2004), most treatments, including cholinesterase inhibitors, are not cost-effective and produce at most minimally relevant improvement. *JAMA* (2003): 289 presented a meta-analysis of twenty-nine trials involving almost eleven thousand patients and basically came to the same conclusion. AD is quite horrific. I recommend prevention as its best cure.

Statin drugs, which lower cholesterol and some inflammation, may theoretically help in dementia prevention. Amazingly, the human brain contains a little more than 20 percent of the body's total cholesterol, although it accounts for less than 2 percent of body mass. Basically, the brain is two-thirds fat, while the circulating blood contains usually only 5 percent fat. Most of this cholesterol is wrapped up in the myelin sheath, the fatty insulation protecting the wirelike nerve cell within. Researchers at the University of California in Los Angeles used MRI to show that myelin degeneration progressed more rapidly and was greater throughout the brains of Alzheimer's patients compared to healthy older adults. Genetically, apo-E lipoprotein mutations may account for the improper release of free radicals that cause the production of the fibrillary tangles and amyloid plaques that typify Alzheimer's. Other research suggests low-dose Advil, a common OTC anti-inflammatory, may also help. There is somewhat conflicting data concerning the benefits of vitamins E and C. These include unknown effective dosing, the safety of higher dosing of E, and the comparison of dietary versus supplemental forms.

One of the best ways to prevent dementia is to prevent getting any degree of hypertension, cardiovascular disease, peripheral vascular disease or diabetes. There are simply too numerous studies to mention backing this up. One of the most common forms of dementia, *small vessel dementia*, is produced when the brain suffers one or a few ministrokes that, depending on which area was affected, may produce insidious, variable cognitive and neurological losses. Anything to help prevent the vessel disease that results from these comorbidities would accordingly prevent these ministrokes and the additional "hits" to the vulnerable aging brain. Recent studies show diabetics are twice as likely to develop AD. Pathologically, both share the deposition of destructive amyloid protein deposits in the affected organ. Given the increase in our aging population, together with the obesity epidemic, personal and social costs will only skyrocket.

Let's get back to some practical knowledge to help you have a healthier mind. Anybody with mental or of mood concerns should undergo a comprehensive history and physical examination including appropriate lab work. As presented earlier, age-related midlife hormonal changes, including lower DHEA, thyroid, and testosterone, cause many cognitive and emotional complaints. In the hormonal chapters, we reviewed how replacing these resulted in improvement. Abnormal cortisol diurnal levels, as presented earlier, can be a player as well. Additionally, B_{12} and folate levels should be checked; this was presented in the supplement chapter. Heavy metal toxicities including lead and mercury should be investigated and treated if positive. Additive toxicities and side effects from medications, both OTC and prescription, should be identified and limited as appropriate. The usual suspects are the anticholinergic or antihistaminergic ones. Rarely, but if clinically warranted, a workup for autoimmune diseases such as multiple sclerosis, or sexually transmitted diseases such as syphilis or HIV, may be necessary. Brain imaging such as MRI or PET/CT may help rule in or rule out a diagnosis. Also infrequent, but nonetheless still a possibility, various types of narcolepsy or even seizures may be considered. Lastly, mood disorders and sleep disturbances can imitate many of the symptoms of dementia or mild cognitive impairment.

Psychiatric evaluation or sleep studies may be necessary to arrive at a definitive diagnosis and appropriate treatment. Sleep disturbances have been known to commonly precede new-onset mood disorders. Two patients I saw last month with complaints of fatigue and memory lapses had previously been seen by many specialists but were offered no real help. Investigation and the initial treatment with my integrative techniques only helped somewhat. Still, we weren't satisfied. However, further conversation revealed possible sleep disturbances that were then confirmed by a positive sleep study indicating sleep apnea. Appropriate CPAP (continuous positive airway pressure) treatment for these two resulted in a marked improvement in their mental, emotional, and cognitive daytime abilities. Excessive sleepiness, a rather new diagnostic term, may be helped by Provigil©, typical ADHD drugs, or some serotonergic antidepressants that raise norepinephrine levels. As you can deduce, the investigation and treatment for mind disorders are vast, and demands an appreciable amount of patience and communication on both the physician and the patient's part.

Reviewing most of the research, I come to the conclusion that there are multiple roads that lead to the various pathologies and resulting presentations of the aging, diseased brain. There are probably some genetic predispositions; but granted, most risk factors mentioned above are almost totally preventable or at least readily treatable if caught early. These would include hypertension, hypercholesterolemia, metabolic disorders, and such mentioned above. Inflammation, hormonal imbalances especially insulin dysregulation, and abnormal oxidative pathways complete the picture. For now, prevention offers the best cure. Also, remember, "If you don't you use it; you'll lose it." Much research reinforces that having a healthy mental attitude along with lifelong cognitive challenges promote a healthier brain.

Lastly, the resulting frailty of older age and its related diseases closely imitates the results from having a physically and emotionally sedentary lifestyle. Most of the elderly that suffer from these many debilitating chronic illnesses actually succumb to the complications of the related immobility more so than the actual diseases themselves. Examples include hip fracture, falls and related trauma, urinary tract infections or sepsis resulting from bedsores, the many pulmonary complications including DVT, pulmonary embolism or pneumonia, and many more. Although there may not be a cure for chronic disease, there are always methods to help prevent frailty and its deleterious consequences. Physical therapy, along with proper anabolic hormonal replacement, including HGH and/or testosterone, has proven beneficial in many of these instances. Proper nutritional guidelines should be followed.

In the future, hopefully a vaccination or more effective drugs will become available for AD. Recently, a DNA-based vaccine used in rats showed promise by reducing plaque deposition. If successful in monkeys, testing on people could begin within a few years. As far as investigational drugs are concerned, one called Flurizan works by decreasing beta-amyloid buildup in the brain. During phase 2 trials, it has been more helpful for those in the early stages of Alzheimer's.

In closing, addressing the progressive physiological and cognitive decline of *normal aging* has become much more complicated because of the current health-care system, the polluted environment, and the sedentary lifestyle of today's society. At best, quantity, but not always quality, of life has been improved. A better focus on *optimal* or *successful aging* would result in an improved *health span*. Proactively preventing age-related decline is much better than reactively treating the many complications of aging. There is an integral mind-body connection here as well. Midlife offers such a *window of opportunity*, and I've certainly presented the means to help achieve this paradigm shift. Realistically, we all must eventually die; however, the goal should be to live a longer yet healthier and more productive life until the very end. Such a goal, called *morbidity compression,* was introduced early in the book and is what I wholeheartedly support. Optimal health is our greatest asset.

```
CAUTION!!
MID-LIFE AHEAD!

CAN BE ROCKY

LAST CHANCE TO
GET HEALTHY!!!
```

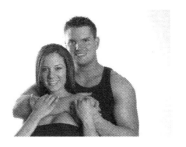

XVI.

Special Topics

Here I will introduce various topics pertinent to midlife men. Some of these were introduced in earlier chapters because of the important roles diet, exercise, inflammation, hormonal replacements, various supplements, and toxins play in the following. Resources will be given for additional information.

A. The Prostate Gland. Originally about the size of a walnut, the prostate's basic job is to add nourishment and some lubricating fluid to the ejaculate. It wraps around the urethra like a small doughnut between the bladder and the penis. Similar to the hormonal changes presented earlier, as we age, the things you wish would get smaller, get bigger; and the things you wish would get bigger, get smaller.

Benign prostatic hypertrophy (BPH) is the term used to describe how our prostates enlarge as we age; it's a fact of life. The amount of BPH varies though. This is a different ball game altogether than *prostate cancer.* The amount of enlargement doesn't predict any risks for cancer, such that an enlarged prostate doesn't increase your risk of prostate cancer. BPH symptoms can start to show up in midlife. Basically, the enlarging doughnut starts squeezing the urethra and slows urine flow.

As would be expected, these are the symptoms:

- decreased urine stream (can't pee over the hood of a car anymore)
- urgency (feeling you have to go urinate again after just going)
- hesitancy (yet having to wait a while to initiate a urine stream)
- dribbling (losing urine after finished)
- pressure or bloating in the pelvic area

By the very nature, BPH is *benign* in its causes; usually it's caused by age. But this is a *diagnosis of exclusion*, meaning when there is any change in your urine, you need to get checked out by a doctor as soon as reasonably possible. Serious causes such as a urinary tract infection, sexually transmitted disease, various stones, inflammation, polyps, and more may be considered depending on the situation.

Commonly in the healthy middle-aged guy, it winds up being *prostatitis*—inflammation and infection in the prostate gland. You still need to get properly checked. Depending on the severity and what's abnormal, you may be prescribed some antibiotics and a drug to help your flow in the meantime. Another frequent cause for these symptoms is medication. OTC or prescribed ones with *anticholinergic* effects may cause dry mouth, constipation, and urinary trouble. Examples would be decongestants and antihistamines, and all common cold and allergy remedies. Ask your pharmacist or doctor about taking any new drug, even OTC ones.

For BPH treatment, there are the *5-alpha reductase inhibitor* class of medications such as Proscar and Avodart we spoke about in the chapter on TRT's side effects. There may be the need for surgical options, as the TURP procedure. The *transurethral resection of the prostate* is basically a Roto-Rooter-like job done under anesthesia. Nowadays, there are laser-assisted surgical options that can be done right in the urologist's office!

In the way of supplements, I must stress a healthy lifestyle, which includes natural sources for vitamins E and C, and drinking a lot of filtered water help out. Eating tomatoes that are naturally rich in lycopene helps. Other supplements such as saw palmetto, nettles leaf, pygeum bark, and pine bark extracts may help too. The lack of unknown quality available and amounts needed of these to do any good go against my unconditionally recommending them. Nonetheless, I find the pharmaceutical grade of these to clinically help the majority of my patients with mild symptoms of diagnosed BPH. I personally don't have signs of BPH, yet I take these daily for prostate health. First, you need the accurate diagnosis to know what's best for you and your prostate. Supplements mostly help *prevent* a disease. They are no substitution for correct medical treatment.

Prostate cancer, the commonest cancer in men, was mostly covered in the TRT chapter, under side effects. Although this book can't be expected to address prostate cancer in detail, it will cover the appropriate screening exams and tests that should be performed. An ounce of prevention is worth a pound of cure, right? As mentioned, it's actually men with *low* testosterone and higher estrogens that constitute the increased-risk population. According to the vast majority of research, TRT doesn't raise PSA or worsen BPH symptoms. Exposure to pesticides and a family history do add to the risk. A healthy lifestyle will help prevent prostate cancer, as reflected by Dr. Dean Ornish's research that showed an anti-inflammatory type diet helps prevent and treat prostate cancer. This was reviewed in the diet-related chapters. At the very least, if you do get a cancer when you get older, you better be in shape to fight it.

Under normal circumstances, an annual screening for prostate cancer should start at age fifty and should include a digital rectal exam (DRE) *and* a prostate specific antigen (PSA) blood test. You need both. If there is a family history, symptoms, or if you're of African American descent, you better start this regimen at age forty. There may be additional tests or imaging studies, as deemed necessary. If on TRT, you have to get the exam and blood work more often. Since hypogonadal men may represent a higher risk group for prostate cancer, the increase, or the velocity, of the PSA should be watched closely.

Many believe that taking prostate supplements containing lycopene, the carotenoid that gives tomatoes their red color, may help them avoid imminent prostate conditions and cancer. Well, again from the There-Is-No-Single-Magic-Bullet Department, animal research suggests eating whole tomatoes may be better than just taking the supplement when it comes to preventing prostate cancer.[223] "The finding strongly suggests that risks of poor dietary habits cannot be reversed simply by taking a pill. We must focus more on choosing a variety of healthy foods, exercising and watching our weight," reasoned one author. I agree. Research presented at the 2006 Annual Meeting of the American Association for Cancer Research found that high serum retinol levels were significantly associated with reduced rates of advanced prostate cancer. However, the source of vitamin A wasn't defined and the association was not significant for milder prostate cancers. In summary,

---

223 S. Clinton of Ohio State University, *Journal of the National Cancer Institute*, November issue (2003).

the convergence of evidence doesn't reveal a specific amount of lycopene that's beneficial, nor does it show if supplementing outperforms dietary sources.

B. Premature Ejaculation (PE). Approximately 30 percent of men between the ages of eighteen to fifty-nine experience PE, or "ejaculating too soon"; and most falsely believe it's a purely psychological or situational problem that usually resolves with time. According to the *DSM-IV* official psychiatric definition, PE is defined as "persistent or returned onset of orgasm and ejaculation with minimal sexual stimulation before, on, or shortly after penetration and before the person wishes it … causes marked distress or interpersonal difficulty … not due to a drug or general medical condition." (As you can see, psychiatric definitions can be quite lengthy. I think if you ejaculate before you can finish reading that sentence, you have PE.) PE can be a lifelong or an acquired condition and is considered one of the most common male sexual dysfunctions. For many obvious and not-so-obvious reasons, the exact definition and prevalence are difficult to pinpoint. Regardless, it can understandably cause substantial distress on many levels to the midlife man and his partner. Thirty percent of men with ED have PE as well.[224]

Because of the reluctance to report and subsequently receive professional help, many sufferers resort to self-help methods, which may make matters worse. Because of the various causes, it takes patience on the part of the patient, his partner, and the physician to come up with solutions. Most of the time, in acquired cases where it hasn't been a lifelong problem, I find PE to be situational. Help by a certified sexual therapist may be a good option for men with a willing long-time partner. Topical treatments include topical anesthetic creams or a Korean herb cream called SS-cream that can be quite difficult to find. There are specific precautions to note. The anesthetic cream requires a condom in order to avoid contact with the partner and has its own spontaneity and logistical problems. Repeated or prolonged use can cause numbness, dermatitis, no ejaculation, or even internal systemic effects including erectile dysfunction.

As far as oral agents are concerned, interestingly enough, PDE5 inhibitors as Viagra may be of benefit to those suffering with ED and PE. As mentioned before, these drugs have their own set of risks and side effects, including flushing and headache. Since most antidepressants cause delayed ejaculation, these are probably the most common pill option used. Again, there are a host of side effects including many undesired physical, sexual, and psychiatric ones. Of these, the

224 T. Lue, "Summary of the sexual recommendations on sexual dysfunctions in men," *J Sex Med* 1 (2004): 6–23.

serotonin selective reuptake inhibitors such as Paxil, Prozac, and Zoloft are the most studied. Dapoxetine is a new related agent specifically developed for PE treatment that may have less undesired psychiatric and sexual dysfunction effects. The good thing is that it may be used *on demand*, i.e., one to three hours prior to the anticipated sex act, as opposed to the others' daily regimen.[225]

I initially offer education and counseling about the male sexual response's four phases and how to slow the progression from sexual plateau to orgasm.[226] If a lifelong condition, I find PE has a lot to do with a man's first usual and lifelong partner. That's right, his hand. As a learned behavior, the adult male's sexual response has its roots in the young adolescent. This was a totally different environment. Here, the teenage boy probably had to secretly, quietly, and quickly ejaculate— say, between commercials of *I Dream of Jeanie*. It's then a mostly physical act with some visual or imaginary components at most. It's quite unidirectional and a fast race to the finish!

So the first task is to (re)discover the partner's role and interactions, and then recognize and prolong the sexual plateau phase. Slow it down some. You know, like in the middle groovy part in *Slow Ride* by Foghat or some of Barry White's soulful tunes. This can take some practice; but hey, with a willing partner, it can be quite fun. Basically, we guys have to realize the road leading to the destination can be more exciting than the final destination itself. It's okay, and even fun in this instance, to ask for directions along the way. Those two things don't usually jive right with the typical perceived male's macho image, but good sex *is* a learned behavior. You have to *become* good at it. Some tricks that may help out in the meantime may include having a *minimal* amount of alcohol, or taking a *low* dose of a decongestant or antihistamine before sex. (I stress *very small* amounts because these have variable effects on different people and may cause some undesired side effects as slowing things up too much, even causing erectile dysfunction or no orgasm at all.) Another nonmedical approach involves the partner *gently and lovingly* pulling down on the scrotum and testes before ejaculation occurs. This typically involves some communication and practice to master.

In summary, PE can be an embarrassing and detrimental concern for the middle-aged man and his partner. But there is help. Many nonmedical and medical treatments are now available to be individualized for your specific situation.

---

225 G. Broderick, W. Hellstrom, and I. Sharlip, "Advances in the premature ejaculation management: treating the aging patient," *Clinical Courier* 23, no. 64 (2006): 1–8.

226 The four stages are excitement, plateau, orgasm, and resolution.

C. Erectile Dysfunction (ED). A lot of this has been covered in earlier chapters focusing on hormones, but I will simply add some practical knowledge and thoughts. Similar to above, ED can be neither primary (lifelong) or secondary (acquired or situational). A simple definition would be that the penis doesn't get hard or stay hard long enough to complete a satisfying sex act for the man or partner. Similar to PE above, it is quite common yet embarrassing to bring up—please pardon the pun. Unlike PE though, ED usually increases with age and can be the first of sign of serious coronary or peripheral vascular disease. Accordingly, ED complaints demand a thorough medical evaluation. As mentioned, diabetes, smoking, and obesity are the biggest risks for *penis attack*—a symptom of peripheral vessel occlusion. A good erection depends on good blood flow to give tumescence, i.e., getting it up.

There are gimmicky ads everywhere with not-so-subtle slogans or taglines, so you would have to live in a bubble or missed every Super Bowl not to know the medical options for ED. These phosphodiesterase-5 inhibitor class drugs include Viagra, Levitra, and Cialis—the cure-all for getting a two-day hard-on. Just what society needs—a bunch of old demented geezers with a heavy! Some tidbits follow:

- Be sure to do Viagra on an empty stomach; it'll be twice as effective. Supposedly, Levitra has no such interaction with food. According to the *PDR*, you can't be on any nitrates or alpha blockers—two common heart, prostate, and/or hypertension medications. The combination can lower your blood pressure too much and can cause serious acute health risks. I add *all* hypertensive medications to this cautionary list. Ask your doctor or pharmacist about this, or you won't know if you're coming or going.

- These PDE-5 inhibitor drugs can cause permanent blindness. (Geez, here we go again with that "blindness thing." As a kid we were told if we masturbated we would go blind. Now as an adult, we've got this threat, again?) This risk is quite real though, and is increased with diabetes, smoking, and hypertension. Unfortunately, these are the very same diseases that cause ED.

- You may want to do an "undressed rehearsal" of sorts the first time you try these pills to see if they agree with you. For example, when I took one of these, I got flushing and a severe headache that made sex prohibitive. You wouldn't want this to happen with someone you're trying to impress on the first encounter.

- If these pills don't work, it's a probable indication of hormonal imbalances, especially low testosterone. As mentioned before in the hormonal chapters, proper TRT has vast systemic effects, not just improving libido and sexual functioning. ED is actually a late symptom of low testosterone. It's as if Mother Nature decreed, "Hey, you're too old and sick now to reproduce. You probably won't be around another twenty years on the planet to help raise that kid!"

Serious medical conditions, previous urologic surgery, and advanced age aside, the following probably represents the most common causes for ED I see in the office:

First would be medications and drugs. OTC decongestants and antihistamines are big players. Alcohol and other sedatives, such as pain pills or sleep aids, can relax things too well. Many other prescription drugs, especially in combination, can compound erection problems. But before you get on or off any medication, even OTC, ask your doctor first. Bring a complete list of *all* the things you ingest.

Second would be *performance anxiety*. Basically, your head, the one on your shoulders, gets in the way. Let's say you had a few too many beers one date and despite wanting to, when it came time to do the deed, you couldn't rise up to the occasion. Naturally, we all would be embarrassed. Well, let's say you were able to patch things up with her and went out another time. You get back to her place, making sure this time not to drink too much. You were a good boy this time. However, during foreplay, you start thinking things like, "What if the same thing happens? What am I going to do? This will be so embarrassing! She'll think I'm a failure and really have something wrong with me. Am I going queer?" Eventually, you become more neurotic than Woody Allen after drinking three Red Bulls. After being privy to all this, your penis says, "Never mind, dude, I'm outta' here!" Eventually, this self-defeating cycle can become ingrained.

Well, don't beat yourself off … errrr … I mean, *up* over it. I hate to say it, but maybe a little alcohol, like *one* drink, may be enough to take the edge off yet not too much to cause impotence. Openly discuss it with your partner and don't take things so hard on yourself. Well, you know what I mean. Even laugh about it. Your humor will disarm the situation, and she'll dig that. If that doesn't work, then you may want to try the following: The next time you're in a romantic situation, explain things and coax your partner into doing everything *except* intercourse. Do all the kissing, rubbing, massaging, oral things, and all. Usually in this situation, since the threat of erection failure or performance is removed, you'll have a big purple throbber!

Third, sheer boredom and relationship problems can contribute to ED. Now, I'm not suggesting you go out and get a new partner for obvious reasons, but someone or something new can dramatically improve ED. Think about it. If *Playboy* magazine used the same model every month, they probably would have gone broke the second or third month, right? Yet, for most of us, a new partner is out of the picture. So we must be inventive. Together, read books or watch videos about sex and romance. Yes, even chick flicks. Become the romantic that you used to be; really listen and be conversive. Stick little love notes around. Try different times or locations; be spontaneous and loving. Many times, libido and sexual performance are a reflection of how we feel about ourselves and each other. If we are in poor health, don't feel good about how we look, or have hormonal imbalances; sex-related difficulties may be a symptom. Maybe your lives are out of balance. At any rate, this could be a sign of deeper physical or emotional problems and likewise demands a thorough investigation and solution. You can visit the American Urological Association's Web site at http://www.UrologyHealth.org for a wealth of knowledge.

D. Hair Loss.

Out of five brothers, I was the only one to lose his hair in his mid-twenties. Lucky me! Actually, the vast majority of us will lose a variable amount of hair as we get older. Seen most commonly, *male pattern baldness* (MPB) is basically a sex chromosome—derived trait with variable expression. So blame your mother's side not your father's. The pattern here is the so-called widow's peak, combined with loss on the very top of the head. Yet, any sort of hair loss should be properly evaluated as there could be other easily treatable causes. These may include stress, nutritional or vitamin deficiencies, thyroid, or other hormonal disorders, even allergies or fungal infections. Although rare, it can also be caused by some serious autoimmune diseases, so get properly checked out by a dermatologist or a good family physician.

There are basically two types of drugs used to treat MPB. One is a topical treatment called minoxidil that is applied twice per day to the scalp. Basically this works by increasing blood flow to the hair follicle. In a much higher concentration and in a pill form, minoxidil is used to treat blood pressure. Originally, the trade name was Rogaine; but it is now available OTC in the generic version for about ten bucks a month. When used as directed, it's quite safe, with minimal, if any, side effects. As far as effectiveness is concerned, realistically you can expect somewhat of an increase in villouslike hair growth. That means some increase in *fine* hair growth at best on the vertex (top) of the head, with basically no effect on the widow's peak, or receding hairline. As for me, I've used it for years in the hope it may retard further hair loss; and what the heck, it's quite cheap.

The other class of treatment is the *alpha-5-reductase inhibitors* which, as explained in the earlier hormonal chapter, help block the conversion of testosterone to dihydrotestosterone, or DHT. This metabolite is believed to be a big player in MPB, and in enlarging the prostate size of aging men, although the latter point can be somewhat debated. Propecia© is the Merck drug trade name used for hair loss and usually comes in one milligram. Proscar©, also from Merck, is manufactured as a 5 mg tablet and is the one used for benign prostatic hypertrophy, or BPH. The generic drug is known as finasteride. A newer drug, Avodart©, may be more selective for the prostate and have less side effects. Because it can affect a developing fetus, these drugs shouldn't be used in or exposed to a childbearing-aged woman. Thus, some reasonable contact precautions should be practiced and are usually included with the package insert. I personally take Proscar daily to help prevent further hair loss and keep lower DHT levels. However, in my case, the hair loss is so global; I doubt the minoxidil and the Propecia are doing much good. But nothing ventured, nothing gained.

Some final tidbits follow on MPB. There are some so-called herbal varieties that claim to be a *natural* form of alpha-5 reductase inhibitors. Again, you run into the issue of non-FDA regulation of OTC supplements, so you never know what you're actually getting. I can't vouch for them. Also, healthy hair must come from a healthy scalp and body, so be sure to pay attention to the latter two. It may be that the earlier you start treatment for hair loss, the better results you obtain. Personally, I use a copper peptide—enriched shampoo-conditioner each day to help keep a healthy scalp.

Lastly, there are newer, more effective hair transplant methods. These include using micrografts and better matching the natural swirls and angles to the hair. This lowers the appearance of the easily detectable *doll's head* appearance from the earlier surgical techniques. I suggest you carefully scrutinize the qualifications and expertise of the surgeon you plan to use, and ask for references. He or she should probably be specializing solely, or mostly, in hair transplantation, and has done a lot of them daily for a long time. This will increase the surgeon's proficiency in dealing with the many inherent variations in order to obtain the perfect cosmetic result. In my particular case, there is just too much of an area to cover to achieve a reasonable aesthetic result. I guess I am left with wearing one of those funky, god-awful T-shirts or ball caps emblazoned with "I'm a solar-powered sex machine!" More on hair loss can be found at the American Academy of Family Physicians' Web site, http://www.familydoctor.org, or from the American Academy of Dermatologists at http://www.aad.org.

E. Depression, Anxiety, and Other Mood Disorders. Of course it
is beyond the scope of this book to cover mood disorders and similar concerns. Suffice to say, if you think you have a mental or emotional problem, please seek help. This could be through your regular primary care physician, a psychologist, or a psychiatrist. As mentioned, middle age has its hormonal changes and stressors that can cause an anxious or depressed personality to then dip into an anxiety or depressive disorder. Basically, if your friends, family, or coworkers express concern, then it's probably becoming more serious and warrants additional attention.

Everybody has various addictions. It just so happens that some addictions are more damaging to the person or to those around him. This depends on the type, severity, and the legality. *Alcohol* is quite common. Often, the alcoholic can hide his addiction quite well early on. However, in middle age, the disease may progress to cause personal, social, and financial ruin. Have you ever had a DUI? Have you had any blackouts? That's when you can't remember how crazy you acted the night before, but your friends do. Have you had more than five drinks containing alcohol in a single day within the past six months? Do you try to schedule your drinking so that nobody knows? If you answered yes to any of these, then there may be a problem. Alcohol is a depressant and, as such, makes any depression or sadness even worse. Although considered a sedative or sleep aid by most, drinking too much alcohol before bedtime paradoxically causes you wake up around 3:00 a.m. and unable to get back to sleep. If you think you, your spouse, or a friend may have a problem with alcoholism or drug addiction, at least discuss it. As any condition, the sooner you get help, the easier it is to get cured. Don't wait to hit rock bottom, please.

Smoking is another. Remember, this was highly associated with ED, guys. If you smoke a pack or more a day, you've built up tolerance. If you have to puff that morning cigarette within a half hour of awakening, you're hooked. With this level of addiction, you may need a nicotine replacement method. These give you the nicotine without the cancer-causing chemicals; and include the various gum, skin patches, and inhalers. Most of these are OTC. Some smokers have had help with hypnotism or low-level laser. Then, there's Zyban©. However, it's an antidepressant that requires a prescription. There's a new drug out called Chantix© that patients have had good luck with. As you can see, there are many options; so ask your doctor, friends, employer, or health planner for input. I find it's really what's *between your ears* that mostly determines how successful you'll be in quitting. No matter what, you have to *want* to quit and have the willpower. You can do it, man!

As alluded to, there are many various addictions. Some people are addicted to shopping, sex, being in control—they're countless. What's *really* been eating you? Of course, there may be heavy metal toxicity, hormonal imbalances, and other metabolic disturbances that may contribute to the difficulty of digging out this hole. There are various FDA-approved drugs that may help, but I find counseling is mandatory for success. This may be short- or long-term. No matter what else you may be doing healthily, if your mental attitude isn't right, you'll never reach your full potential.

We are, in fact, bombarded daily by today's society about things that really shouldn't matter so much. As mentioned before, most people desire peace in their lives. However, that peace must ultimately come from *within*. To paraphrase the Bible, the spirit must overcome the desires of the flesh.[227] Sure, your body is going to crave food, alcohol, sex, or cigarettes, but your spirit is going to have to over-come the material temptation. Nothing on God's green earth beats that feeling! Is your spirit going to win every time? Of course, it will not. But you have to try your best. I feel successful if I'm making the same mistakes, but less often and not as severe. World peace is impossible. But any peace must start within you. Once achieved, spread this love to your spouse and family. From there, work on togeth-erness in the neighborhood, as in times past. Get involved in the community and church. Be the example for peace. Like the song goes, "Let there be peace on our Earth and let it began with me." When it comes down to it, you're really only responsible for your own actions, not others. Choose peace, brother!

If you think you or your spouse may suffer from a mental disorder, again please seek help. There are many links and responsible Web sites that have question-naires and information about diverse mental disorders such as bipolar, borderline personality, anxiety, and others. There's a page on the symptoms of depression and such links in the appendix. You can also visit the National Mental Health's Institute's Web site at http://www.nimh.nih.gov and find out more. Please discuss this information with your doctor.

---

227 The Bible is really the original "self-help book." Catholics celebrate Lent, the forty days before Easter, by giving up something that the flesh craves, and replacing it with thoughts or actions of peace and love.

F. Pain Pills Decrease Testosterone Levels. I also see quite a few MAGs in my practice having quite a physically demanding job or suffering from chronic pain related to old sports injuries. Mostly, they complain of back pain. Often, they've been prescribed opioid-like drugs such as Lortab, Percocet, Vicodin, or even OxyContin from a pain clinic. These injuries have severely limited their level of activity, and they're now experiencing that loss of muscle mass and increase in visceral fat typically seen in older hypogonadal men. Based on my initial training, I would blame this sarcopenic obesity solely on their inactivity and stress-related snacking. I never fully appreciated the connection here until I read a report in 2003 by Dr. H. Daniell given at the annual meeting of the Endocrine Society.[228] The researcher stated, "The risk of sustained, long-term treatment with opioids is that permanent damage such as osteoporosis or testicular atrophy may result … long-acting opioids creating a vicious cycle because these drugs cause a drop in testosterone which in turn increases pain sensitivity and then eventually necessitates a higher dose of the pain medication." Low T additionally can bring the previously mentioned symptoms such as low libido, erectile dysfunction, fatigue, hot flashes, depression, and anxiety.

Bingo! As I learned more about andropause, I began to check these MAGs' T levels based on the severity of symptoms, visceral fat, and variable metabolic derangements. Lo and behold, most were T deficient. Clinically, once on TRT, they improved on many levels. Most back pain sufferers would be expected to benefit the usual increases in muscle mass and strength and the decreases in fat and weight seen in men undergoing TRT. Many were able to wean down the pain pills. TRT was only part of the integrative approach I used though. Depending on the circumstances, many got referrals to specialists such as anesthesiologists, neurosurgeons, acupuncturists, and chiropractors. Complementary supplements such as Sam-E and fish oil were often given a try, for example.

Of course, low T didn't *cause* their back pain to begin with. Yet, the use of opioids is known to lower androgen levels; this is fairly well documented. The syndrome is now called opioid-induced androgen deficiency, or OPIAD. Three years after that initial report mentioned above, Dr. Daniell did conclude TRT improved many of these symptoms. Yet, a certain degree of hypogonadism could have pre-

228 Dr. Daniell, clinical professor of medicine at the University of California–Davis. Opioids offer chronic pain relief at expense of testosterone, a poster presented to the 2003 Endo Society on baseline subjects. H. W. Daniell, "Open-label pilot study of testosterone patch therapy in men with opioid-induced androgen deficiency," *Journal Pain* 7, no. 3 (2006): 200–10.

existed or have been acquired after the pain and opioids came into the scene. Less physical activity results in increased visceral fat and less muscle mass. This would secondarily lower T levels further, thereby increasing payload on the back and resulting in increased pain and strain. Regardless if androgen deficiency preceded or followed opioid medication for chronic pain relief, it makes sense to consider TRT for improved body composition, higher pain threshold, improved mood, and overall improvement of many related conditions. Doctors and patients need to have an increased index of suspicion of andropause in these challenging, yet frustrating instances. Treat the patient, not just the disease! More help may be found at the National Institute of Neurological Diseases and Stroke's Web site at http://www.ninds.nih.gov.

Chapter 15. MAG reviews the information and decides a supplement containing phosphatidylcholine and phosphatidylserine will help out his mind. His blood pressure, fasting glucose and cholesterol indices are much favorable now. He knows that by keeping these diseases at bay, he's preventing heart and brain disease later in life. He also was concerned of some hair loss. His DHT was a little high after TRT, so he starts Propecia, 1 mg per day. He doesn't suffer as much from ED or PE since being on the program, and he's getting closer with his wife.

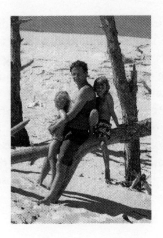

XVII.

Summary

If you want to beat Mother Nature, you must first learn to play her game!

Often unappreciated until it's too late, optimal health is truly the biggest asset you can achieve. Investing wisely and routinely in your health should be job 1. On the other hand, if you take a reactive, come-as-it-may approach, your health will become your biggest liability. When you get old, you'll either have a credit or a debit. *You* can make it happen!

Midlife presents the excellent *window of opportunity* to take a more preventive, proactive stance. It's a time when you enjoy being at the "top of your game" and focusing on being a good provider, yet may be putting your own health last. As a result, many early warning signs of disease are already underway, but may be ignored or undetectable by traditional means. Making matters worse, today's health-care system is mostly a self-perpetuating, reactive, sickness-based model that's expensive and unjust. Health insurance companies are raking in profits by cherry-picking beneficiaries while leaving fifty million stranded. Shamelessly, less than 5 percent of today's U.S. health-care dollars is spent on preventing of disease. Is it any wonder our health-care expenses are skyrocketing? Adding to this *perfect storm*, we baby boomers are reaching Medicare age at the same time our teenage kids are getting adult-onset diabetes. They do grow up quickly, don't they? Dude, it's time for a health-care revolution! Don't sit back and wait for the government to lock you up in an old folk's home one day. Take a stand, man! Get proactive and become free of disease now. As the '60s mantra stated, "You're either part of the solution or part of the problem!" It's really how healthy we are in midlife that determines how well we are in our golden years. We're not going to take getting older and sicker lying down, are we, brother?

If you truly want to fight the aging process, you must first learn the tricks of the enemy. Why do some of us age better than others? Of course, having good genes is a great head start. However, these genes will only help you the first half of life, mostly. After that, it's the lifestyle you lead from midlife on that determines how well you'll do. Genetic manipulation itself is a still a long way off; however, a healthy lifestyle can help naturally *repress* the bad genes and *express* the good ones. Secondly, there's the "wear and tear" or degeneration that takes its eventual toll. Again, a healthy lifestyle helps keep Father Time in a kinder mood. As covered in the supplements chapter, many antioxidants and fish oil may help limit his getting (free) radical on us. Hopefully, we can boost the repair of such universal damage. "Aging is a disease which can be prevented or reversed. We need not be prisoners of our genetic destiny!"[229]

As if those two methods aren't enough to age us, Mother Nature, being a woman, has a much more secretive, complex, personal way of doing her duty. She indeed has a love-hate relationship with us men. On one hand, she's allowed us to reproduce our entire life. Yeah! On the other, we don't live as long as women—that's a bummer. Maybe she's trying to make up for all the hassles we put women through. Who knows? Much as a soap opera villain, Mother Nature slowly but methodically whacks us guys out by using the age-related hormonal changes described earlier. The aging hormones—insulin and cortisol—increase. The youthful hormones—DHEA, pregnenolone, testosterone, HGH, and thyroid—variably decrease. As Austin Powers would exclaim, "There goes our mojo, baby!" With these changes, visceral fat, acting as a medusa with all its tentacles, increases our risks for most age-related diseases. Like the rust on an aging ship, or the waves beating against the shoreline, it's her *modus operandi.*

When it comes down to aging, the hormones you wish would go up go down. And the ones you wish would go down go up! Recent research stated aging male veterans with low testosterone levels had a seventy-five increased mortality rate in five years. Just how much testosterone and human growth hormone drop as we

---

229. Denam Harman, 1954.

age is quite variable. These decreases lead to increased risk for frailty syndrome and sporting more visceral fat. This *apple shape* then starts a cascade of metabolic events ultimately leading to diabetes, hypertension, hypercholesterolemia, and much more. These ultimately snowball into increased risks for heart disease, stroke, cancers, dementia, and many other age-related diseases.[230] Research shows that when these hormones are properly replaced in those suffering from such deficiencies, symptoms improve and risks for these problems are greatly lessened.

When *biologically identical hormonal replacement* is appropriately and routinely monitored by those experienced, most of the literature reports no increased risk of cancer. For if you wish to beat Mother Nature, I believe you must first learn to play her game. Using only partial hormonal replacements or using artificially manufactured ones seem to only upset her. We all know it's *not nice* to fool Mother Nature! All the hormones must work in concert with each other for life's symphony to get a standing ovation when done.

There's indeed no magic bullet to decrease insulin and cortisol, you have to do this the old-fashioned way—the proper *diet* and *exercise* we recommended. Most of the pros and cons of all the popular diets were covered. There is no one diet that works for everyone, but this book helped you separate fact from fiction. Yet, by selecting healthier fats, carbs, and protein, you can simply improve many disease risks. This should only be a part of a comprehensive approach to one's health. Although staying away from the higher *glycemic index* carbs helps immensely, eating fats from a fish or a plant and avoiding processed meats are also important. Eat to live, don't live to eat, remember?

There's also no getting around routine exercise! Sorry. "If you don't use it, you'll lose it." We do lose 1 percent of muscle mass per year and gain that amount in fat, unless we're more proactive. Men do get osteoporosis—no bones about it. Get a balanced, safe program going. You need from a half hour to an hour of intense physical activity daily. Don't forget, spend one-third of your exercise time stretching. Much as paying your bills each week, you have to regularly invest in yourself to have a healthy reserve when you age. If not, you may find yourself overdrawn. The penalty here is worse than any NSF charge. Give time to your health—your biggest asset!

---

230. L. Yan, "Midlife body mass index and hospitalization and mortality in older age," *JAMA* 295 (2006): 190–8.

What we're talking about is more than just *life span*; *it's about health span.* The quality of life matters most when it really comes down to it. Think, if you had only one vehicle to last you your whole life, would you abuse it? You wouldn't wait until something breaks to check it out. Of course not! You would make darn sure it wouldn't rust. You would change the oil regularly and use the best gas so your engine doesn't prematurely wear out. Well, your body is, in fact, the *only* true vehicle you're stuck with your whole life. As they say, "An ounce of prevention *is* worth a pound of cure. Unfortunately, most guys take much better care of their cars than themselves. But the focus shouldn't just be on how *long*, it's really how *well* we live that matters most.

There's no one magic pill or diet that works for everyone. It's the beneficial synergism of all we've reviewed that culminates in optimal health. Besides what's mentioned above, some people may have additional hang-ups. Remember, drink lots of filtered water. Learn better coping mechanisms and get good rest—it's a concrete jungle out there! If you still don't feel quite right, possible *food allergies, specific vitamin deficiencies, or heavy metal toxicities* may be playing a role and warrant investigating. It appears the environment we're living in today is more toxic than ever.

Obviously, one's own health is very personal and highly individual. As such, no two people have exactly the same concerns, problems, goals, nor do they respond the same to particular therapies. It takes patience from the experienced, qualified physician and commitment from the patient. When you have the knowledge and you take charge of your own health, *you* are in the driver's seat and can control the direction you're headed. The destination should be *optimal* aging, as opposed to just *normal* aging with its many complications and disabilities.

Last but certainly not least, there is the profound *mind-body-spirit connection* that must be nourished to make all these worthwhile. I always say the best self-help book is the Bible. For if your spirit isn't flourishing, what good is life? Most Western-educated physicians aren't trained in most of these modalities. The whole reactive system is basically a sickly-based, pill-and-scalpel-pushing model. Yet as I said many times before, "Your best health insurance is to be healthy in the first place." I hope to lead you on the right path and provide you with some sound information. Additionally, resources were given for you to do some investigating on your own. Midlife for us guys is the time to do this—to invest in our health; you'll never regret it. That's probably the best gift we can give ourselves, as well as to our family and loved ones.

In life, you have to think out the box—the pine box, that is! Check the appropriate box:

- I am going to age *normally*, suffer all its related complications and spend my last few years on Earth in a very dependent, debilitated way.

- I am going to be proactive about obtaining optimal health and invest daily in this most important asset. I plan to *live* until the day I die.

Coming soon, *The Midlife Health Guide for Women*

MAG is now trimmer and the happiest ever. He knows he needs the proper follow up and repeat lab-work to monitor his success and safety.

Afterword

So what would be Dr. Chris Rao's prescription for a healthier America? The current health-care system is very expensive, unjust, and upside-down. Less than 5 percent of health-care dollars is spent on prevention. For example, if I were to list *weight loss* or *smoking cessation counseling* as a reason for a patient's office visit, most insurances including Medicare would deny payment because, according to their rules, the visit wasn't *medically necessary*! Yet, ten years later, the same overweight smoker would be rushed to the local hospital and receive emergent coronary bypass, carotid endarterectomy, abdominal aortic aneurysm repair, or be hospitalized for a heart attack or stroke. Meanwhile, the personal and social costs of this illogical and reactive system are steadily climbing.

But glance at any financial section in the newspaper and you'll see that big health insurance firms such as Aetna, United, Humana, and others are making record profits. They certainly aren't hurting in all this; the government allows them to simply pass on their costs. This results in today's unaffordable insurance premiums in order to offset those who continually abuse what little health they have left. Why do over fifty million Americans have no health insurance? These companies can cherry-pick their beneficiaries and drop those at higher risk. Most Americans will have to survive until they reach Medicare age to get any medical attention. By that time, midlife is over, and multiple diseases are already well entrenched. It's too late to prevent them; it's only damage control then. We all pay more in the end.

Similar to the behavioral change an individual must do to become healthy, the government must now change its thinking and direction when it comes to delivering health care or it will truly become a terminal case. Despite having one of the most expensive health cost per capita, America ranks well below many less-affluent countries when it comes to the quality of health care and prevention. It's a worldwide embarrassment. As a reflection of this irony, instead of giving our future generations some inheritance and financial security as our parents did for us, we'll unfairly overburden them with debts they didn't create.

Unfortunately, I see no light at the end of the tunnel. To paraphrase an old Chinese saying, "It takes an adequate doctor to treat a disease. It takes a good doctor to prevent a disease from coming back. However, it takes a *great* doctor to prevent a disease in the first place." Unfortunately, insurance firms and the government don't grasp this wisdom. There are more expensive drugs than ever to merely treat the many complications of aging. Recently, instead of trying to bargain with the major drug firms for cheaper drugs, as all insurance companies do, Medicare Part D is lining the pharmacies' pockets in a feeding frenzy. Wyeth-Ayerst, the makers of Premarin (an artificial women's hormone that increases inflammation) and Provera (a fake, kerosene-based progesterone that is banned in most parts of the world), is trying their best to stop the sales of all bioidentical hormonal replacements—a much more natural option. Of course, the many doctors who profit off performing procedures on the very sick have no complaints either. The cardiothoracic surgeon is not sorry to hear you need a bypass, or is the hematologist-oncologist going to cry because you now have cancer. It's business as usual; that's how they make their living. God bless them for being there when most needed though. But as opposed to being paid to treat sick people, I much prefer to be rewarded for preventing sickness.

One way to contain costs would be to ration health care, as most of the industrialized world has done. Let's see … assume I'm a politician running for office. My platform is to raise the age for Medicare eligibility to seventy years and increase taxes to offset the increased costs. Anyone who's smoking, overweight, or an alcoholic won't get immediate services. As elsewhere in the world, you'll have to be put on a waiting list to get any tests or elective surgeries. Oh, and you'll have a drug formulary with an annual cap. In the good side, all Americans will now have health care. This would actually lower costs and taxes in the long run. What lobbyists or special-interest group do you think would support me—the AARP or the insurance companies? Of course, they would mount an all-out counter-attack. I would be politically dead in the water. Rationing health care, as the rest of the world has done, will never fly in America. So what can we do?

Well, instead of giving a disincentive to the unhealthy, why don't we have incentives for all to get healthier? We were taught in school that positive reinforcement beats negative reinforcement, right? My plan would give a tax credit to those who don't smoke, don't have any traffic accidents or tickets, and are within their proper weight. But wait, what about those of you that smoke or overweight now? In these instances, the government would support smoking-cessation and weight-loss measures. If a smoker attended a smoking-cessation class, she would get credit. Likewise, if the overweight attended a weight-loss program and lost 10 percent of his weight, he would get a tax break or refund check. Similar programs can be made for drug addiction, alcoholism, teen pregnancy, etc. This makes for good logic, as preventing these will cost a lot less in the long run, personally and socially. Maybe the government needs to invest more in wellness centers, as opposed to treating the more expensive outcomes of a sedentary lifestyle. It may seem odd at first to have the government so involved with these programs, but most health problems and costs are deeply rooted in societal problems. It beats building more prisons as a solution. We basically reap what we sow.

Additionally, the government should provide *all* preventative care to *all* ages, no matter what their economic status. Many countries such as France believe in this concept—and it makes sense. We don't have to reinvent the wheel here, guys. It just takes putting some common sense into action. As I stated before, the only way to keep health-care costs down is to have an overall healthier nation. As it stands now, many poor and middle-class families are uninsured and waiting for Medicare to pay for needed health care. By that time, it's often too late for prevention. Others who are financially sound would be put in the poor house if disease was ignored or discovered too late. All society pays when somebody gets too sick to be productive or goes broke because of their doctor bills. Therefore, if somebody was up-to-date on all their preventative care for their particular age group, they also get a tax credit. Bamm! For example, a fifty-year-old woman that undergoes her government-reimbursed gynecologic exam, colonoscopy, and preventative physical examination would also get a tax refund. She saves, and society as a whole saves. The same would be for young children and men of all ages, of course. A healthier society is a more competitive, satisfied workforce. There's also the reduced tax burden of an antiquated, reactive health-care delivery system. That's a tax refund check for everybody! America would be proud.

Lastly, here are some other suggestions:

- Free prophylactics and sexually transmitted disease treatments from doctor's offices and pharmacies, as appropriate.
- Government-sponsored addiction, marriage, anger management, gambling, and anxiety/depression counseling.
- Gas stations and especially drugstores (that are supposed to help you stay well, right?) couldn't sell cigarettes, alcohol, or junk food anymore. Taxes would go way up on those items to realistically offset the damages they cause society. (These would still cost less than bottled water.)
- People would be required to have a license to carry a gun. They would have to prove knowledge and maturity when it came to firearms and not

have a criminal record. Likewise, there would be a tax to offset society's expense of having some of these guns getting into the wrong hands.

- There would also be government-sponsored TV and radio ads promoting health, and the schools would have standard curricula that teach our young the responsibility for their own health. Trans fats and junk food would be banned.

- Health-insurance firms would not be allowed to cherry-pick and profit off the healthiest individuals. They would have reasonably set profit margins with any remainder going into health promotion or government-subsidized programs. Those health plans with the best record for prevention would get additional tax breaks. Responsibility for adults' own health would be promoted through the expanded use of pretax medical savings accounts, long-term care plans, and government-subsidized health plans that focus more on prevention.

- Lastly, there would be a big push to outlaw toxins and to establish incentives to keep a cleaner environment. No more pesticides, either. Well, that's a few of the biggies on my wish list.

All the above makes common sense; just take a look at the costliest, commonest diseases out there. When we are faced with increasing costs, combined with an overall sicklier, more demanding population stuck in an unfair health-care system that has many gaps and holes, this is the only direction for a cure. No Band-Aid fixes allowed. We baby boomers need to pick up the protest signs, wear our head bands, and shoot the peace sign again. We should demand adequate health care for all and emphasize prevention. Our mantra should be this new paradigm shift and to buck the old government system. The revolution is at hand—being free of disease!

Index-Glossary

Most terms are described in the book when necessary, with resources and references given. Given the integral nature of health, it is difficult to focus on only one topic or aspect at once, i.e., present fish oil's benefits and not to discuss arthritis and the heart.

- acrylamide. A toxin found in many snack foods. See fluids and toxins chapter.
- addictions. See special topics chapter under mood disorders.
- Addisonian crisis. Failure of the adrenal gland to produce its hormones involved with sugar, sex and salt balance, can be lethal.
- ADHD. Attention deficit, hyperactivity disorder, adult types. See supplements chapter and special topics chapter.
- adipokines. Fat molecules that further metabolic disturbances.
- Adrenopause. Mild, age-related failure of the adrenal gland.
- advanced glycation end products. Cancer-causing and inflammation-causing compounds resulting from glycosylation.
- age-related macular degeneration (ARMD). Leading cause of blindness in America.
- AICR. American Institute for Cancer Research (http://www.aicr.org)
- AIDS/HIV (acquired immunodeficiency syndrome/human immunodeficiency virus). A gradually debilitating, ultimately lethal disease marked by frailty and immunocompromise that is caused by a virus-using RNA.
- alpha lipoic acid. A fatty acid that may help the brain and nerves. See supplement chapter.
- Alzheimer's disease. A progressive inflammatory and degenerative disease of the brain. Coined by Dr. Alzheimer.
- American Institute for Cancer Research. Profit-free organization helping cancer research.
- andropause. The syndrome of low testosterone in men and women. See testosterone chapters.
- anxiety mood disorder. See special topics chapter.
- anxiety. See stress and sleep chapter.

- apoptosis. Programmed cellular death.
- Armour thyroid. The trade name thyroid drug, a combination of T3 and T4. See thyroid chapter.
- arthritis. The age-related wear and tear degeneration of the joints.
- atherothrombosis. The formation of plaques and vessel blockages.
- Atkins diet. Low-carb diet pioneered by Dr. Atkins. See weight loss chapter.
- atrial fibrillation. An irregular heartbeat, causing increased risks of stroke.
- Avandia. A newer, better drug used to treat younger healthier diabetics.
- bariatric surgery. Risky surgery that removes portions of the gastrointestinal tract. See weight loss chapter
- Beck's Depression Inventory. A questionnaire that helps measure symptoms of depression. See appendix.
- benign prostatic hypertrophy (BPH). Benign enlargement of the prostate. See special topics chapter under prostate.
- bioidentical hormonal replacement. The optimal physiological replacement of the exact original hormone your body originally created, given in the modality that closely mimics what nature originally intended. See introduction to men's hormones chapter.
- body burden. How much and how many toxins the body accumulates over a lifetime.
- body mass index (BMI). A measure of being overweight. See weight loss chapter.
- borage oil. Source of omega-3 fatty acid. See supplement chapter.
- BPH (benign prostatic hypertrophy). Noncancerous enlargement of the prostate seen as men age. See special topics chapter.
- BRCA 1 cancer gene. An inherited gene that increase risks for breast cancer
- carbohydrate blockers. Compounds that may plot the absorption of carbohydrate. See weight loss chapter.
- carbs (carbohydrates). A food group basically consisting of carbon and hydrogen, responsible for energy source and complex carbohydrates, proteoglycans, and aminoglycosides, for more complex functions including immune and fertility functions, about 4 kcal per gram. See chapter 3.

- carcinogenesis. The formation of a cancer in the first place.
- cardiac output. How much blood the heart pumps, a result of stroke volume times heart rate.
- chelation. The process of scavenging the body of heavy metals. See supplement chapter.
- Chromium. Supplement that may help glucose metabolism. See supplement chapter.
- chronic fatigue syndrome. A vague collection of symptoms—usually achiness, tiredness, depression, and more—that has nebulous causes.
- chronic pain. See special topics chapter.
- colon cancer. Cancer of the rectum.
- congestive heart failure. Failure of the heart as a pump, starting off as early diastolic failure, mostly caused by coronary artery disease.
- COPD. See emphysema.
- coronary artery disease. Plaques and blockages of the heart vessels.
- coronary calcium scoring. A noninvasive measure of risks for coronary disease
- cortisol. Produced by the adrenal gland and responsible for the fight-or-flight stress response.
- CRAN diet. Calorie restriction but adequate nutrition diet. See calorie restriction but optimal nutrition diet. See also weight loss chapter.
- CRP-hs (C-reactive protein-high specificity). A serum marker for vessel inflammation and a better predictor of heart disease then cholesterol. Try to keep under one.
- cystic fibrosis. A progressive disease of the lungs in children.
- Cytomel. The trade name for T3 thyroid drug. See thyroid chapter.
- Dash diet. High fiber diet promoted by Dr. Dean Ornish. See weight loss chapter.
- Dean Ornish. Promoter of natural methods to reduce inflammation and risks for coronary disease and prostate cancer. See DASH diet.
- dementia. Forgetfulness. There are many stages and forms of dementia.
- depression. See special topics chapter.
- depressive mood disorder. See special topics chapter.

- DHA (docosahexaenoic [fatty] acid). Tends to help neurological systems.

- DHEA. A sex steroid important for men and women; a precursor to testosterone and other sex hormones. See hormonal chapters

- dihydrotestosterone (DHT). A metabolite of testosterone responsible for benign prostatic hypertrophy and male pattern baldness.

- DMSA. A compound used to rid the body of heavy metal. See supplement chapter.

- DNA (deoxyribosenucleic acid). The double-helix molecules found in the nucleus that are basically the blueprints for the cell, isolated by Watson-Crick in the 1970s.

- Eicosanoid pathway. The metabolic pathways of good anti-inflammatory fats and the bad pro-inflammatory ones. See DHA and EPA types.

- emphysema. Nonreversible, smoking and age-related obstructive disease of the lungs.

- EPA (eicosapentaenoic [fatty] acid). Tends to be more anti-inflammatory in nature, overall.

- erectile dysfunction (ED). The inability to obtain and sustaining an erection. See special topics chapter.

- estrogen (estradiol is one form). The woman's major sex hormone, also increases in older men. See hormonal chapters.

- fat blockers (Orlistat). Blocks the absorption of fats. See weight loss chapter.

- fats. Includes oils, unused sugar that gets stored inside the fat cell. High insulin levels keep the fat locked inside. Consume fats from plant and fish sources. About 10 kcal per gram and you should consume 30 g or less of fat daily, mostly from mono- and polyunsaturated types. See chapter 3.

- fatty acid metabolism, lipoxygenase, and cyclooxygenase pathways of inflammation. See diet chapter, under fish oil, figure in chapter 3.

- fen-phen. Appetite suppressant combination. See weight loss chapter.

- fertility. The quality of reproducing.

- Fiber. Nondigestible cellulose, important for a bowel health. See diet chapter.

- fibromyalgia. An inflammatory condition causing muscle and tendon aches.

- fish oil. Please see diet and supplement chapter for the many benefits of fish oil.

- flaxseed. A beneficial source of fat and fiber. See supplement chapter.

- Flurizan. A new drug. See special topics chapter.

- folate (folic acid). Necessary B vitamin for heart, blood, and neurologic health. See supplement chapter

- food pyramid per the FDA. A schematic describing what should be the proper types and proportions of a diet.

- free testosterone. The relatively 2 percent of total testosterone that is active. See testosterone chapters.

- ginkgo biloba. A supplement that may help with symptoms of forgetfulness. See supplement chapter.

- gluconeogenesis. The formation of new glucose by the liver.

- Glucophage. A newer, better drug used to treat younger healthier diabetics.

- glucosamine sulfate and chondroitin sulfate. Supplement that may help joints. See supplement chapter.

- glycemic index. A measure of the sugar spike occurring in the blood after a particular food's ingestion. Glucose is given a value of 100. You should prefer to consume foods that have a glycemic index under 50.

- glycosylation. The abnormal sugarcoating of cellular and tissue components resulting in inflammation and degeneration.

- green tea. Along with black tea and white tea contain catechins, a class of antioxidants.

- *H. pylori.* A bacteria that cause gastric ulcers.

- hair loss, male pattern baldness. See special topics chapter.

- HDL. The healthy cholesterol, keep above 50.

- health span. How well you live, not just how long you live.

- homocysteine. A metabolite that probably plays a role in heart, bone, and other parameters of one's health. See supplement chapter.

- human growth hormone (HGH). The so-called antiaging elixir produced by the pituitary that is then converted into the IGF superfamily by the liver. See IGF-1. See also HGH chapter.

- Hypertension. Elevated blood pressure

- IGF superfamily. The many different forms of converted HGH that represent the yin and yang of its effects. See HGH chapter and illustration.

- IGF-1. Intrinsic growth factor-1 subtype used to measure HGH levels; converted from HGH by the liver.

- inflammatory bowel syndrome (ulcerative colitis, Crohn's disease). Moderate to severe sensitive, inflamed bowels.

- inositol. A flush-free form of niacin. See supplement chapter.

- insomnia. See stress and sleep chapter.

- insulin. A complex protein molecule created by the beta cells of the pancreas involved with the glucose balance between the blood, liver, and muscle cells. This is elevated in the type 2 adult-onset diabetic, although absent in the type 1 diabetic.

- iron. Needed by the red blood cell to carry oxygen.

- irritable bowel syndrome (IBS). Mildly sensitive, inflamed bowels.

- jet lag. See stress and sleep chapters.

- L-carnitine. Supplement that helps fat metabolism and body composition. See supplement chapter.

- LDL. The lousy cholesterol, keep under 70.

- Lead. Another heavy metal causing multiple derangements. See fluid and toxin chapter.

- leaky gut syndrome. Inflamed bowels that allow the inappropriate absorption of macro molecules that may cause other metabolic and immune dysfunction. See supplement chapter.

- liposuction. Plastic surgery procedure that removes peripheral fat. See weight loss chapter.

- lithium orotate. A supplement that may help symptoms of depression. See supplement chapter.

- Macrobiotic diet. Fad complex carbohydrate diet. See weight loss chapter.

- Male-pattern baldness. See special topics.

- melatonin. Produced by the pineal gland; important for nocturnal and diurnal rhythms; helps you sleep; also antioxidant. See stress and sleep chapter.

- Mercury. A heavy metal causing central and peripheral nerve damage. See fluids and toxins chapter.

- Meridia. Appetite suppressant. See weight loss chapter.

- metabolic syndrome. A totally preventable, currently epidemic disease caused by improper lifestyle characterized by obesity, cholesterol abnormalities, metabolic disturbances including diabetes, and hypertension.

- mitochondria. The organelle in the cell responsible for energy production.

- morbidity compression. The goal of trying to limit disability and dependence at the end of life.

- morbidity. Death

- mortality. Sickness

- MUFA, PUFA. Monounsaturated and polyunsaturated fatty acids, respectively. These are from plant and fish sources and are anti-inflammatory in nature.

- myeloperoxidase. An enzymatic compound acting as a reactive oxygen species. See current and future research chapter.

- niacin. B_6 vitamin responsible for increasing HDL and decreasing triglycerides. See supplement chapter.

- NSAIDs. Nonsteroidal anti-inflammatory drugs that can cause ulcers.

- opioid-induced androgen deficiency (OPIAD). See special topics chapter.

- osteopenia. The early stages of bone loss.

- osteoporosis. Brittle bones.

- P53 gene and cancer. One of the many cancer-causing genes.

- Parkinson's disease. A progressive degenerative and inflammatory disease of the brain that results in tremor, frailty, and, eventually, death.

- PBDEs. Another toxin. See fluids and toxins chapter.

- PCBs. A plastic toxin that is ubiquitous.

- PC-SPES. Banned prostate support supplement.

- performance anxiety. When the brain gets in the way of the penis. See special topics chapter.

- pernicious anemia. "Bad" anemia caused by B_{12} and folate deficiency.

- phentermine. Appetite suppressant. See weight loss chapter.

- pregnenolone. An important sex steroid precursor that is involved with immune and mood balance. See hormonal chapters.

- premature ejaculation. Too early of a climax with ejaculation. See special topics chapter.

- primary prevention. The early treatment of risks for a disease before that disease actually happens, i.e., being overweight.

- primrose oil. Source of omega-3 fatty acid. See supplement chapter.

- probiotic. A supplement containing a mixture of beneficial symbiotic bacteria that may help many allergic, infectious. and immune conditions. See supplement chapter.

- progeria. A disease of premature aging presumably caused by a mutated gene(s).

- progressive resistance training (PRT). See exercise chapter.

- prostaglandins, mediators of inflammation. See fatty acid metabolism.

- prostate cancer screenings. See special topics chapter under prostate.

- prostate specific antigen (PSA). A screening blood test for the prostate. See special topics chapter under prostate.

- prostatitis. Inflammation and infection of the prostate. See special topics chapter.

- protein. Food group consisting of amino acids, the building blocks of many important structures, hormones, chemical messengers, and other important compounds. About 4 kcal per gram and you should consume about 0.8 g per kilogram of your weight per day. See chapter 3.

- Proteoglycans, a.k.a. aminoglycans. Complex carbohydrates used in joint, immunity, and fertility functions. See diet chapter, fiber section.

- Provigil. A drug used to treat daytime sleepiness, ADHD, and fatigue. See special topics.

- quercitin. Antioxidant found in onions and apples.

- ratcheting effect. The phenomenon of making more, larger fat cells with yo-yo dieting, i.e., losing weight and regaining it back many times over.

- reactive oxygen species, a.k.a. free radical. Unstable substances within a cell that scavenges electrons from neighboring structures and causing them damage.
- receptor complex. When the enzyme binds with the receptor site causing a reaction to occur.
- relative risk. A measure of risk.
- resveratrol. Antioxidant found in wine, grapes, and nuts. See future in current research chapter.
- rheumatoid arthritis. A complex, systemic immune disorder affecting the joints.
- Rimonabant. Cannabinoid receptor blocker. See weight loss chapter.
- Sam-E (s-adenosyl methionine). Supplement that helps support liver, mind, and joints. See supplement chapter.
- sarcopenia. The loss of muscle mass.
- sarcopenic obesity. The body composition of lost muscle mass and increased fat mass.
- secondary prevention. The treatment of an established disease to prevent its complications, i.e., hypertension.
- sex hormone binding globulin (SHBG). The compound that carries inactive forms of estrogen and testosterone.
- silymarin. The active ingredient and milk thistle that helps support the liver.
- sleep disturbance (insomnia). See stress and sleep chapters.
- small vessel dementia. A form of dementia caused by vessel disease and "mini" strokes.
- smoking, nicotine addiction. See special topics chapter under mood disorders.
- St John's wort. A supplement that may help symptoms of depression. See supplement chapter.
- Synthroid. A trade name thyroid drug, mainly T4. See thyroid chapter.
- tertiary prevention. The treatment following an acute worsening of a disease in order to prevent its recurrence, i.e., using drugs to treat a person after a heart attack.

- testosterone. The male sex hormone that has universal, systemic effects; also important for women. See hormonal chapters.
- Thyrolar. Combination T3-T4 thyroid drug. See thyroid chapter.
- triglycerides. The ugly cholesterol, keep under 100.
- uric acid. Higher levels associated with coronary disease only, elevations found in gout—and inflammatory condition of the joints.
- vitamin C. Ascorbic acid. See supplement chapter.
- vitamin D. Important for cardiac, bone, and immune system health. See supplement chapter.
- vitamin E. A tocopherol. See supplement chapter.
- xenohormone. A nonhuman hormone, or a toxin, that mimics a human hormone and has different, unknown ill effects.

APPENDIX

Meal Ideas

Breakfast

* Natural (old fashioned) oatmeal (cooks quickly in microwave!), 1 egg white, 1 Tbsp natural almond butter

1 Whole egg, 2 egg whites, scrambled in small amount of butter, apple slices, 1 Tbsp organic peanut butter

* Natural oatmeal, sliced apple, cinnamon, 3 Tbsp fresh ground flaxmeal

Cottage cheese, chopped apples, pears, raw almonds, 1 Tbsp ground flaxseeds

* Poached organic omega-3 eggs (*Eggland's Best*), 1 slice whole grain rye toast with butter

Chicken breast, cubed, black beans, salsa, ¼ chopped avocado

Plain yogurt, berries, small handful of raw nuts

Smoked salmon (lox) on thick tomato slices, capers, olive oil, 1 apple

3 Egg white omelet, chopped green peppers, onions, 1 Tbsp guacamole

2 Slices lean ham, 2 slices low-fat cheese, 2 slices tomato, 2 slices avocado

* 1 Hard boiled egg, 1 slice pumpernickel toast with 1 Tbsp. almond butter

* Natural oatmeal, 1 scoop vanilla protein powder, 1 cup blueberries, 1 handful walnuts

Assorted imported low-fat cheese, sliced cucumber, olive oil, 5 dried apricots

1 Scoop protein powder, water, 1 cup frozen berries, 1 Tbsp. organic peanut butter

* 1 Scoop protein powder, 1 cup skim milk, ½ banana, 1 Tbsp. natural almond butter

1 Whole egg, 2 egg white omelet with spinach, feta cheese, 4 Calamata olives

1/8 Cup almond milk, 1 cup ground almonds, 1 tsp. blueberries, 1/8 cup ground flaxseeds

2 Eggs cooked in 4 tsp. olive oil, topped with 2 Tbsp. Hollandaise sauce, 4 sliced Calamata olives

½ Chicken breast, ½ cup plain yogurt, berries, 1 Tbsp. flaxseeds

1 Whole egg, 2 egg whites, scrambled in small amount of butter, apple slices, 1 Tbsp organic peanut butter

Smoked salmon spread with 1 oz. low-fat cream cheese, rolled and speared with Calamata olives on a toothpick

1 Whole egg, 2 egg white omelet, 1 oz. Sausage, mushrooms, 4 Calamata olives

*Indicates a high carbohydrate option. Try to avoid these during the 1st 2 weeks and no more than 3 times a week thereafter. Or save for AFTER exercise.

<u>Lunch & Dinner</u>

Turkey burger, tomato, low-fat cheese, mustard, relish, wrapped in lettuce, side salad, olive oil & vinegar

White meat turkey, Dijon mustard, spinach Caesar salad

Roasted turkey, steamed broccoli, mustard vinaigrette, seasonings to taste

Broiled lamb chop, cooked asparagus, spinach salad, balsamic vinaigrette dressing

1 Chicken breast on 2 cups spinach, 4 Calamata olives, 4 oz. guacamole, 2 Tbsp. olive oil and vinegar dressing

Cottage cheese, low glycemic fruit salad, 2 Tbsp. pecans

Curried shrimp on 2 cups mixed salad greens, 4 slices avocado, 2 Tbsp. balsamic vinaigrette dressing

Beef soup with lentils, celery, onions, cabbage, spinach or mixed green salad with ½ cup chicken or tuna salad

Broiled salmon on ½ cup spaghetti squash with tomato sauce, grilled vegetables, oregano, thyme, garlic

* Chicken, shrimp or beef stir fry, onions, peppers, water chestnuts, ½ cup brown rice

Avoid sweetened sauces (use sesame/peanut oil and rice vinegar)

1 Grilled chicken breast, pesto sauce, steamed spinach, rosemary, green salad, olive oil dressing

1 Chicken breast, rosemary, ½ cup black eyed peas, roasted onions, garlic, spinach salad

Large mixed green salad, small can tuna or 1 grilled chicken breast, chopped veggies,

Olive oil dressing with lemon, blue cheese crumbles

Salmon burger patty: 6 oz. chopped salmon, onions, dill, 1 egg, ¼ cup ground sesame seeds

Sautéed in skillet with 1 Tbsp. butter, served with small Caesar salad

Broiled salmon, 1 cup spaghetti squash, tomato sauce, oregano, thyme, garlic, grilled vegetables

* Albacore tuna pockets: celery, red onion, olive oil mayo, lemon juice,

Herb seasonings stuffed into sprouted wheat pita pocket

Filet mignon, mushrooms sautéed in butter and garlic, Caesar salad

Beef soup with lentils, celery, carrots, onion, cabbage, spinach or mixed green salad, ½ cup chicken or tuna salad

* London broil, green beans, ½ sweet potato, low-fat sour cream, Caesar salad

* Marinated broiled flank steak, ½ baked sweet potato, steamed squash, green salad, raspberry vinaigrette dressing

Indicates a high carbohydrate option Try to avoid these during the 1ˢᵗ 2 weeks and no more than 3 times/week thereafter. Or save for AFTER exercise.

Lunch & Dinner

* Broiled red snapper or grilled tuna, steamed broccoli, tomato soup, ½ baked yam

Shrimp or scallops, snow pea pods, onions, bean sprouts, broccoli, stir-fried in 3 Tbsp. peanut oil

Salmon, grilled onions, green salad, balsamic vinaigrette dressing

Sautéed giant garlic shrimp, 1 Tbsp. salsa, mixed green salad, ½ avocado, 4 strips jícama

6-8 Pieces brown rice sushi or sashimi with fish, shrimp, crab, green tea, seaweed salad, egg drop soup

Tuna steak, juice of ½ lime, ¼ cup ground hazelnuts, herb seasonings, 1 Tbsp. softened butter,

(Patted onto all sides of the fish), broiled

Crab and avocado salad: 1/3 cup chopped celery, ½ lb. cooked fresh crab, 1 Tbsp. olive oil mayo

1 tsp. cumin, ½ tsp. turmeric, 1 Tbsp. capers, juice of ½ lemon, ½ medium avocado,

Seasonings to taste, 1 bunch watercress with stems removed (Makes 2 servings)

Albacore tuna broccoli custard: ½ lb fresh chopped broccoli, 4 oz. tuna, 1 egg, ¾ cup milk,

¼ Cup grated low-fat cheese, 2 Tbsp. lemon juice, seasonings

Mix together and bake at 375ºF for 35 minutes

Spinach and cheddar casserole: sauté 2 minced garlic cloves in 1 Tbsp. olive oil, 2 lb. spinach

Cook 5 minutes, then add 2 Tbsp. pine nuts, ½ cup grated low-fat cheddar cheese

Lightly brown in broiler (Makes 2 servings)

* 1 Cup split pea soup, 1 slice pumpernickel toast, 1 Tbsp. cashew butter, ½ cup steamed yellow squash

Ricotta and leek frittata: sauté ½ inch pieces of leek in ½ Tbsp. butter

Mix and cook with 1 ½ Tbsp. ricotta cheese, seasonings, 4 organic eggs,

Place under broiler for 2 minutes to grill top golden brown

Cucumber and tomato salad with mozzarella: mix 1 Tbsp. extra virgin olive oil, 1 Tbsp. olive oil,

2 Tbsp. lemon juice, fresh parsley, dill, garlic, onion, 1 diced tomato,

1 cup diced cucumber, ½ cup mozzarella

* Indicates a high carbohydrate option Try to avoid these during the 1st 2 weeks and no more than 3 times/week thereafter. Or save for AFTER exercise.

Snacks

To increase metabolism & maximize energy throughout the day, it is recommended to eat a small meal about every 4 hours. Snacks between these meals should be minimized.

If the time between meals is longer than 4 hours, increase the snack size accordingly.

Edamame	1 Tbsp. nut butter on celery sticks	Macadamia nuts
Almonds	Hazelnuts	Walnuts
1 Small can tuna (in water)	Pumpkin seeds	Cashews
1-2 Hard boiled eggs	Low-fat cheese cubes	Cottage cheese
Protein shake (add nuts)	Plain yogurt & fresh berries	Meat with mustard/horseradish
1 *Wasa* cracker & 1 oz. cheese	Low glycemic fruit & nut butter	Smoked fish (salmon/lox)

Beverages

Water
Tomato juice or green vegetable drinks
Herbal teas: chamomile, ginger, peppermint, green tea, etc. with cinnamon stick

Quick & Easy
Ham and cheese salad
Broiled fish and vegetables
Broiled/grilled hamburger (no bun)
Poached eggs
Tuna fish (no bread)
Chef's salad
Omelet with green peppers or spinach
Chicken Caesar salad

Avoid

High glycemic foods	Refined carbohydrates	Hydrogenated oils
White rice	Bagels	Margarine
White potatoes	Bread	Processed meats
Sugar	Crackers	Additives
Alcohol	Cookies	Artificial colors and flavors
NutraSweet (aspartame)	Pretzels	

Salad Dressings

• An olive oil (good fat) dressing is the best choice.

• *Newman's Own* is a good brand, which is found on the inner aisles of most grocery stores.

• Avoid salad dressings made with hydrogenated oils.

• Avoid fat-free dressings. Usually when fat is removed sugar is added to make up for the lack of taste. Read your labels!

• If you like creamier salad dressings (saturated fats), try those that are found in the refrigerated section of the grocery store, such as *Marie's* or *Lighthouse*.

• Ask for dressing on the side and dip your fork in it, rather than the dumping it on the salad.

Omega-3 Eggs

• Free range or nest eggs from chickens that have been fed flaxseeds, such as *Eggland Best*.

• The eggs actually contain omega-3 fats, a healthy essential fat.

• Regular eggs are still good, especially if you eat fish frequently or are taking omega-3 supplements.

Free Range/Organic

- Refers to the lack of chemicals present in the growing of a plant or raising of an animal.

- Free range animal meats contain a better ratio of good to bad fats compared to traditionally raised animals that are raised in small pens and fed grains to fatten them up faster.

- Non-organic meats contain certain amounts of antibiotics and bovine growth hormone. Hormone-free animal foods and dairy are recommended if you have access to them and can spare the greater expense.

- Non-organic fruits and vegetables can contain pesticide chemicals. Always wash your fruits and vegetables thoroughly.

Food Allergies

- If you experience symptoms that include but are not limited to the following, you may have a food allergy: chronic congestions, chronic post-nasal drip, eczema, gastrointestinal distress and foggy head.

- To test if you have a food allergy, keep a food diary, recording the foods eaten and any symptoms. Eliminate those foods that most often precede the symptom for at least two weeks. If symptoms are alleviated, continue to avoid the food.

- Wheat is the most common allergen. Whole grains are always the best option but very difficult to find–most grain products are processed into flour. Some uncommon but tasty alternatives are amaranth and quinoa.

- For those with gluten intolerance, avoid foods from the acronym B.R.O.W.: Barley, Rye, Oats and Wheat. A list of other foods that should be avoided can be provided upon request.

- Other common food allergens include: dairy, soy, nuts (especially peanuts), corn and shellfish.

Adapted from Cenegenics Medical Institute ©.

Glycemic Index

Vegetables

Parsnips	97
Baked Potato	85
Pumpkin	75
Beets	64
Corn	55
Sweet Potato	54
Yams	51
Carrots	49
Green Beans	40
All Lettuces	< 30
Cauliflower	< 30
Eggplant	< 30
Onions	< 30
Radishes	< 30
Yellow Squash	< 30
Water Chestnuts	< 30
Sauerkraut	< 30
Tomatoes	15

Fruit

Watermelon	72
Pineapple	66
Cantaloupe	65
Raisins	64
Mango	56
Banana	54
Kiwi	53
Grapefruit Juice	48
Grapes	46
Orange	44
Peach	42
Plum	39
Apple	38
Pear	37
Apricots, dried	31
Grapefruit	25
Cherries	22

Sweeteners

Maltose	105
Glucose	100
Sucrose (table sugar)	64
High Fructose Corn Syrup	62
Honey	58
Fructose (fruit sugar)	22
Stevia	3

Dairy Products

Tofutti	115
Ice Cream, full fat	61
Yogurt, sweetened	33
Skim Milk	32
Soy Milk	30
Whole Milk	27
Yogurt, plain	14

Grains and Cereals

French Bread	95
Instant Rice	90
Cornflakes	83
Pretzels	81
White Bread	78
Waffles	76
Cheerios	74
Bagel	72
Shredded Wheat	69
Wheat Bread, high fiber	68
Stoned Wheat Thins	67
Grapenuts	67
Couscous	65
Hamburger Bun	61
White Rice	58
Pita Bread	57
Muesli	56
Brown Rice	55
Special K Cereal	54
Oatmeal, slow cooking	49
Rye Kernel Bread	46
Pita Bread, stone ground	45
All-Bran Cereal	42
Spaghetti, white	41
Spaghetti, protein enriched	27

Legumes

Baked Beans, canned	48
Pinto Beans	39
Chickpeas	33
Black Beans	30
Kidney Beans	29
Lentils	29
Peas, dried	22
Soy Beans	18

Other Foods

Dates	103
Jelly Beans	80
Rice Cakes	77
Vanilla Wafers	77
French Fries	75
Graham Crackers	74
Pizza, cheese	60
Popcorn	55
Chocolate	49
Olives	18
Nuts	15-30

Most Common High Glycemic Offenders:

Alcohol – Beer and drinks made with juice, soda or sugar

Candy – All types

Dried Fruits – Except apricots

Frozen Yogurt – Pure sugar & carbs with no fat or protein to slow the rate of absorption

Sugar-Sweetened Beverages – *Coke, Sprite, Snapple,* bottled teas, spritzers

Sugar – On coffee, tea and on cereal

Tubers & Roots – Parsnips, potatoes, beets, etc.

Watermelon

Refined Foods – Cereal, breads, cookies, rice/rice cakes, crackers

Eat only those carbohydrates that are 45 or lower on the glycemic index. Always eat carbs in combination with protein, fat or fiber in order to slow the rate of digestion and, therefore, the glycemic index of that carb.

Avoid white potatoes. Tropical fruits are higher in sugar. Omit the simple carbs, and note the tips on the upper right. Adapted Cenegenics(c)

FOOD LIST (This is great to bring when shopping)

Good Choices

Meats & Proteins
- The leaner, the better
- Best cooking methods: baked, broiled, grilled, steamed
- Free range, hormone & additive-free preferably

Chicken—Skinless
Eggs—Omega-3 enriched, free range
Fish—Ocean fish, not farm-raised or fresh water fish
Lamb
Lean Beef—*Coleman, Boar's Head* (less than 5 times/week)
Legumes—Lentils, dried beans, dried peas, etc.
Shellfish—Crab, shrimp, lobster (less than 2 times/week)
Tuna or Chicken Salad—Made with small amount of canola mayo
Turkey—Skinless

Vegetables—Low Glycemic
Asparagus
Broccoli/Cauliflower
Cabbage
Cucumber/Squash/Zucchini
Green Beans
Leafy Greens (Endive, Spinach, Collard Greens, etc.)
Sweet Potatoes/Yams
Tomatoes

Fruits—Low Glycemic
Apples
Berries
Dried Apricots
Grapefruit/Oranges/Citrus Fruits
Peaches/Pears

To Avoid

Meats & Proteins
Fast Food
Fatty Meats
Fried Meats
Poultry skin

Vegetables—High Glycemic
Baked Potatoes
Beets
Carrots
Corn
Parsnips
Pumpkin

Fruits—High Glycemic
Bananas
Dried Fruit (Dates, Raisins, Prunes, etc.)
Fruit Juices
Mangoes
Melons (Cantaloupe, Honeydew, Watermelon)
Pineapple

FOOD LIST

Good Choices	To Avoid

Good Choices

Dairy
• Organic, imported and low-fat preferably
Butter—Better to cook with
Cheeses (less than 5 times/week)
Cottage Cheese—Low-fat
Cream Cheese—Low-fat
Half & Half—Small amounts (in coffee?)
Milk—Skim or 1%
Yogurt—Unsweetened

Starches
• No more than 3 times/week
100% Rye/Pita/Pumpernickel/Protein Enriched Bread (1 slice)
Oatmeal—Old Fashioned/Natural/Steel-Cut
Pasta—Legume, Artichoke, Spinach, Soy, Egg
Rice—Wild or Brown
Sweet Potatoes/Yams
Wasa Crackers—Made with whole grains and good fats

Good Fats
• Oils should be organic, cold or expeller pressed
Avocados
Nuts—Almonds, Cashews, Macadamias, Raw
Salmon
Sardines
Sesame Oil
Tuna
Canola Oil—*Newman's Own*
salad dressing uses canola oil
Flaxseed Oil—*Spectrum,*
Udo's Choice, Barleens
Olive Oil

} COOK SLOW AND LOW!

To Avoid

Dairy
• Bovine growth hormone & antibiotics used
2% or Whole Milk
Cheeses—With hydrogenated oils, artificial colors and flavors
Cream & Whipping Cream
Fat-Free Products
Margarine
Yogurt—Fat-free or Sweetened with NutraSweet

Starches
• Packaged variety usually made w/hydrogenated oils
Baked Goods—Pies, Cookies, etc.
Bread—Bagels, Rolls, Croissants, etc.
Crackers
Oatmeal—Instant
Pasta—White, Wheat
Potatoes—White, Red, Instant
Pretzels
Rice—White, Instant, Rice Cakes

Bad Fats
Corn Oil
Donuts
Fried Foods
Hydrogenated/Partially Hydrogenated Oils
Lard
Margarine
Palm Oil
Peanut Butter—With added sugar and hydrogenated oils
Safflower Oil
Shortening
Vegetable Oil

© Cenegenics

Daily Food Log

- Eat a balanced meal or snack about every 4 hours
- Protein: roughly the size of the palm your hand
- Low glycemic veggies should make up the majority of your carbs – at least a fist full of veggies per meal is ideal
- Fruit can be eaten after a meal in place of a desert to satisfy a sweet craving
- Do not eat fruit or high glycemic carbs (GI > 45) without a protein or fat to slow absorption
- Allow higher glycemic carbs as side portions only or within the hour after exercising
- Fat: a closed handful of raw nuts, ¼ avocado, 1-2 Tbsp. of olive oil, etc.
- Enjoy one free day per week!

Day 1		Day 4	
Breakfast	? Protein:	Breakfast	? Protein:
	? Veggie/Fruit:		? Veggie/Fruit:
Time:	? Good Fat:	Time:	? Good Fat:
Snack	? Protein:	Snack	? Protein:
	? Veggie/Fruit:		? Veggie/Fruit:
Time:	? Good Fat:	Time:	? Good Fat:
Lunch	? Protein:	Lunch	? Protein:
	? Veggie/Fruit:		? Veggie/Fruit:
Time:	? Good Fat:	Time:	? Good Fat:
Snack	? Protein:	Snack	? Protein:
	? Veggie/Fruit:		? Veggie/Fruit:
Time:	? Good Fat:	Time:	? Good Fat:
Dinner	? Protein:	Dinner	? Protein:
	? Veggie/Fruit:		? Veggie/Fruit:
Time:	? Good Fat:	Time:	? Good Fat:
Day 2		**Day 5**	
Breakfast	? Protein:	Breakfast	? Protein:
	? Veggie/Fruit:		? Veggie/Fruit:
Time:	? Good Fat:	Time:	? Good Fat:
Snack	? Protein:	Snack	? Protein:
	? Veggie/Fruit:		? Veggie/Fruit:
Time:	? Good Fat:	Time:	? Good Fat:
Lunch	? Protein:	Lunch	? Protein:
	? Veggie/Fruit:		? Veggie/Fruit:
Time:	? Good Fat:	Time:	? Good Fat:
Snack	? Protein:	Snack	? Protein:
	? Veggie/Fruit:		? Veggie/Fruit:
Time:	? Good Fat:	Time:	? Good Fat:
Dinner	? Protein:	Dinner	? Protein:
	? Veggie/Fruit:		? Veggie/Fruit:
Time:	? Good Fat:	Time:	? Good Fat:
Day 3		**Day 6**	
Breakfast	? Protein:	Breakfast	? Protein:
	? Veggie/Fruit:		? Veggie/Fruit:
Time:	? Good Fat:	Time:	? Good Fat:
Snack	? Protein:	Snack	? Protein:
	? Veggie/Fruit:		? Veggie/Fruit:
Time:	? Good Fat:	Time:	? Good Fat:
Lunch	? Protein:	Lunch	? Protein:
	? Veggie/Fruit:		? Veggie/Fruit:
Time:	? Good Fat:	Time:	? Good Fat:
Snack	? Protein:	Snack	? Protein:
	? Veggie/Fruit:		? Veggie/Fruit:
Time:	? Good Fat:	Time:	? Good Fat:
Dinner	? Protein:	Dinner	? Protein:
	? Veggie/Fruit:		? Veggie/Fruit:
Time:	? Good Fat:	Time:	? Good Fat:

Most Unhealthy Day

Meal/Snack (Time)	Food	Portion size or estimation	Leave blank for our comments
Breakfast Time: ____	Skipped -	Ø	Don't skip!
AM Snack Time: ____	Coffee Rice cakes, Juice	sml	Protein, Carb better No Rice Cake!
Lunch Time: ____	Bagal Salad, sml		No Protein
Midday Snack Time: ____	Coffee, candy		needs boost then crashes
Dinner Time: ____	Small Salad Chicken Potato chips		No chips- Do yam, Veggie.
PM Snack Time: ____	Popcorn		
Before Bed Snack Time: ____	Yogourt tea		- Plain white add fruit - Nuts. No caffeine @ bed- Time.

Please note any specific problem foods you consistently overeat, including the frequency (i.e. daily, weekly, or monthly). Anxious then tired afternoon
Alc: ~~nua diet bttl~~ ~~stilling~~

Note situations, moods, or occasions that cause you to eat or drink more than you should.
stressed at work, home
can't sleep.
exercise, melatonin before bed.

It's not good to skip meals and needs more complex carbs----more veggies and fruits. Also, add stress-reducing exercise, and better sleep, no caffeine before bed! Watch the glycemic index of foods.

Exercise Summary

1. On a regular basis, over the last 3 months, indicate the number of days per week you performed the following activities.

    a. Aerobic exercises (swimming, walking, jogging, cycling, stationary bike) _____

    b. Structured resistance training exercises _____

    c. Structured strength building (strenuous calisthenics) _____

    d. Structured stretching exercises, either alone or with an exercise program _____

    e. Strength building sports, such as gymnastics, martial arts, wrestling _____

    f. Hard physical labor for at least one hour per day (i.e. lifting, pushing, heavy tool operation) _____

    g. Strenuous housework _____

    h. Gardening, including strenuous digging _____

2. If you do aerobic exercise, how long is your average workout? _____

3. What is the intensity of your aerobic exercise?

☐ Very Light	Stretching
☐ Light	Includes some movement as in leisure walking
☐ Moderate	Continuous movement causing increase in heart rate (brisk walking, leisure swimming)
☐ Heavy	Continuous movement involving fluctuation in intensity from moderate to heavy with significant increases in heart rate
☐ Very heavy	Continuous movement causing heaving breathing, sweating, marked increases in heart rate, etc. (swimming laps, interval training, running, cycling, stationary bike, spin cycling, etc.)

4. Do you walk, jog, or run on a regular basis? ☐ Yes ☐ No

    a. If yes, how many times per week? _____

    b. What is the average number of miles per workout? _____

5. During the last year, have you experienced any injuries? Yes No

    a. If yes, please describe your injury?

       _____

       _____

       _____

    b. Did this injury occur as a result of exercising? ☐ Yes ☐ No

    c. Did this injury cause you to modify or stop your exercise regimen? ☐ Yes ☐ No

    d. If yes, for what period of time did you stop exercising? _____

6. Please describe your current aerobic exercise program. Include type, duration, and intensity.

    _____

    _____

    _____

    _____

    _____

    _____

7. Please describe your current flexibility and/or stretching program (i.e. yoga, tai chi, stretching and toning classes, martial arts, brief stretching after aerobics or weights) Include type and duration.

    _____

    _____

    _____

    _____

    _____

8. Please describe your current resistance/strength training exercise program i.e. free weights, weight machines, body pump classes, water aerobics, etc. (discuss type, duration, intensity).

    _____

    _____

    _____

    _____

    _____

Fitness Activity Assessment

Question	Yes	No
Do you enjoy exercising?		
Have you ever been a member of a health club? If yes, for how long?		
Are you currently a member of a health club?		
Have you ever worked with a personal trainer? If yes, for how long?		
Did you enjoy it?		
Are you still with a personal trainer?		
Do you have any exercise equipment at home (bike, treadmill, free weights, etc.)? If yes, please list:		
Are you presently receiving physical therapy? If yes, please describe:		
If exercise is not part of your weekly routine, please explain the reasons.		

HOLMES-RAHE LIFE CHANGES SCALE

Please review the events below. Beside each one, indicate the number of times each event occurred in the past year only.

Event	Number of times in past year
Death of a spouse	
Divorce	
Marital separation	
Law suits	
Jail term	
Death of a close family member	
Personal injury or illness	
Marriage	
Fired from work	
Marital reconciliation	
Retirement	
Change in health of a family member	
Pregnancy	
Sexual difficulties	
Gain of a new family member	
Business readjustment	
Change in financial state	
Death of a close friend	
Change to a different line of work	
Change in number of arguments with spouse	
Mortgage over $500,000	
Foreclosure of mortgage or loan	
Change in responsibilities at work	
Son or daughter leaving home	
Trouble with in-laws	
Outstanding personal achievement	
Spouse began or stopped work	
Began or ended school	
Change in living conditions	
Revision of personal habits	
Trouble with the boss	
Change in work hours or conditions	
Change in residence	
Change in schools	
Change in recreation	
Change in exercise program	
Change in social activities	
Change in sleeping habits	
Change in number of family get-togethers	
Change in eating habits	
Vacations	
Religious holidays	
Minor violations of the law	
Major violations of the law	

Holmes & Rahe (1967), Holmes-Rahe life changes scale. Journal of Psychosomatic Research, Vol. 11, pp. 213-218.

Body Mass Index Table

	Normal						Overweight					Obese										Extreme Obesity														
BMI	19	20	21	22	23	24	25	26	27	28	29	30	31	32	33	34	35	36	37	38	39	40	41	42	43	44	45	46	47	48	49	50	51	52	53	54
Height (inches)												Body Weight (pounds)																								
58	91	96	100	105	110	115	119	124	129	134	138	143	148	153	158	162	167	172	177	181	186	191	196	201	205	210	215	220	224	229	234	239	244	248	253	258
59	94	99	104	109	114	119	124	128	133	138	143	148	153	158	163	168	173	178	183	188	193	198	203	208	212	217	222	227	232	237	242	247	252	257	262	267
60	97	102	107	112	118	123	128	133	138	143	148	153	158	163	168	174	179	184	189	194	199	204	209	215	220	225	230	235	240	245	250	255	261	266	271	276
61	100	106	111	116	122	127	132	137	143	148	153	158	164	169	174	180	185	190	195	201	206	211	217	222	227	232	238	243	248	254	259	264	269	275	280	285
62	104	109	115	120	126	131	136	142	147	153	158	164	169	175	180	186	191	196	202	207	213	218	224	229	235	240	246	251	256	262	267	273	278	284	289	295
63	107	113	118	124	130	135	141	146	152	158	163	169	175	180	186	191	197	203	208	214	220	225	231	237	242	248	254	259	265	270	278	282	287	293	299	304
64	110	116	122	128	134	140	145	151	157	163	169	174	180	186	192	197	204	209	215	221	227	232	238	244	250	256	262	267	273	279	285	291	296	302	308	314
65	114	120	126	132	138	144	150	156	162	168	174	180	186	192	198	204	210	216	222	228	234	240	246	252	258	264	270	276	282	288	294	300	306	312	318	324
66	118	124	130	136	142	148	155	161	167	173	179	186	192	198	204	210	216	223	229	235	241	247	253	260	266	272	278	284	291	297	303	309	315	322	328	334
67	121	127	134	140	146	153	159	166	172	178	185	191	198	204	211	217	223	230	236	242	249	255	261	268	274	280	287	293	299	306	312	319	325	331	338	344
68	125	131	138	144	151	158	164	171	177	184	190	197	203	210	216	223	230	236	243	249	256	262	269	276	282	289	295	302	308	315	322	328	335	341	348	354
69	128	135	142	149	155	162	169	176	182	189	196	203	209	216	223	230	236	243	250	257	263	270	277	284	291	297	304	311	318	324	331	338	345	351	358	365
70	132	139	146	153	160	167	174	181	188	195	202	209	216	222	229	236	243	250	257	264	271	278	285	292	299	306	313	320	327	334	341	348	355	362	369	376
71	136	143	150	157	165	172	179	186	193	200	208	215	222	229	236	243	250	257	265	272	279	286	293	301	308	315	322	329	338	343	351	358	365	372	379	386
72	140	147	154	162	169	177	184	191	199	206	213	221	228	235	242	250	258	265	272	279	287	294	302	309	316	324	331	338	346	353	361	368	375	383	390	397
73	144	151	159	166	174	182	189	197	204	212	219	227	235	242	250	257	265	272	280	288	295	302	310	318	325	333	340	348	355	363	371	378	386	393	401	408
74	148	155	163	171	179	186	194	202	210	218	225	233	241	249	256	264	272	280	287	295	303	311	319	326	334	342	350	358	365	373	381	389	396	404	412	420
75	152	160	168	176	184	192	200	208	216	224	232	240	248	256	264	272	279	287	295	303	311	319	327	335	343	351	359	367	375	383	391	399	407	415	423	431
76	156	164	172	180	189	197	205	213	221	230	238	246	254	263	271	279	287	295	304	312	320	328	336	344	353	361	369	377	385	394	402	410	418	426	435	443

Source: Adapted from *Clinical Guidelines on the Identification, Evaluation, and Treatment of Overweight and Obesity in Adults: The Evidence Report.*

Understanding the Symptoms of Depression*

For major depression, you may experience five or more of the following for at least a two-week period:

- Persistent sadness, pessimism.
- Feelings of guilt, worthlessness, helplessness or hopelessness.
- Loss of interest or pleasure in usual activities, including sex.
- Difficulty concentrating and complaints of poor memory.
- Worsening of coexisting chronic disease, such as rheumatoid arthritis or diabetes.
- Insomnia or oversleeping.
- Weight gain or loss.
- Fatigue, lack of energy.
- Anxiety, agitation, irritability.
- Thoughts of suicide or death.
- Slow speech; slow movements.
- Headache, stomachache and digestive problems.

For dysthymia (minor, but long-term depression), symptoms are less intense and fewer in number, but long-lasting.

Notify your doctor, family members, and seek help if you have the following:

- You or a loved one have suicidal thoughts, or have other signs of either major depression or dysthymia; help is available.
- You are considering alternative or complementary treatments. It's important that your doctor be aware of all aspects of your treatment.

There is a difference between feeling down occasionally and having a depressive illness. If things get to where feeling blue affects you personally, your relationships or job performance, then there's a problem. If you feel you can't lift yourself out of your misery, seek profesional help. The symptoms of depression can be elusive and vague. If there are any concerns, talk to someone.

*Adapted from WebMD and DSM-V. There are descriptions and symptoms for other mood cocerns as anxiety, bipolar, alcoholism and more on their Web sites.

Screening Tests for Men: What You Need and When

Screening tests can find diseases early when they are easier to treat. Health experts from the U.S. Preventive Services Task Force have made recommendations, based on scientific evidence, about testing for the conditions below. I added or modified the ones below with an asterisk. Talk to your doctor about which ones apply to you and when and how often you should be tested. For more information about USPSTF recommendations and Put Prevention Into Practice, go to the Agency for Healthcare Research and Quality Web site at: http://www.preventiveservices.ahrq.gov.

- **Obesity:** Have your body mass index (BMI) calculated to screen for obesity. (BMI is a measure of body fat based on height and weight.) You can also find your own BMI with the BMI calculator from the National Heart, Lung, and Blood Institute at: http://www.nhlbisupport.com/bmi/. Get an estimation of your visceral fat.*

- **High Cholesterol:** Have your cholesterol checked regularly starting at age 35. If you are younger than 35, talk to your doctor about whether to have your cholesterol checked if:
  - o You have diabetes.
  - o You have high blood pressure.
  - o Heart disease runs in your family.
  - o You smoke.

- **High Blood Pressure:** Have your blood pressure checked at least every 2 years. High blood pressure is 140/90 or higher.

- **Heart Disease: Get and EKG starting at 35 years old and get a stress test if abnormal, at risk, or any symptoms relating to the chest or breathing.***

- **Glaucoma:** Get regular eye exams starting at 40 years old.*

- **Lung Cancer: No guidelines published but if at risk, at least do a chest X**-Ray-talk to your doctor.

- **Colorectal Cancer:** Have a test for colorectal cancer starting at age 50. Your doctor can help you decide which test is right for you, but I recommend you get a colonoscopy. If you have a family history of colorectal cancer or any symptoms, you may need to be screened earlier.*

- **Prostate Cancer:** Get a rectal exam and a PSA blood test each year after age 50. Start at age forty if Black or at increased risks. Ask your doctor when you may not need these any more.*

- **Testicular Cancer:** Starting as a teen, examine your testicles monthly for any lump larger than a pea or any enlarging masses or tenderness. Call your doctor if any penile discharge, blood in the urine, or pain when urinating.*

- **Diabetes:** Have a test for diabetes if you have high blood pressure or high cholesterol.

- **Depression:** Your emotional health is as important as your physical health. If you have felt "down," sad, or hopeless over the last 2 weeks or have felt little interest or pleasure in doing things, you may be depressed. Talk to your doctor about being screened for depression.

- **Sexually Transmitted Infections:** Talk to your doctor to see whether you should be tested for gonorrhea, syphilis, chlamydia, or other sexually transmitted infections.

- **HIV:** Talk to your doctor about HIV screening if you:
  o Have had sex with men since 1975.
  o Have had unprotected sex with multiple partners.
  o Have used or now use injection drugs.
  o Exchange sex for money or drugs or have sex partners who do.
  o Have past or present sex partners who are HIV-infected, are bisexual, or use injection drugs.
  o Are being treated for sexually transmitted diseases.
  o Had a blood transfusion between 1978 and 1985.

- **Abdominal Aortic Aneurysm:** If you are between the ages of 65 and 75 and have ever smoked (100 or more cigarettes during your lifetime), you need to be screened once for abdominal aortic aneurysm, which is an abnormally large or swollen blood vessel in your abdomen.

- **Bone Density: Get a baseline DXA bone scan starting at age fifty or earlier if at risk or symptomatic.***

- **Dental: Get regular dental examinations and cleanings, twice per year.**

- **Vaccinations:** The Centers for Disease Control and Prevention provide more information on immunizations at: http://www.cdc.gov/nip/recs/adult-schedule.htm.

Screening Test Checklist

Take this checklist with you to your doctor's office. Write down when you have any of the tests below. Talk to your doctor about your test results and write them down here. Ask when you should have the test next. Write down the month and year. If you think of questions for the doctor, write them down and bring them to your next visit.

Test	Last Test (mo/yr)	Results	Next Test Due (mo/yr)	Questions for the Doctor
Weight (BMI)				
Cholesterol Total:				
HDL (good):				
LDL (bad):				
Blood pressure				
Colorectal cancer				
Diabetes				
Sexually transmitted diseases				
HIV infection				
Miscellaneous				

More Information

For more information on staying healthy, call the AHRQ Publications Clearinghouse at 1-800-358-9295, or send an E-mail to: ahrqpubs@ahrq.hhs.gov.

Adapted from AHRQ, and USPSTF.
* I added these based on my readings and professional opinion.

NOTES:

Resources

Below are some resources you may find helpful. As discussed, there are some quacks out there, so try to get your information from reliable sources, i.e., those government or university based.

http://unisonproyouth.com/ My Web site for Unison Pro-Youth Medical Institute. My CV and e-mail address is there. You'll get a newsletter, if you sign up, and regular, pertinent news updates.

http://www.cenegenics-drrao.com/ My Cenegenics Affiliate Web site and information gateway on most that's discussed in the book. There are great references, too.

http://www.metagenics.com/ This form has a great reputation for GMP, pharmaceutical-grade supplements and reliable information.

http://www.mqrx.com/ Ditto, per above. These two are my favorite source for supplements.

http://www.inetsupermall.com/life_extension.htm This site has information, though they push too much of their own stuff.

http://intl-jcem.endojournals.org/ The *Journal of Clinical Endocrinology and Metabolism.* A lot of peer-reviewed facts on health subjects are found.

http://www.hormonecme.org/default.asp This is similar to the above listing, though more for doctors' level of understanding.

http://www.fda.gov/ The USFDA Web site with great reference and tools to stay healthy, and it's free!

http://www.webmd.com/ A reliable resource for doctors and the public.

http://www.aafp.org/online/en/home.html The American Academy of Family Physicians homepage, a great starting point for information.

http://www.aicr.org/site/ The America Institute for Cancer Research homepage is a great resource for diet, exercise, and ways you can help prevent carcinogenesis in the first place. Also, it's a good resource for cancer survivors.

http://content.nejm.org/ This is the homepage for the *New England Journal of Medicine*. Although geared toward doctors, you probably can do a search and find reliable information on practically any topic.

http://www.nih.gov/ This is the National Institutes of Health homepage. You can find ways to keep a healthy weight and to calculate your Body Mass Index at http://www.nhlbisupport.com/bmi/.

http://jama.ama-assn.org/ This is the homepage for the American Medical Association and *JAMA,* their most highly respected journal. Although this site is geared for doctors, you probably can do a search and find reliable information on practically any topic.

http://www.mayoclinic.com/ This is the Mayo Clinic's homepage. There's also a lot of reliable, useful information available here.

http://www.fda.gov/ This is the official web site for the Food and Drug Administration. Here you will find a wealth of reliable information on pollution, diet (different ethnic food pyramids) supplements, exercise, and more.

You can add your own search results below for future reference:

Edited by Reiza S. Dejito

Reviewed by Elmer J. Mangubat

978-0-595-42176-3
0-595-42176-8

Lightning Source UK Ltd.
Milton Keynes UK
UKHW010433210220
359064UK00002B/651